An Introduction to Epidemiology

An Introduction to Epidemiology

Michael Alderson

Chief Medical Statistician
Office of Population Censuses and Surveys

SECOND EDITION

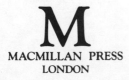

MACMILLAN PRESS
LONDON

First edition 1976
Reprinted (with corrections) 1977, 1980, 1982
Second edition 1983

Published by
THE MACMILLAN PRESS LTD
London and Basingstoke
Companies and representatives throughout the world

ISBN 0 333 35014 6 (hard cover)
      0 333 35015 4 (paper cover)

Filmsetting by Vantage Photosetting Co Ltd
Eastleigh and London
Printed in Hong Kong

Contents

Preface

Epidemiology has three main aims: to describe the distribution and size of disease problems in human populations; to identify aetiological factors in the pathogenesis of disease; to provide the data essential for the management, evaluation and planning of services for the prevention, control and treatment of disease. In order to fulfil these aims, three rather different classes of epidemiological study may be mounted.

(1) Descriptive studies concerned with observing the distribution and progression of disease in populations;
(2) Analytical studies concerned with investigating hypotheses suggested by the descriptive studies;
(3) Experimental or intervention studies concerned with measuring the effect on the population of manipulating environmental influences thought to be harmful, or by introducing in a controlled way preventive, curative and ameliorative services.

This book describes the various approaches that can be made in following such paths of investigation.

Since routine mortality and morbidity statistics may provide background information for many studies and may be the sole source of data for some, two chapters are devoted to these issues. There follow chapters on the use of cross-sectional, retrospective and prospective studies, with examples in each of particular studies, the principles involved and some of the advantages and disadvantages of the different approaches. A further chapter deals with intervention studies, including preventive, clinical and medical-care trials. There then follow chapters dealing with the application of epidemiology to three very different topics: medical-care studies, genetics and occupational hazards. The final chapter provides some general comments on study design and the derivation of inferences from empirical data. For the second revision of this book the last three chapters are new additions to the text; chapters 4 and 5 have been rewritten, while all the others have been extensively revised.

Considerable emphasis is placed on study design in each chapter and attention is also paid to methods of analysis and the interpretation of data, particularly to certain statistical techniques that are used predominantly in the field of epidemiology. The intention is to indicate the relevance of these approaches, and to provide a guide to the literature and textbooks on statistics for readers wishing to explore these aspects further. The examples of published work that are quoted have been chosen to illustrate the methods of epidemiology. It is hoped that each example will help to stimulate interest in the subject, but no attempt has been made to provide a comprehensive cover of all the findings of epidemiological studies. The examples deal predominantly with the methods used in the study of chronic disease, the main field of work of epidemiologists in developed countries, together with an application of these methods to medical-care studies.

Epidemiology will be one of the sources of fresh data that may be of concern to everyone involved in the health-care field, whether these data relate to aetiology, means of prevention or modes of delivery of health care. It is suggested that many entrants into the health-care field (doctors, nurses, administrators and ancillary staff) should have some appreciation of the role of epidemiology and the underlying methods used in order to be able to read published work and interpret it. It is also hoped that a clear exposition of the various approaches used in epidemiology may stimulate a wider range of individuals to carry out their own, however limited, studies. In addition to the general acceptance that undergraduates should be introduced to this subject, there is a growing tendency to acknowledge that administrators in the health service should be trained in disciplines such as epidemiology. It is hoped that this book will provide a basic introduction to the subject suitable for this general readership who may not wish to study the subject any further. In addition the text should act as a useful basis for a more detailed course suitable for those entering into community medicine, and should also provide guidance for individuals in any branch of medicine who wish to carry out their own studies.

The stimulus to write this book came from the involvement in the teaching of medical and other students in the health field. This was reinforced by individuals bringing a range of fascinating problems for discussion. Each of these problems from the different branches of medicine has indicated the growing interest of many individuals working in the health service to carry out their own projects. It is hoped that this book will give assistance to such persons. These people are not named in the text, but a debt of gratitude is owed to them for the way in which the presentation of practical issues has stimulated thought. Hubble* drew attention to the relatively fine dividing line that separates plagiary from correctly attributed quotation, and original thought. It is obvious that the bulk of the ideas in this text have been distilled from contact with many colleagues over the past twenty years; in particular a debt of gratitude is owed to Robert Wofinden, Jerry Morris and Alwyn Smith. It is a pleasure to acknowledge the help from staff in the Medical Information Unit of Wessex Regional Health Authority, and the Division of Epidemiology in the Institute of Cancer Research.

I am most grateful for the help given by Elizabeth Horne, Senior Editor, Medical Books, and Steven Redwood, Production Services Manager, both of The Macmillan Press Ltd, and of Richard Powell, Editorial Consultant, in the preparation of this new edition.

Southampton, 1983   Michael Alderson

*Hubble, D. (1974). Personal view. *Br. med. J.*, **3,** 623

1 The Role of Epidemiology

Epidemiology may be defined as the study of the determinants of the incidence and prevalence of disease. This relatively simple definition has some extremely widespread implications. It immediately suggests that epidemiology may be used to identify the cause of disease, but it must be remembered that it is most unusual that there is a single cause for a disease without any other confounding or intervening factors playing a part. Thus the examination of the causation of disease may involve investigators in an extremely wide range of studies unravelling a complex tangle of factors. The consideration of factors influencing the prevalence of disease adds a different perspective to the role of epidemiology; the prevalence of disease (the measure of the extent to which a disease exists in a population at a point in time) is a combination of the incidence of the condition, the cure rate and the fatality from this condition. In order, therefore, to study the determinants of the prevalence of a condition, information about the incidence, the natural history of the disease and the impact of the health-care system on the disease is required. This involves studying the cause of disease, the identification of disease patterns, the population's attitudes to disease, their tendency to seek cure, the range of care provided and the impact of such care on the disease. The above definition thus acknowledges the activities of epidemiologists in a range of studies throughout the medical-care field in examining the functioning of the health-care system and its impact on the health of a population.

1.1 Who Practices Epidemiology?

There is a very small but steadily growing proportion of the total manpower in the health field identifying themselves as trained epidemiologists. Although many of the studies discussed in this book have been carried out by 'professional epidemiologists', it is important to point out that many studies have been done by individuals working primarily in other branches of medicine. Recently, classic work has been carried out in general practice and by hospital staff. Pickles (1939) described a whole series of studies carried out in a rural practice in the Yorkshire dales. By the use of relatively simple methods relying on careful documentation and analysis of observations, he provided unique contributions on the spread of a number of infectious diseases. Fry (1966, 1974) has patiently documented the health problems of patients in an urban practice and reported on the natural history of a range of acute and chronic diseases. A major extension of such work in general practice has been the large-scale study on oral contraceptives involving 23 000 users, an equal number of controls and records provided by 1400 general practitioners whose activity was co-ordinated by Dr Clifford Kay (1974). Gregg (1941) noticed a change in the proportion of children

1

referred to his clinic in Australia with certain eye defects; this stimulated him to initiate studies on the association between material rubella and congenital abnormality of the subsequently born child. More recently Burkitt (1962), while working as a surgeon in East Africa, was responsible for the identification of a new form of malignant disease; he then launched studies of its epidemiology.

These examples are arbitrarily selected from a wide range of studies that have been carried out by clinicians either in the primary medical-care or in the hospital field. They indicate that there is no need to consider that epidemiology is a branch of medical science only practised by a restricted group of specially trained individuals. Over the past few years increasing emphasis has been placed on the need for administrators in the health service to be trained in disciplines such as epidemiology. This is an indication of the acceptance of the application of these techniques to the study of medical problems and the contribution that such studies can make to the management and planning of the delivery of health-care services.

The points argue for a wide range of individuals being familiar with the general principles of epidemiological studies. Epidemiology will be one of the sources of fresh data that will be of concern to everyone in the health field whether these data relate to aetiology, means of prevention or modes of delivery of health care. It is on these grounds therefore that all categories of health-service staff should have some appreciation of the role of epidemiology and the underlying methods in order to be able to read published work and interpret it. The medical field undergoes continuous change and therefore the most important aspect of training is not the accumulation of facts, but the acquisition of the ability to accept fresh information, and judge whether the findings warrant change in practice.

Apart from facilitating the interpretation of other people's findings, it is possible that a description of the methods of epidemiology may stimulate the use of these techniques by a wider range of individuals. Some of the work discussed in later chapters has been carried out using the minimum of facilities. Useful studies can be done either by examining the routinely available data, or by collecting a restricted amount of information and analysing this in a relatively simple way; the resources required for many worthwhile studies are slight compared with research in other fields. The emphasis is mainly on the need for careful planning and consideration of the issues involved, the collection of observations of known accuracy and the careful interpretation of such material.

1.2 Development of Epidemiology

The foundations of epidemiology were laid in the nineteenth century, when a few classic studies made a major contribution to the saving of life. This work was particularly concerned with infectious diseases. However, even at that time there was an awareness of the need to look at the influence of the environment. Other studies early in the nineteenth century demonstrated the influence of occupation on morbidity and mortality, and also the effect on health of the general environment and social conditions. Thackrah (1832) produced a lengthy book on the effects of arts, trades and professions on health, while Chadwick (1842) in his report on the sanitary condition of the labouring population in Great Britain discussed the influence on health of drainage, ventilation, overcrowding in dwellings, low income and poor diet.

A misconception that has lingered too long is that epidemiology is primarily concerned with infectious diseases. From the start it was recognised that the onset of disease can be due to an infective agent; this was associated with an awareness of the important influence of physical, emotional, social and genetic factors. In developed countries the majority of health-care problems now stem from chronic disease and the bulk of the examples in the following chapters are related to studies on chronic disease. The basic techniques for studying infectious disease are similar. However, due consideration must always be given to the relative influence of the prime aetiological agent, the 'vehicle' for transmitting it, the associated factors affecting risk of development of a disease and the host's reponse to the disease.

1.3 Four Categories of Study

Epidemiology involves four different categories of study. The first one is descriptive: for example, 'Who gets heart disease?' National data have been used to examine the mortality from heart disease in different countries in relation to some of the characteristics of the individuals who died and other basic items available in the mortality data (for instance the fatality rates in relation to age, sex, time of year and secular trend). This limited material has then been supplemented by population surveys, which have looked at the prevalence of identified heart disease.

A second category of study is hypothesis testing, for instance exploring the question 'Does diet influence heart disease?'. National mortality rates have been contrasted with estimates of intake *per capita* of various nutrients. This has been followed by the examination of the reported diets of persons with heart disease and of control subjects. A more precise examination may occur with the measurement of the habitual diet in a large number of subjects and their follow up to determine which individuals develop heart disease in relation to initial categorisation of diet.

If the descriptive and hypothesis-testing studies point to a particular factor being of importance in the development of the disease, these studies may be followed by a third phase—an intervention study. For example, work has been carried out to test whether an actual alteration of diet in individuals has any effect on the incidence, recurrence rate or fatality from heart disease.

These three main categories of epidemiological study may each require, as a preliminary phase, a fourth and rather different approach—that is, a method study. As with any other research work, before embarking on a definitive study there may be a need to refine the techniques required in the applied study. For example, in order to examine the diet of a large number of individuals, there is the need to develop a technique for assessing diet that is reliable and valid, and yet sufficiently simple to be applied in the field to a large number of subjects.

Method studies involving the development of data-collection techniques may also lead to improved disease categorisation. For example, epidemiological, clinical and pathological work has indicated that Hodgkin's disease may be a heterogeneous collection of conditions. The ability to distinguish between these types of Hodgkin's disease may be a necessary preliminary to aetiological studies (MacMahon, 1966). Other work may suggest that a 'condition' does not really exist. Examination of the X-rays of 132 subjects with dysphagia by eight observers resulted in variation of between 6 and 59 per cent of the subjects being reported as having a web (Elwood and Pitman, 1966). This suggests that the Patterson–Kelly syndrome may be nothing more than a variation in observers' interpretations of barium swallows.

1.4 Need for Numeracy

Considerable emphasis is placed on study design in each of the chapters and attention is also paid to the methods of analysis and interpretation of collected data. Epidemiology is essentially a multidisciplinary approach, and in particular relies heavily on numerical techniques. Each chapter ends with brief consideration of some of the relevant statistical techniques. This is not intended to serve as a text of statistical techniques, but merely to indicate the relevance of statistical method and in particular to emphasise those methods that are of special use in epidemiological studies. Some of the techniques, such as the calculation of relative risk or proportional mortality, are not generally dealt with in the standard books on statistics. These techniques are therefore given more emphasis, and only the most cursory mention is made of those statistical approaches that have been fully dealt with elsewhere. One of the reasons for including the sections on statistics is to indicate the specific methods appropriate in the various categories of epidemiological study. This should facilitate communication between the research worker and the statistician. It must be emphasised that when statistical advice is required, this should be sought at an early stage in planning a study and not when the material has all been collected and an attempt is being made to interpret it. Armitage (1971) has suggested that 'statisticians are in too short a supply to act as collaborators in more than a fraction of all statistically orientated studies in medical research'. There is a need therefore for those mounting epidemiological studies or attempting to interpret the work of others to appreciate the relevance of certain statistical techniques in the handling of material.

The advent of the microprocessor makes it increasingly likely that many epidemiologists will have access to calculating facilities that can directly handle the range of statistical tests usually required. Rothman and Boice (1979) have set out in a clear fashion the algebra and program listings for the range of conventional tests in a form suitable for use in a handheld programmable calculator. The statistical sections in each of the chapters in this book provide a guide to the relevance of the various techniques and some of the problems of application and interpretation of results. These aspects are more important to the general reader than the details of the method of calculation.

1.5 Different Approaches to the Consideration of Epidemiology

Epidemiology could be considered under the applications it may have, such as the definition of disease groups, the unravelling of primary and associated aetiological factors in the causation of disease, and the delineation of the natural history of disease. Another approach is to describe the findings of epidemiology in relation to disease entities, such as malignant, heart and respiratory diseases. A third approach is to describe the methods of epidemiology, illustrating these by the different categories of use (thereby indicating some selected findings from the application of such methods).

This is the approach that has been used in this book, but this should in no way suggest that a study of the methods of epidemiology in isolation is of merit. The approach has been deliberately chosen, however, in an attempt to interest a wide range of individuals in the use of such methods, whatever their particular field of work. In this book, there has not been any attempt to provide a comprehensive account of the findings of epidemiology in relation to every major category of disease problem. This is chiefly because the approach selected only provides a discussion of the findings as part of a consideration of particular problems of study design and interpretation of results; also it is felt that the findings of epidemiology cannot be looked at in isolation. For instance, when considering malignant diseases, epidemiology can provide background information and some extremely interesting pointers to the causes of various malignant diseases and the steps that can be taken to prevent these diseases. Even the descriptive data on the disease in question requires support from clinical and pathological studies to indicate the specific nature of the condition. A discussion of the natural history of the disease should not really be divorced from the consideration of the various methods of treatment for each particular malignant disease, and a detailed assessment of the outcome of treatment. Such an approach calls for integrated topic teaching rather than the isolated presentation of the findings of epidemiological studies. Factual information is provided in a number of books (see further reading lists) on the epidemiology of particular diseases, and data are being augmented all the time by fresh studies reported in the literature.

Even in the absence of any clear knowledge of the underlying cause of disease, epidemiology may help to unravel the 'vehicle' responsible for the transmission of the disease (whether this is due to infection, exposure to physical and/or chemical factors, or is genetically determined). Such studies are pursued not merely to add to the general body of medical knowledge, but in the hope that the relationship between aetiology and the development of the disease may be sufficiently clarified that preventive measures can be suggested. For many conditions, whether these are acute or chronic diseases, there is a growing awareness that the individual's level of recognition of diseases varies. In medical-care studies an important aspect of the work involves not only identifying the determinants of disease, but also the factors associated with seeking care. Such studies lead to a consideration of who gets treatment and the results of treatment. A standard treatment given to a number of patients with a disease of particular severity results in a variation in response; epidemiological methods may be used to identify the factors associated with this variation in response. Such information may be useful in improving the selection of patients for each type of treatment. The techniques used for the examination of the results of treatment are closely aligned to some of the general methods of epidemiology and are covered in chapter 7. Work on the examination of the natural history of the disease and of response to the treatment requires measurement of outcome of such care. Such studies may be part of a general examination of the functioning of the health service. This involves consideration of facilities required for care, variation in type of care provided, factors affecting uptake of care and the outcome from such care. Attention is paid to these issues in the final chapter of the book.

Many of the examples given in the following chapters relate to classic examples of particular studies. These have been chosen because they illustrate the particular methods used and not in order to give a systematic catalogue of the various findings of epidemiological studies. A number of the examples stem from the personal experience of the author; again these have been used as an indication of method rather than having been selected because of the specific value of their findings. Some of the problems discussed will be well known to the general reader, while others relate to problems affecting a relatively small segment of the population and involving quite rare diseases. Although the chapters do not provide a systematic or comprehensive documentation of the findings of epidemiology over the complete range of health problems, relatively generous provision of cross-references in the index goes some way to overcoming this issue.

References

Recommended reading

Armitage, P. (1971). *Statistical Methods in Medical Research*, Blackwell, Oxford
Osborn, J. F. (1979). *Statistical Exercises in Medical Research*, Blackwell, Oxford
Pickles, W. N. (1939). *Epidemiology in Country Practice*, Wright, Bristol
Rothman, K. J. and Boice, J. D. (1979). *Epidemiologic Analysis with a Programmable Calculator*. N.I.H. Publication 79–1649, Washington

Other references

Burkitt, D. (1962). *Postgrad. med. J.*, **38**, 71–9
Chadwick, E. (1842). *Report on an Enquiry into the Sanitary Condition of the Labouring Population of Great Britain* (reprinted 1965, University Press, Edinburgh)
Elwood, P. C., and Pitman, R. D. (1966). *Br. J. Radiol.*, **39**, 587–9
Fry, J. (1966). *Profiles of Disease*. Livingstone, Edinburgh
Fry, J. (1974). *Common Diseases: Their Native Incidence and Care*. Medical and Technical Publishing, London
Gregg, N. M. (1941). *Trans. ophthal. Soc. Aust.*, **3**, 35–46
Kay, C. (1974). *Oral Contraceptives and Health—Interim Report on the Oral Contraception Study of the Royal College of General Practitioners*. Pitman Medical, London
MacMahon, B. (1966). *Cancer. Res.*, **26**, 1189–200
Thackrah, C. T. (1832). *The Effects of Arts, Trades and Professions*. Reprinted 1957, Livingstone, Edinburgh

2 The Use of Mortality Statistics

Mortality returns have been collected in England and Wales since 1839, and an annual publication of statistics produced. Soon after their introduction they were used in a number of special studies on the cause of disease. Hill (1955) suggested that perhaps the most important feature in Snow's argument about the transmission of cholera was his adept handling of the vital statistics for London, which were provided by the Registrar General in the mid-nineteenth century. Since then, these statistics have continued to serve as a ready source of background information for many health problems. Partly because of their extensive history, they form a suitable starting point for the consideration of the methods of epidemiology. Their use is chiefly as a constant source of descriptive material, although subsection 2.2.3 provides an example of their use in hypothesis testing. An additional reason for commencing with a consideration of mortality statistics is that they provide an introduction to the consideration of the steadily expanding range of morbidity statistics now becoming available in both developing and developed countries.

2.1 Basic Example of the Use of Mortality Statistics

A dense fog engulfed the Greater London area during the four days, 5 – 8 December, 1952. Although the fog was exceptionally severe, its grave effects were only recognised as information was accumulated from a number of sources. Newspapers carried stories about the fog, and a heavy demand for hospital beds was noted. The public appeared to expect that the main mortality would occur in the elderly; only those intimately concerned with deaths, such as coroners and registrars of deaths, were able to realise, and then only on a local basis, the true extent of the mortality. Not until all the death certificates had been assembled and analysed did the excess mortality become apparent. The figures were immediately made known to Parliament by the Minister of Health. On 18 December, in answer to a written question, the Minister replied that the number of deaths from all causes occurring in Greater London during the week ending 13 December had been 4703; this compared with 1852 in the corresponding week of the previous year. It was suggested that the cold weather had caused some of the increase in the number of deaths, but that a large part of the increase must be attributed to the fog. Since the Minister of Health replied in writing, there was no discussion and no reference was made to the need for a special study. However, the information produced an immediate reaction and it was apparent that the problem of preventing further disasters of this nature was urgent. It was decided that a special study, concentrating primarily on the fatalities, and in particular a statistical investigation of the material available to the Registrar General, would try to discover the factors responsible for the increased mortality.

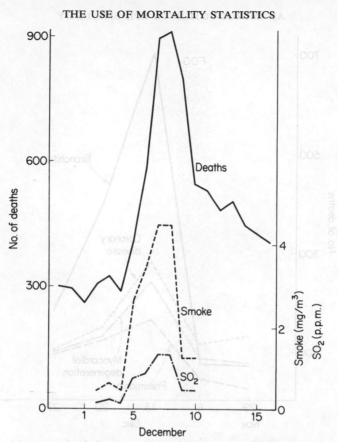

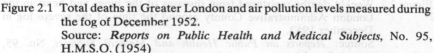

Figure 2.1 Total deaths in Greater London and air pollution levels measured during the fog of December 1952.
Source: *Reports on Public Health and Medical Subjects*, No. 95, H.M.S.O. (1954)

Figure 2.1 presents a clear indication of the link between the level of atmospheric pollution and the number of deaths recorded daily during the fog. Atmospheric pollution was measured at the monitoring station at County Hall in London. Data are shown for the total suspended matter in the air and the atmospheric concentration of sulphur dioxide. Two years after the fog a report was published (Ministry of Health, 1954), which provided a detailed analysis of the cause of death before, during and after the period of the fog. The striking feature of this analysis was that the major rise in deaths was ascribed to bronchitis, there being 9.3 times more deaths from this cause in the week of the fog compared with the preceding week. The total deaths increased over this period by 2.6 times. Apart from motor-vehicle accidents and suicides, every other specific cause examined had shown some rise. Data are presented graphically in figure 2.2 for selected causes of death that showed a major change over the period of, or immediately after, the fog.

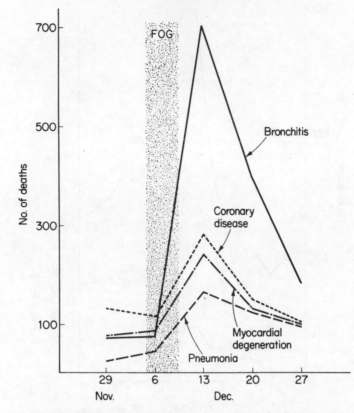

Figure 2.2 Weekly deaths registered from diseases of the lungs and heart in the London Administrative County around the time of the severe fog in December 1952.
Source: *Reports on Public Health and Medical Subjects*, No. 95, H.M.S.O. (1954)

Because there were a number of stations throughout the London Administrative County routinely monitoring atmospheric pollution, it was possible to compare indices of atmospheric pollution against the mortality rates in individual boroughs. Using available meteorological data, it was also possible to look at the relationship of the fog to temperature. There was a noticeably greater increase in the number of deaths in the eastern and northern parts of London, where there was the highest concentration of atmospheric sulphur dioxide. The report pointed out that social and occupational factors normally play an important part in determining mortality, and the effects of these might well have been accentuated under the adverse climatic conditions. The report also commented that some of the deaths occurred in elderly persons who were unlikely to have travelled far from home, but the increased death rate in some of the outer areas might have been among those who worked in the centre of London. The ratio of deaths in the week of the fog to those in the previous week was as high for those aged 45–64 as for those aged 75 and over. Comparison with data for the preceding year suggested that the number of deaths in excess of those that would normally have been expected during the first three weeks of December was between 3500 and 4000. This tragedy, and the factual report on its extent and cause, was followed by a growing interest in the control of atmospheric pollution—but discussion of this is somewhat removed from the main purpose of this chapter. However, it is of interest to note that in 1962 there was again a 'fog' in London; though the SO_2 levels were as high as in 1952, only about 750 additional deaths were observed. Ten years later there was a further minor episode with some rise of SO_2 but no appreciable increase in deaths. Waller (1981) has drawn attention to the reduction in concentration of benzo(a)pyrene in air in Central London in 1949–73, the reduced mortality from lung cancer in males aged 60–64 between 1951 and 1973 in Greater London and in rural districts in England and Wales, and the diminution in relative disparity in mortality rates for the areal statistics.

The above example relates to an acute episode that caught the public attention. The impact was sustained by the presentation of data that provided a clear description of the extent of the problem (the locality affected, the duration, the groups in the population involved and the specific causes of death). This was by no means the only source of data on the effects of air pollution; statistics of mortality due to chronic bronchitis in relation to social class and occupation, time of year, trends over many years and place of residence have all contributed to the study of this issue. The various ways in which mortality data can be handled are now discussed in greater depth.

2.2 Principles

The value of data on cause of death has been appreciated since the publication in 1662 of Graunt's classic work *Natural and Political Observations upon the Bills of Mortality*, which indicated the influence of living and working conditions on death rates in London (see Greenwood, 1948). The present system of registration of deaths in the United Kingdom dates from the Births' and Deaths' Registration Act 1836; although this did not become subject to penalty for noncompliance until 1874. Mortality data are derived from the medical certificate of the cause of death issued by a medical practitioner, together with the information given to the registrar by the informant. The practitioner completes the regulation form, in the first part of which he records the disease or condition directly leading to death, giving antecedent conditions if appropriate. In the second part he indicates other significant conditions contributing to the death, but which were not related to the disease or condition actually causing death. The informant is expected to provide the following information about the deceased: the name, sex, marital status, the maiden name of married women, the date and place of birth, his or her final occupation, and usual address of the deceased, together with the date and place of death.

This information is transcribed by the registrar into a draft entry of death registration, and a copy of the form is sent to the Office of Population

Censuses and Surveys (O.P.C.S.), where the data are coded by trained and supervised staff. The underlying cause of death is coded, using a standard manual prepared by the World Health Organisation (W.H.O.). The address of the deceased is stored as the post code, which provides specific indication of the locality of residence. The sex, marital status, place of death, type of certifier and the circumstances of certification are also classified. These data, together with the dates of birth and death, are punched, verified and entered into a computer system; an edit program checks the data prior to these being fed on to master tapes.

The master file is used to produce the output tabulations from which the tables in the annual reports are printed. The annual reports produced from this material are extremely comprehensive, but not every possible analysis is routinely carried out. It is, however, possible to approach the Registrar General and obtain specific unpublished information from the computer file. This means that theoretically any combination of two, or more, factors recorded within the system can be studied. In particular the material can be examined for variations in mortality between different categories of people, between different places at a particular time, or for one place at different times. These are the three classic axes on which analyses are performed. Examples of use of data to explore these aspects are given in the next subsection.

However, before providing further examples of the use of mortality statistics, it is necessary to consider briefly the various ways in which such statistics may be presented. All the data presented so far have involved simple counts of deaths, whether the deaths have occurred on one day, in one week, by specific cause or according to age. Contrasts have been made from period to period, again just by looking at the relative change in the number of deaths occurring. Many analyses of mortality data require more than just an examination of the number of deaths. Particularly when making comparisons of one place with another, or over a long time, it is necessary to take into account the size of the basic population among which the deaths are occurring. The simplest use of population data is to produce a 'crude mortality-rate', which is usually presented as the number of deaths occurring in a given period per 1000 population at risk. The published national data on mortality use the count obtained of the population at the census in order to provide the denominator for the calculation of such rates; the O.P.C.S. produces a mid-year estimate of the population for each year between the censuses. (The source of population estimates is discussed in subsection 3.1.9.)

The next subsection discusses the major variation in mortality by age and sex (see figure 2.3). A corollary of this variation is that there is little use in comparing the crude mortality-rate for two populations that differ widely in the proportion of the elderly or of the sexes. There is a relatively simple mathematical technique for overcoming this difficulty and producing a Standardised Mortality Ratio (S.M.R.). This technique corrects for the distribution of the population by age and sex, and produces an index that enables one to compare the mortality occurring in two different populations (see subsection 2.5.4 for a discussion of the method of calculation of the S.M.R.).

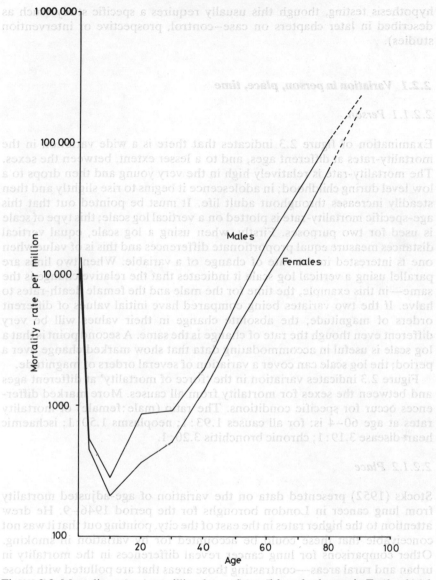

Figure 2.3 Mortality-rates per million for males and females by age in England and
Wales during 1980.
Source: DH3 No. 7, *Mortality Statistics; Cause.* O.P.C.S. (1982)

In general, routine statistics and results from surveys can be used for
either descriptive or analytical (hypothesis testing) purposes. The following
three subsections provide examples of these different activities. The examination of the data by person, place, time provides the basic descriptive
material; this may lead on to the intermediate activity of generating
hunches. In certain circumstances the routine data may actually be used for

hypothesis testing, though this usually requires a specific study (such as described in later chapters on case–control, prospective or intervention studies).

2.2.1 Variation in person, place, time

2.2.1.1 Person

Examination of figure 2.3 indicates that there is a wide variation in the mortality-rates at different ages, and to a lesser extent, between the sexes. The mortality-rate is relatively high in the very young and then drops to a low level during childhood; in adolescence it begins to rise slightly and then steadily increases throughout adult life. It must be pointed out that this age-specific mortality-rate is plotted on a vertical log scale; this type of scale is used for two purposes. Firstly, when using a log scale, equal vertical distances measure equal proportionate differences and this is of value when one is interested in the rate of change of a variable. When two lines are parallel using a vertical log scale it indicates that the relative change is the same—in this example, the time for the male and the female death-rates to halve. If the two variates being compared have initial values of different orders of magnitude, the absolute change in their values will be very different even though the rate of change is the same. A second point is that a log scale is useful in accommodating data that show marked change over a period; the log scale can cover a variation of several orders of magnitude.

Figure 2.3 indicates variation in the 'force of mortality' at different ages and between the sexes for mortality from all causes. More marked differences occur for specific conditions. The ratio (male:female) of mortality rates at age 60–4 is: for all causes 1.93:1; neoplasms 1.50:1; ischaemic heart disease 3.19:1; chronic bronchitis 3.20:1.

2.2.1.2 Place

Stocks (1952) presented data on the variation of age-adjusted mortality from lung cancer in London boroughs for the period 1946–9. He drew attention to the higher rates in the east of the city, pointing out that it was not conceivable that these could be accounted for by variation in smoking. Other comparisons for lung cancer reveal differences in the mortality in urban and rural areas—contrasting those areas that are polluted with those with a cleaner atmosphere. In this country there is about a twofold difference in mortality for areas of high atmospheric pollution compared with the smoke-free rural areas. International comparisons of mortality have also been carried out, but these are beset with a number of problems making the interpretation of data difficult. In general, it appears that mortality due to lung cancer is high in those countries with a high consumption of cigarettes, but these are often the countries that also have a high level of atmospheric pollution.

It should be noted that analyses by 'place' may involve either within country or international comparisons. Various systems exist throughout the world for the certification of cause of death and the statistical tabulation of the material, the present state of such systems being related to the development of the country and its system for health care. From 1921 to 1939, the League of Nations published a series of annual epidemiological reports; this is now the responsibility of the World Health Organisation (W.H.O.) who publish *World Health Statistics Annual* (prior to 1962 titled *Annual Epidemiological and Vital Statistics Report*). One of the three annual volumes contains vital and other medical statistics (the data for figure 2.8 came from this source). There is also a quarterly report, with the same title, which contains articles with detailed analyses on special subjects.

There are various ways in which geographical material may be handled; one is by plotting the events, or rates, on maps, so that the spatial distribution and association with geochemistry and other environmental aspects may be considered. However, as Shaper (1981) has emphasised, there is a need for caution in mapping, as the number of events and preferably the range of variation from chance should be carefully considered.

2.2.1.3 Time

During the first half of the twentieth century the death-rate from lung cancer steadily rose and by the late 1940s the mortality statistics suggested that there had been a dramatic rise in the number of deaths from this cause in the United Kingdom. Lung cancer particularly affects the older section of the population and it was necessary to standardise the mortality data in order to take into account changes in the age structure of the population. Analysis confirmed that there had been a steady rise in the death-rate due to lung cancer, which was independent of the change in the age structure.

Some doubt was raised about the accuracy of the data: it was questioned whether the rise was due to an improved quality of diagnosis, associated with the introduction of X-ray examination and other techniques (Heady and Kennaway, 1949). However, figure 2.4 shows the rise in mortality-rate has been much more marked in males than in females; it seems unlikely that the diagnosis has become so much more accurate for the male patient. (A more complex examination of the time trends in mortality from lung cancer is discussed in subsection 2.5.1, which indicates how the effects of age, sex and calendar period can be simplified.)

The very dramatic change over a relatively short space of time, as shown in figure 2.4, suggests that some environmental factor might be responsible. Careful thought was given in the late 1940s to the possible factor that could have been associated with the observed rise in mortality due to lung cancer. Attention was focused on atmospheric pollution, and consideration was given to the effect of pollution from burning coal (particularly that burnt in open-grate fires) and the increasing pollution due to the internal-combustion engine, whether run on petrol or diesel fuel. Another source of atmospheric pollution considered (in the micro-atmosphere) was cigarette smoke. More specific studies were required to explore this issue further, particularly involving case–control or prospective studies.

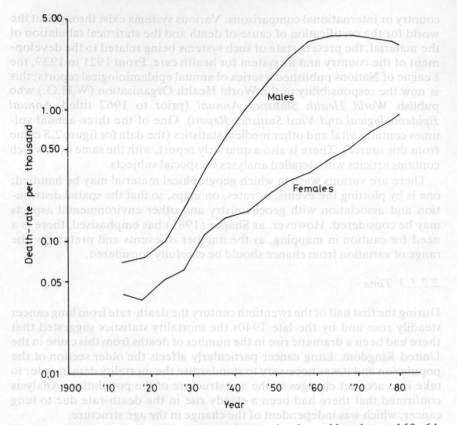

Figure 2.4 Lung cancer mortality-rates per thousand males and females aged 60–64
in England and Wales, 1911–80.
Source: Case and Pearson (1957); Alderson *et al.* (1981)

2.2.2 Generation of hunches

The probing of mortality patterns by person, place, and time will rarely be
used solely for descriptive purposes. The identification of variation immediately leads on to the questions: Why do middle-aged males have a
higher risk of fatal ischaemic heart disease than females? Why has the rise in
death-rate from this condition continued in England and Wales but halted in
the United States, with even recent evidence of a decline there?

The generation of hunches is perhaps the most tantalising aspect of
mortality data. Many workers using the material available hope that an
examination of the data will lead directly to fresh knowledge. In the early
part of the nineteenth century Dr William Farr, the first medical statistician
to the Registrar General, was deeply involved in setting up a system for
collecting, handling and interpreting the material in England. Farr (1840)
wrote

Diseases are more easily prevented than cured, and the first step to their prevention is the discovery of their exciting causes. The Registry will show the agency of these causes by numerical fact and measure the intensity of their influence and will collect information on the laws of vitality with the variation in these laws in the two sexes at different ages and the influence of civilisation, occupation, locality, season and other physical agencies, either in generating disease and inducing death, or improving the public health.

The previous section has discussed how mortality data have been of use in examining the gradual onset of an epidemic of lung cancer. A different study in which mortality data have been of use in exploring the aetiological factors in disease is the work of Aird and his colleagues (1953). These workers were aware of the well-documented fact that mortality due to stomach cancer varied according to locality, and was highest in the north and west of England. At the same time they were familiar with the variation in distribution of blood groups; there was a higher frequency of blood group O in persons living in the north of England. To test the hunch that there was an association between stomach cancer and blood group O, they examined the blood group of patients with stomach cancer in different parts of the country. Results showed that there were fewer patients with blood group O than with blood Group A—in fact, just the opposite finding to the one that they had expected from mortality data.

Although this study resulted in an unexpected finding, it serves as a simple example of how the consideration of basic mortality data can give rise to ideas about the possible causation of disease, which can then be followed up by special study. The above example also reflects the fact that mortality data cannot be expected to produce a whole series of fresh ideas on the causation of disease. It requires an alert mind to notice variation in the patterns of mortality and react to these with positive ideas of the factors that may be behind the variation. There is then the need to suggest ways in which these tentative hypotheses may be tested. This issue is discussed more fully in chapter 11, while the following subsection indicates the possible contribution from mortality statistics.

2.2.3 Testing hypotheses

Mortality statistics can also be used to test hunches derived from other sources. A good example of this work is the recent rise and fall in asthma mortality that has occurred in this country. One of the earliest indications of a particular problem was a report from a clinician (McManis, 1964), who had observed sudden death in a few patients who had received injections of adrenaline after inhalations of another bronchodilator. The following year, Greenberg (1965) pointed out the dangers of excessive use of similar drugs in bronchial asthma. Following sporadic case reports of fatalities, information became available to the Committee on the Safety of Drugs (C.S.D.) whose medical field workers had established strong circumstantial evidence of the harmful side-effects of pressurised aerosols. Inman and Adelstein

(1969) examined the trends in asthma mortality for an eleven-year period (1958–68) in relation to the use of pressurised aerosols containing bronchodilators. In the period 1961–6 they noted a rapid growth in the sales of pressurised aerosols and a considerable increase in asthma mortality. The latter was particularly apparent in children aged ten to fourteen, among whom there was a sevenfold increase in asthma mortality. In June 1967, the C.S.D. issued a warning to all doctors in the United Kingdom about the possible hazards of pressurised aerosols if used excessively in the treatment of asthma. Figure 2.5 demonstrates that from about this time there was a significant fall in the number of deaths from asthma.

Although this circumstantial evidence was strongly suggestive, it did not amount to proof that excessive absorption of bronchodilators from pressurised aerosols was responsible for the epidemic. In fact, there were some unexplained geographical variations that could not be readily dismissed. Scotland, Ireland, New Zealand and Australia shared in the experience of England and Wales. However, the United States, Canada and the Netherlands were not affected, and only a small increase was noted in other parts of Europe and in Japan (Fraser and Doll, 1971). It was reported, for instance, that although the epidemic had not occurred in the United States, there had been large sales of aerosols there. A report by Stolley (1972) went a long way to clarify the situation. He demonstrated convincingly a significant positive correlation between increased mortality from asthma and the national sales of those aerosols that delivered a concentrated dose. Neither Canada nor the United States had licensed the more concentrated preparations and neither country had experienced the epidemic of asthma death.

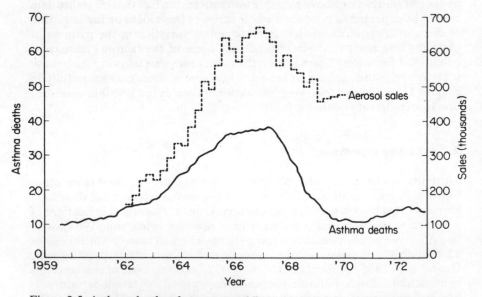

Figure 2.5 Asthma deaths of persons aged five–thirty-four compared with sales and prescriptions of asthma preparations in England and Wales for 1959–68. Sources: Inman and Adelstein (1969) and *Registrar General's Statistical Reviews for England and Wales 1969–73*

Therefore, a careful examination of the mortality data helped to support the basic contention obtained from clinical studies. This contention became much more firmly supported when examined in relation to data about sales of aerosols and the type of aerosol used in the different countries. Neither a case–control study, nor a prospective study, was thought suitable to examine this issue and a change in clinical practice appears to have been accompanied by an abatement of the problem.

2.2.4 Monitoring the public's health

Routine mortality data can be used to monitor the state of public health, and this was one of the uses that Farr (1840) suggested more than 130 years ago. By examining the overall mortality, corrected for age, of a population over a period of time, one can get an index of the force of mortality. Perhaps of more interest is the examination of age-specific mortality-rates.

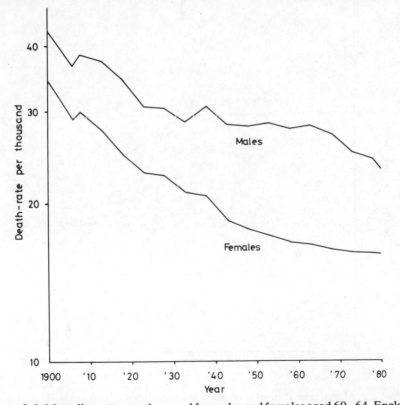

Figure 2.6 Mortality-rates per thousand for males and females aged 60–64, England and Wales, 1900–80.
Source: *Registrar General's Statistical Reviews for England and Wales, 1900–73*; *Mortality Statistics: Cause, England and Wales*, DH2, 1974–80

An example is provided in figure 2.6, which shows the trend in mortality rates for males and for females aged 60–64 in this country during the present century. A remarkable difference in trend is observed, the mortality of the middle-aged male being nearly as high now as it was at the beginning of the century. For the female there has been a slow, but steady, decline during the past fifty years. This seems to indicate that advances in medical knowledge and the generally greater availability of health-care services have been unable to improve the health of the male section of the population. These data are compatible with the suggestion that changes in the way of life of the middle-aged male during this century have been harmful to health—smoking, lack of exercise, obesity and diet have been suggested causes.

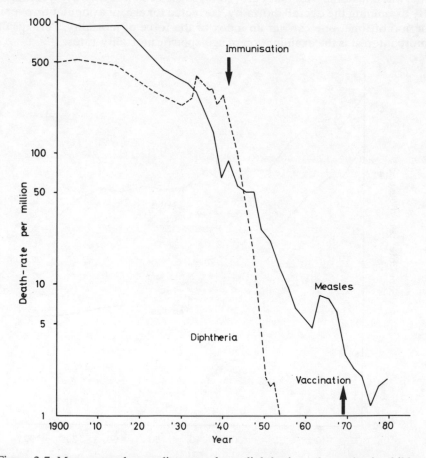

Figure 2.7 Mean annual mortality-rates from diphtheria and measles in children under fifteen in England and Wales, 1900–80.
Source: *Registrar General's Statistical Reviews for England and Wales, 1900–73; Mortality Statistics: Cause, England and Wales*, DH2, 1974–80

So far two separate approaches to the use of mortality data have been presented: the provision of a description of the well-being of the total population; and the quantification of the specific force of mortality affecting certain segments of the population. Mortality data may also be used to throw light on the effects of public-health programmes. One such programme introduced during the early part of the Second World War was the scheme for immunisation against diphtheria. Treatment of an acute attack of diphtheria was introduced in about 1870, by the use of sera derived from patients who had recovered from the infection. Between the World Wars a method of active immunisation against the disease was developed, but this was only launched nationally in the United Kingdom in 1940.

Figure 2.7 shows the pattern of mortality in young children since the latter part of the nineteenth century. It can be seen that the mortality due to diphtheria declined steeply after the introduction of prophylactic immunisation. The contrast, however, with measles is not as great as might be expected when one bears in mind the fact that immunisation against measles has only just been introduced. This topic will be discussed further in the subsection on evaluation of the health services (8.1.6).

2.2.5 Validity of mortality statistics

All routine data-collection systems are open to the challenge that the material is not completely accurate; this is particularly a problem in the case of mortality data. It is suggested that there is a potential error at each link in the chain of events between the diagnosis of the cause of death by the clinician and the publication of routine mortality data:

$$\text{diagnosis} \rightarrow \text{certification} \rightarrow \text{coding} \rightarrow \text{processing} \rightarrow \text{interpretation}$$

A number of studies have been carried out to determine the accuracy of the diagnoses of fatal conditions and the quality of certification. Although a clinician may be clear in his own mind about the diagnosis, he does not always record this clearly on the death certificate in a way that can be appropriately coded. Coding the data may create difficulties, particularly where there is some doubt about the interpretation of the entry on the death certificate. The processing system may introduce some errors, especially at the data-input stage. The final source of error is during interpretation (or misinterpretation) of the analysed material. Specific studies have been used various approaches:

(1) Comparison of clinical diagnoses against autopsy findings (Heasman and Lipworth, 1966; Cameron and McGoogan, 1981);
(2) Production of a certificate from dummy case histories (Reid and Rose, 1964; Diehl and Gau, 1982);
(3) Review of complete case-histories against the death certificate (Alderson, 1965; Clarke and Whitfield, 1978);
(4) Duplicate coding of the death certificate (Wingrave et al., 1981).

A review of these studies suggested that there were appreciable errors (perhaps 20 per cent being minor and 5 per cent involving shift of the diagnosis from one body system to another); despite such errors it was concluded that mortality statistics could be interpreted with caution (Alderson, 1983).

2.2.6 Classification of disease

As long ago as 1853, following the first statistical congress, Farr in England and D'Espine in Switzerland were asked to prepare lists of diseases suitable for a classification. Though a combined list was revised over the next thirty years, the classification was not generally adopted in different countries. However, at the end of the nineteenth century the first revision of the International Classification of Diseases (I.C.D.) was agreed and its adoption gradually extended to more countries; decennial revisions were instituted. Since 1946 the W.H.O. has been responsible for these revisions; the sixth, introduced in 1948, had the dual purpose of classifying diseases as well as causes of death. The ninth revision, of 1978, introduced a dual classification of certain diagnostic statements which contain information about both aetiology and manifestation (where the latter is important in its own right). For example, mumps encephalitis can be coded both to mumps—the primary aetiological classification—and to encephalitis, which is the important manifestation relevant to medical-care issues. Such dual codes are distinguished in the I.C.D. by a dagger (†) and an asterisk (*) (e.g. mumps encephalitis is coded 072.1† and 323.4*).

Various rules have been introduced since 1900 to formalise the selection of the primary or underlying cause of death, when the certificate mentions two or more conditions present at the time of death. Virtually all national mortality statistics are derived from underlying-cause coding. However, periodically suggestions have been made that all conditions mentioned should be coded and analysed; this would give quite a different perspective to the importance of various conditions. For example, an appreciable number of deaths are associated with diabetes, in addition to those where the diabetes is thought to be directly responsible for the death. Using deaths for the United States for 1976, Chamblee and Evans (1982) examined the ratio of mentions to underlying codes for various diseases. They highlight diabetes as a major cause of death, which is also 'mentioned' in many other death certificates. The extreme were 'symptoms and ill-defined conditions' which were mentioned over twelve times for every death coded to this as the underlying cause.

One of the difficulties in using the I.C.D. is that medical knowledge may advance fairly rapidly for certain conditions; together with changes in medical terminology, this can pose problems for coding with a relatively inflexible international classification. One consequence of this is the pressure to change and update the I.C.D. at periodic revisions; this may then lead to alteration in structure of sections of the classification or changes in the rules of selection of underlying cause that create discontinuity in the long-term trends in certain statistics. There are also conflicts due to the wide range of users and uses of the I.C.D.; the classification is meant to be suitable for coding mortality statistics for any country in the world (including those where a majority of deaths are not medically certified). At the same time, there are very different interests represented by users coding routine morbidity data in national data systems (such as discussed in the next chapter), and research workers collecting extensive particulars about a relatively small number of patients with specific conditions.

2.3 Advantages and Disadvantages of Mortality Statistics

As has already been mentioned, the routine collection of mortality data commenced in the middle of the nineteenth century, and since then material has been collected for virtually every death occurring in the United Kingdom. The reason for the introduction of the registration of deaths was not purely to collect mortality data of interest to the medical profession—in fact the registration was introduced for different reasons. The recording of the cause of death was only introduced as an amendment of the initial Bill while it was passing through the House of Lords. Since the material has to be collected for other legal and demographic purposes, the actual cost of obtaining mortality data is relatively low, compared with some routine data that will be discussed in the following chapter.

The W.H.O. has been responsible for sponsoring and encouraging the collection of accurate mortality statistics throughout the world, and the majority of developing countries now have some system for the recording, collection, processing and production of mortality data. The developed countries produce annual publications covering various aspects of the material, and the data are usually presented in such a way that comparisons can fairly readily be made between countries. This extends the value of the material, and enables one to probe the data in some of the general ways indicated above.

All sets of routine data have certain disadvantages, however, that need to be borne in mind. With any data-collection system there is always concern as to whether a complete set of data is collected and processed. As has already been mentioned, the vast majority of deaths are registered and the cause of death obtained for each registered death. (In this country there are approximately 500 000 deaths a year, and only about 100 persons are believed to disappear and possibly die without a death certificate being obtained. The majority of deaths are certified by the practitioner attending the patient, or by the coroner in cases of doubt or a violent death.)

Many routine data-collection systems suffer from delay in data collection, but owing to the legal requirement to register the death and the establishment of registrars responsible for handling this material, there is a steady flow of data into the central processing system. Copies of the basic material are currently made available to the District Medical Officer. Very simple weekly analyses of the data are produced by O.P.C.S, and there is a more extensive quarterly report, but the principal analyses are published annually in the Registrar General's *Statistical Review* (now Annual Reference Volumes in the DH series). The mortality data for one complete calendar year is published two years later, but owing to the relatively slow change in mortality data from year to year this means that the national data are usually available within an acceptable time period.

Another problem in handling routine mortality data is that it is not generally applicable to all medical problems. Some conditions have a high mortality rate and the death occurs quickly; for such diseases mortality data can provide a fairly accurate quantification of the problem. Other diseases have a much longer natural history and a variable mortality, and the longer the natural history the less information mortality statistics can provide about the causative factors in the disease. In such circumstances, the mortality data can indicate the age at death and the variation in the mortality between the sexes, in different places and at different times; one cannot immediately interpret these findings as being associated with differences in causative factors. This is particularly so if the case fatality varies in relation to some of these factors. If, for example, the incidence of a particular disease is higher in women, but the proportion of women surviving is greater, theoretically there would be a higher mortality rate in males, which would tend to hide the fact that the actual condition is more common in females.

A further aspect of this problem is that there are many conditions that create considerable discomfort to patients (and, incidentally, a considerable workload to the health-care services) and yet rarely figure in the mortality data. An extreme example of this is the common cold; this is responsible for virtually no deaths. A more severe disease, that causes considerable incapacity and pain, is established arthritis; again the mortality is low, and the routine mortality data are of limited value in a study of arthritis.

Many routine data-collection systems are relatively inflexible, and there is little facility for introducing new items into the system and processing these alongside the original standard particulars. This is particularly true of mortality data, for the basic items mentioned in section 2.2 have hardly altered over the past 100 years. Flexibility can only be provided by a special study of additional material collected independently of the vital statistics system.

Another general point that can occur in the interpretation and use of routine data is that many of the potential users of the material can have some inbuilt objections to the acceptance of the data. There is often a tendency to disregard studies based on mortality data, because of an over-awareness of the potential inaccuracy of the material. By stressing the inaccuracy people may fail to realise how data pooled for a country can still show very important trends—such as has been discussed in relation to the testing of hypotheses on the danger of the use of aerosol bronchodilators (see subsection 2.2.3). The fluctuation in the mortality rates due to asthma in the past decade or so, when examined at national level, is consistent with the rise and fall of the hazard due to the over-use of these aerosols. However, this information has been achieved with data that are of a variable level of accuracy. An important point to bear in mind is that by examining national material some of the problems of interpretation have been reduced owing to the cancelling of random errors.

Moriyama (1982) discussed the advantages and disadvantages of continuous vital registration systems and the contribution that can be made from the combination of surveys and indirect estimation techniques as an alternative in developing countries. He suggested these other approaches should not be regarded as an adequate long-term substitute for death registration.

2.4 Extensions of the Use of Mortality Data

This section describes some of the different methods of manipulating mortality data; some of the approaches have already been foreshadowed earlier in the chapter, but aspects of method are now covered.

2.4.1 Analyses by additional characteristics of the deceased

Some of the material already discussed has involved analyses by sex and age. Additional items available are marital status, occupation, social class and place of birth. Some countries have other items available such as religion. Providing denominators are available from national sources, mortality rates can be calculated and the results examined for variation. It must be remembered, when considering the following brief examples, that such statistics are of value in demonstrating that differences exist, rather than explaining why this should be so.

2.4.1.1 Marital status

It has been known since the eighteenth century that there was an increased risk of breast cancer in nuns (Ramazzini, 1713). Hems (1980) used mortality statistics to demonstrate that the age-specific rates in England and Wales were higher in the single than the married. This leads on to mechanisms that might be involved, including the influence of hormonal changes associated with pregnancy.

2.4.1.2 Occupation

Though this is one aspect of use of mortality statistics and warrants mention in this section, a description of the method and uses of the data is given in the chapter on occupational studies (subsection 10.1.1.1).

2.4.1.3 Social class

An extension of the study of occupational mortality was the development of a more general classification for analysing health experience. Stevenson (1923) divided the population into eight social groups, and tabulated the infant mortality in each of these. This scheme was soon modified to produce the five social classes (coded in accordance with the Registrar General's Classification of Occupations), which are still used to examine mortality (and morbidity) data. The present classification distinguishes the following:

I Professional; II Intermediate; IIIn Skilled non-manual; IIIm Skilled manual; IV Partly skilled; V Unskilled. As an example of the relationship with mortality, there still remain in England and Wales (O.P.C.S., 1982a) and Scotland (Registrar General, 1982) appreciable differences in the infant mortality between the social classes, despite the decreasing rates experienced by all subgroups of the population. The relationship of social class to various measures of mortality and morbidity has been discussed at some length in a report of the Research Working Group (1980); this included a review of the difficulties of using an occupation-based index of social class.

2.4.1.4 Migrants

In aetiological studies a recurring topic of interest is the separation of environmental from genetic influences. One preliminary approach has been the international comparisons of mortality rates. These comparisons are, however, subject to bias owing to variations in diagnostic habit and certification practice in different countries (Reid and Rose, 1964). Around the time of a national census it is possible to use as denominator a count of the population according to place of birth, or length of time in the country in the case of migrants. This has enabled a number of studies to be carried out on the death rates of those born abroad. When the mortality rates in the country of birth are very different, but the rates of long-stay immigrants are similar to those of the 'native' population, it has been suggested that environmental factors are of greater importance than genetic ones (Dean, 1959; Haenszel, 1961; Krueger and Moriyama, 1967; Stenhouse and McCall, 1970). Kallner and Groen (1968) studied the mortality from coronary heart disease and cerebrovascular accidents among immigrants to Israel. Migrants from Turkey had a coronary mortality almost as high as those from Europe and America, while the rates for the Yemenite Jews were very low. The authors stressed the exploratory nature of such studies, but discussed how the material could be used to advance knowledge and assist in the planning of further studies.

2.4.1.5 Race or religion

In some countries the census and the mortality records may identify individuals from different races or religions. Using such material it is thus possible to contrast the age- and/or sex-specific mortality rates for the different racial groups within the country. The prime example is the United States; since the early part of this century, the annual mortality statistics could be separately tabulated for : White, Negro, Indian, Chinese, Japanese, and other—though the majority of published tables only distinguished white and other.

2.4.2 Collation

Morris and his colleagues (1961, 1962) examined the mortality data for eighty-three county boroughs of England and Wales. Specific causes of death as well as total deaths were studied for middle-aged men and women in relation to contemporary estimates of total hardness and calcium content of local drinking water. At the same time an intensive search was made of social and other environmental factors to see if these confounding factors could explain the highly significant negative association between water hardness and cardiovascular mortality. A further study (Crawford et al., 1968) reported on the mortality data for the sixty-one largest county boroughs in England and Wales using information collected around the time of the 1961 census.

Crawford and her colleagues (1971) observed a favourable effect on cardiovascular death-rates in those towns where the water had become harder, and an unfavourable effect in the towns where the water had become softer. Such a natural experiment provided a more positive probe into the relationship between water hardness and mortality. A further important issue is that these studies of mortality data only provide a preliminary examination of a complex problem, and have then to be followed up with detailed studies using other approaches. For example, pathological and biochemical studies on autopsy material have been carried out by Crawford and Crawford (1967); clinical and biochemical studies of men living in hard- and soft-water areas have been reported by Stitt et al. (1973).

Such studies bring together mortality statistics and data from other statistical sources on various factors associated with the population from which the deaths have been obtained. (Similar studies can be carried out using morbidity data, and this is dealt with in subsection 3.4.1.) The important point about collation studies is that the two sets of data being brought together must both relate to the same population; comparisons can be made within a country, for example, looking at the distribution of mortality and occupation by locality. Other comparisons may be between countries contrasting the differences in the two variates (mortality and environmental index) for a range of countries. Another approach takes the same geographical population, and then examines the relative change in the two indices over time.

The environmental data may relate to any factor which is thought to be associated with the risk of the disease being studied, and for which population data are available (e.g. air pollution; various chemical constituents of water; dietary intake by nutrient; consumption of alcohol, cigarettes, or drugs; various indices of industrial production). In comparison with the mortality statistics, the 'environmental' data may be much less specific; information may be only available on a crude per capita basis.

At its simplest the data may consist of two variates for each of the geographical units and one very simple presentation is to plot a scatter diagram, as in figure 2.8. This clearly indicates a fairly crude relationship between per capita intake of fat and mortality rate from breast cancer in fifty countries; the higher the fat intake, the higher the mortality rate. This relationship may also be shown by plotting the data graphically on maps.

In addition to the visual methods of presentation of the data the relationship between two or more variates may be examined statistically. The data for figure 2.8 have also been used to calculate a correlation coefficient (this is the index of association which is further described in subsection 2.5.5).

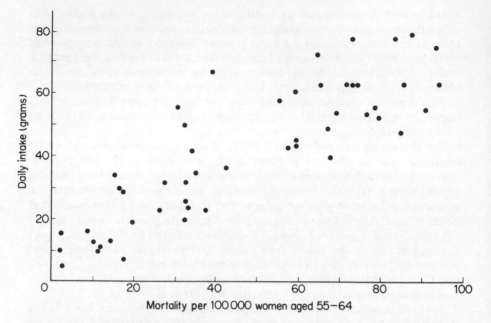

Figure 2.8 Breast-cancer mortality for women aged 55–64 in 1970 plotted against *per capita* daily intake of fat in 1960 for various countries.
Source: *World Health Statistics Annual* (1970); *Food and Agricultural Organisation Production Year Book* (1970)

Such statistical testing of the data can also determine whether the results are likely to have occurred by chance.

The main advantage of a collation study is that it should be relatively cheap and quick; this is because it is using data from published statistics. It is also possible to examine situations where there are wide contrasts—wide variation in mortality, or in environmental factors. This is because the method uses different countries, or within a large country will cover zones where there are major variations. Obviously, because routine data are being used, the items are likely to be relatively crude, while there may be errors or biases in the basic data. Errors in the mortality and environmental data tend to reduce the chance of picking up a genuine relationship. If a country with a high mortality for a particular condition also has a very efficient system for documenting environmental data, which tends to record high levels, a bias will be introduced. Migration can be a source of bias, particularly for within-country analyses. There may be a tendency for the infirm (or the fit) to migrate to certain areas of the country; this can distort the mortality patterns, especially for diseases with long latent intervals. Polissar (1980) used data on United States migration, age-distribution of cancers by site, and latent intervals, to evaluate the loss of power in geographical collation studies. Long latent intervals, cancers affecting children and younger adults, and use of counties instead of states (i.e. smaller rather than larger geographical areas) all militated against the identification of an environmental risk.

It must be borne in mind that collation studies are using population data and therefore average values of both mortality and environmental factors for the selected populations. This is very different from collecting discrete measures on individuals (in either case–control or prospective studies). It is even conceivable that a direct relationship at the population level may hide a genuine indirect relationship as far as individuals are concerned within the populations. For example, there is a positive association between increased intake of fat in different countries and increased mortality rate from colo-rectal cancer. However, measurement in individuals has suggested that a lower blood cholesterol is associated with a higher risk of colo-rectal cancer.

An important issue is that of multiple comparisons. In one study of mortality from different cancers and dietary intake, over 4000 correlation coefficients were generated (Knox, 1977). There is immediately a problem of interpreting any correlation coefficient where p is < 0.01; by chance, 1 in 100 of such correlations might reach this level of significance. This is discussed further in subsection 11.3.2.

2.4.3 Linked data

A major fresh venture began in England and Wales with the selection of a 1 per cent sample of respondents from the 1971 national census. Event data were assembled into a cohort file, including births to sample parents, cancer registration, psychiatric hospitalisation of over two years duration, emigration and death. The sample was enhanced by 1 per cent of identified immigrants as well as 1 per cent of all births. A recent report (Fox and Goldblatt, 1982) presents a wide range of results from mortality of the cohort in 1971–5; this included analyses by economic activity, household structure, housing characteristics, area of residence, internal migration and immigration.

Further discussion of linked studies is provided in subsections 3.4.2 and 3.4.4.

2.4.4 Use of basic data for special studies

So far in this chapter discussion has been restricted to the use of published mortality data derived from death registration. The basic information available on death registration may, however, be used directly for two separate purposes: (1) to initiate case–control studies, or (2) to provide an end-point in prospective studies. Thus the material may be used to identify individuals dying from a given disease, and to initiate a study of these subjects (perhaps by examination of medical records, or by questioning their next of kin). Such a study starting from the death-registration information is further discussed in subsection 5.2.1.1. The second use of the data is where a follow-up study is being carried out on a large number of individuals thought to be at risk of a particular disease. The nominal role of those being followed up may be matched against the lists of deaths and the death notification data.

This use of the routine material as an end-point in follow-up studies will be
discussed in subsection 6.4.1.

2.5 Statistical Techniques

2.5.1 Graphical cohort analysis

Figure 2.9 shows the death-rate according to age for males suffering from
lung cancer; the data are from the pooled mortality-rates for a recent
five-year calendar period (1966–70). The graph shows that the mortality-
rate is low in the young; it then appears to climb to a peak in late middle age,
but falls in the elderly. This figure has been deliberately chosen, because it
has to be interpreted with caution. Men, whose ages ranged from about
twenty to eighty, contributed to the graph. These data represent the
death-rates among different generations, who have been born during a
period of change in the world's history and exposed to very different
environmental and social circumstances during their lives.

An American worker (Frost, 1939) showed that it was instructive to look
at mortality due to tuberculosis for patients born in successive decades; his
approach was generalised by Case (1956a, 1956b). The latter worker drew
attention to the need to study different 'cohorts' of the population, particularly when considering malignant disease or conditions for which the inci-

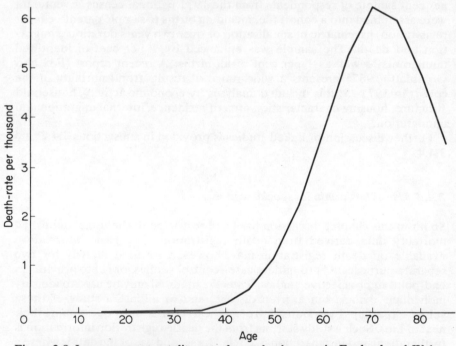

Figure 2.9 Lung-cancer mortality-rate for males by age, in England and Wales,
1966–70.
Source: *Registrar General's Statistical Reviews for England and Wales*,
Part 1 Tables, H.M.S.O. (1968–72)

dence or mortality rate can change fairly rapidly over a relatively short time. Case pointed out that this peak in age-specific mortality was a reflection of different trends in the various birth-cohorts; replotting the 'age contours' for different birth-cohorts removed the peak in mortality. Trends in age-specific mortality may be plotted in various ways and it is now thought instructive to use two contrasting ways with the x-axis relating to (1) year at death, and (2) year of birth. Figure 2.10 (a) and (b) show lung-cancer mortality for males in England and Wales. The curves are derived from the

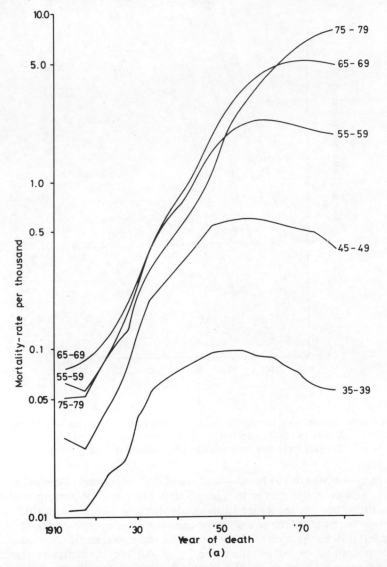

Figure 2.10a Age-specific mortality-rates for lung cancer in males in England and
Wales 1911–80, plotted by year of death.
Source: Case and Pearson (1957); Alderson *et al.* (1981)

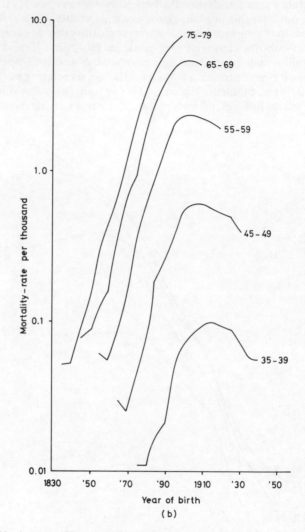

Figure 2.10b Age-specific mortality-rates for lung cancer in males in England and
Wales 1911–80, plotted by year of birth.
Source: Case and Pearson (1957); Alderson *et al.* (1981)

same data—deaths in 1911–80—and are of similar general shape in the two
figures; however, the curves in figure 2.10b are not all superimposed one
above the other (as the older individuals dying in the same period were
obviously born before the younger ones and have their points plotted further
to the left). Both the figures show a peak in the age-specific data for males
35–9 up until 65–9, but not for those 75–9. An important aspect of such a
pair of figures is to check whether any inflections in the curves occur more
nearly in a vertical line above the year of death, or year of birth; this
facilitates consideration of whether the change in mortality trend has

affected different age-groups at the same time or has affected different birth-cohorts. This has implications for the possible causal effects (e.g. some external environmental effect may alter the risk of disease in all age-groups at the same time, while change in behaviour often occurs in a birth cohort, or generation). Case (1956b) clearly demonstrated that succeeding birth-cohorts in England and Wales had higher rates of lung cancer mortality; there is now evidence in the most recent data of a decline in rates for cohorts born in the early part of this century.

2.5.2 Statistical distinction of cohort and period changes

Because of the interest in distinguishing cohort- from period-changes in mortality patterns, statistical methods have been explored in addition to the rather subjective interpretation of graphical material. Recent work suggests that there is now an acceptable method for distinguishing the three components of trend data—age, period, and cohort effects. One approach to this, by fitting various mathematical models to the data, has been described by Hakulinen and Pukkala (1982). Barrett (1973) described other work, illustrated with examination of material for cervical cancer; Osmond et al. (1982) have extended this work and reported their findings for a number of malignancies. The actual statistical method, which is beyond the scope of this section, has been discussed in Osmond and Gardner (1982).

These techniques are also suitable as a basis for projection of trends in mortality, with the development of models that incorporate estimates of the future changes in both exposure to risk and results of intervention. Hakama (1980) has described some results; though he was using cancer incidence rather than mortality data, the underlying statistical concepts are the same. Once the approach extends beyond the very simple linear projection of trends, and incorporates both (1) extrapolation of cohort and secular trends, and (2) estimates of possible future changes, the general field of mathematical modelling is being entered. An example of some of the techniques of modelling (though applied to a very different topic) is given in subsecton 8.5.2.

There are other special applications of cohort data. For instance, Manton and Stallard (1982) used a stochastic compartment transition model to estimate the distribution of morbidity of stomach cancer in the United States population, based on cohort-mortality data and a model of tumour growth.

A rather simpler system is that now utilised for routine mortality data for England and Wales; this examines the age- and sex-specific deaths and death rates by cause over a ten-year period and applies a test for trend that indicates whether there has been a significant increase or decrease in the statistics (see O.P.C.S., 1980).

2.5.3 Do differences in numbers of deaths or death-rates mean anything?

The first example given in this chapter was of a marked rise in the deaths around the time of the major London fog in 1952. Anyone looking at the figures presented would immediately conclude that there had been some association between the fog and the change in the number of deaths. If the fluctuation in the deaths had been lower, there might have been doubt at some point as to whether the fluctuation was just 'chance', or was a true association (or even a cause-and-effect relationship). The data presented could not in fact prove that there was a cause-and-effect relationship, but the first point to be established is whether the fluctuation of deaths was greater than could have occurred by chance.

This is a field in which certain statistical techniques can be used. These techniques stem from work particularly in France, in the eighteenth century, when there was considerable interest in studying games of chance. For example, if over a ten-year period there were on average twenty-five deaths per year from a particular disease in a certain town in England, one would not expect that there would be exactly that number of deaths each year; the number would fluctuate a little. Statistical method can indicate how widely this number could vary. Once in forty years, the number of deaths might be higher than the average figure plus twice the 'standard error', and once in forty years lower than the average figure less twice the standard error. Where the number of deaths in an area is very small compared with the population at risk, an approximate estimate of the standard error of the deaths can be derived from the square root of the number of deaths. Thus, with an average figure of twenty-five deaths the estimate of the standard error is five and twice the standard error is ten. One would expect, therefore, the number of deaths over a twenty-year period to fluctuate between the limits of fifteen and thirty-five with only two values beyond these. This gives a rough rule-of-thumb test that helps in interpreting some of the differences that occur from year to year. Table 2.1 sets out the method of calculation.

Table 2.1   Calculation of the approximate 95 per cent confidence limits of an annual number of deaths

---

95% confidence limits = average annual deaths $\pm 2 \times$ standard error
                      = average annual deaths $\pm 2 \times \sqrt{}$ average annual deaths
                      = $25 \pm 2\sqrt{25}$
                      = 15 to 35

When comparing the deaths in different populations one would not normally be looking at the number of deaths but at the death-rates, and similarly one can calculate a standard error of a death-rate. This standard error is the death-rate divided by the square root of the number of deaths. Usually some indication of the range of chance difference between two local death-rates is required. The appropriate statistical figure in this situation is twice the standard error of the difference between the two rates; this can be calculated fairly readily as follows

$$2 \times \left[\frac{(\text{death-rate in town A})^2}{\text{number of deaths in A}} + \frac{(\text{death-rate in town B})^2}{\text{number of deaths in B}} \right]^{1/2}$$

The important point about presenting the statistical method for examining the difference in the number of deaths, or death-rates, is to indicate at an early stage in the text that there are a series of techniques available that assist in the interpretation of such factual material. It is important to be aware of the problem of interpreting differences in figures. The mortality from all causes in the country, or in large towns, is based on very large numbers of events and the fluctuation in such large numbers is relatively small. The opposite extreme occurs when studying specific causes of death in small subgroups of the population—such as the deaths in the first year of life for specific local authorities; infant deaths are relatively rare and therefore the rates are based on small numbers. The smaller the number of events on which the rates are based the greater the proportional fluctuation that may occur by chance. It is important to use the appropriate statistical techniques for examining differences in such rates before jumping to the conclusion that environmental or other factors have changed and have had a specific effect on the rates. Rosenbaum (1963) published three nomograms, which are of value in assessing the significance of rates per 1000 for (1) providing confidence limits to a rate, (2) comparing two rates based on different samples and (3) comparing two rates based on distinct elements in the same sample.

An important general point to be remembered is that by comparing many pairs of numbers of deaths or rates the likelihood of a chance finding of a 'significant' difference is increased. This must be borne in mind when considering mortality data and all the other sets of data that will be described later.

This issue is discussed further in section 11.3.2.

2.5.4 Standardisation

Reference has already been made in a preceding section to the need to take into account the age distribution of different populations before directly comparing their death-rates. A number of the figures on mortality that have been presented have indicated the close relationship between mortality and age. A simple method is required for comparing the force of mortality in different localities where the proportion of the elderly varies. One approach to this problem is to examine the mortality by specific age-groups. Although this enables direct comparisons to be made irrespective of any variation in age distribution, it can result in the presentation of a large amount of material (if, for instance, the age-specific mortality rates for fifteen five-year age-groups are examined). This creates a problem in the preparation and presentation of the material, and the sheer number of separate sets of data creates difficulties in the interpretation.

Standardisation is a technique that may be used for producing an index of mortality, which is adjusted for the age distribution in a particular group being examined. One approach is to apply the age-specific rates for a 'standard' population to the age-specific numbers of individuals in the study population and then to derive an expected figure for the numbers of deaths. Table 2.2 indicates the general method; the data are taken from a report on

Table 2.2 Calculation of standardised mortality ratio for two occupational groups

(a) Original data 1959–63

Occupation	Number in occupational group	Observed deaths	Crude death-rate/1000 *per annum*
Farmers, foresters and fishermen	705 910	20 973	5.9
Armed forces	301 120	4 282	2.8

(b) Calculation of expected number of deaths

Age	Annual death-rates/1000 men, England and Wales	Farmers, foresters, fishermen		Armed forces	
		Number in occupation	Expected deaths* 1959–63	Number in occupation	Expected deaths* 1959–63
15–24	1.028	134 560	691.6	165 030	848.3
25–34	1.118	124 100	693.7	73 240	409.4
35–44	2.411	132 220	1 593.9	42 250	509.3
45–54	7.072	160 110	5 661.5	15 930	563.3
55–64	21.710	154 920	16 816.6	4 670	506.9
Total expected deaths			25 457.3		2837.2

* Expected deaths = number in occupation × national age-specific rate × 5. An annual death-rate is being used and the expected deaths are required for the period 1959–63 (that is, 5 years).

(c) Calculation of standardised mortality ratio

$$\text{S.M.R. farmers, foresters, fishermen} = \frac{20\,973}{25\,457.3} \times 100 = 82$$

$$\text{S.M.R. armed forces} = \frac{4282}{2837.2} \times 100 = 151$$

occupational mortality for the period 1959–63 (Registrar General, 1971).

If the observed mortality, after taking into account the age distribution of the specific population, is the same as that expected, a S.M.R. of 100 will be obtained. If the mortality is high a figure of greater than 100 will be obtained, while if the mortality is low a corresponding reduction in the S.M.R. will occur. The crude mortality-rate for farmers was 5.9/1000 men *per annum*, and for the armed forces 2.8/1000 men *per annum*. This suggests a lower mortality in the armed forces. However, table 2.2 (b) shows that there are very few men in the older age-groups in the armed forces and an age correction produces an S.M.R. of 151 compared with that for farmers of 82 (see table 2.2 c). Standardisation for age thus indicates a considerably lower mortality for the farmers. The mathematics involved are relatively simple; however, the important point at this stage is to grasp the broad outline of the approach and appreciate the indications for standardisation and the situations in which it should be applied. A matter of judgement is whether to use age-specific rates or age-standardised rates for comparative purposes. The main consideration is the number of age groups for which a comparison is required; thus when comparing the mortality in different towns, to present the results of fifteen five-year age-groups would create difficulties, and it would be more appropriate to use age-standardised rates. The other extreme is consideration of the medical problems of a subgroup of the population defined by age, such as infancy or middle age. In this kind of situation, it is more appropriate to use age-specific rates. Even when making use of an S.M.R. it is advisable to check the age-specific rates for consistency. Kilpatrick (1962) discussed the problem of standardising in a situation where an occupation has raised mortality at one end of the age range, and a low mortality at the other. Any index such as an S.M.R. will be misleading in such a situation. Alderson (1981) has reviewed a variety of indices and concluded that the indirectly calculated S.M.R. is most suitable as the general technique.

The approach described in table 2.2 is known as indirect standardisation. It is more generally suitable, since it uses rates based on the standard population; this method has the advantages that these rates are usually easier to obtain than age-specific rates for the study population, and being based on larger numbers, they are less subject to chance variation and produce a better estimate of the S.M.R.

In the example in table 2.2 three sets of data were used: (1) the number of men in the occupational group (obtained from the census), (2) the number of observed deaths in the occupation (a count of the deaths in the period 1959–63, where the occupation was coded to the particular category of interest), and (3) the annual age-specific death-rates for all men in England and Wales (obtained from the national mortality statistics). Providing equivalent data are available, the process of standardisation can be applied to other factors affecting mortality, or to other measures of outcome, and this is perhaps best explained by presenting specific examples. As well as being associated closely with age, mortality bears an association with the social-class distribution of the population. At the time of a census, data is collected on the age distribution and social-class distribution of inhabitants in each local authority area; it is therefore possible to apply the class-specific mortality-rates to the social-class distribution of towns and obtain a mortality rate corrected for the distribution. With a little extra computation an S.M.R. corrected for both age and social class can be obtained. A parallel example of such an application is in the examination of the mortality for different industries in which the proportion of managerial, clerical and manual workers varies. The mortality for these industries could be standardised by the distribution of staff in the different occupational grades.

Some years ago perinatal mortality for different localities was presented as the rate per 1000 live plus stillbirths. However, because of the known association of risk of perinatal death and birthweight, it was suggested that data for localities should be standardised for the distribution of birthweight in each locality (Chalmers *et al.*, 1978). More recently, it has been considered that such an index—though preferable to 'crude rates'—may lose some of the information, and that the preferable statistics are birthweight-specific rates excluding deaths from congenital malformations (MacFarlane *et al.*, 1980).

Examination of the case fatality-rate for patients treated in hospital for a given condition, such as appendicitis, is a different example. Some hospitals, by virtue of their catchment area, may receive and treat a far higher proportion of emergency admissions; it is reasonable to expect that the cases treated as emergency ones have a higher case fatality-rate. Thus, one could either look at the case fatality-rate solely for the emergency cases in two different hospitals, or one could correct the overall mortality for the proportion of emergency and of routine cases that are treated.

These examples indicate that the use of standardisation in the correction of mortality rates for age distribution is not the only application in the medical-care field; it is just a well-known example of the use of a technique that can be of benefit in a number of different studies. The general technique of standardisation has been introduced in this chapter on mortality statistics, because this is an area in which it is frequently applied and it is the field in which the technique was originally developed. There are many other situations in which the general procedure may be applied. Standardisation may be appropriate to remove the effect of age, sex and/or social class as in the preceding examples, or the procedure may be used to adjust morbidity, admission or consultation rates, or lengths of stay in hospital. Kalton (1968), using a mathematical approach, discussed the general use of standardisation to remove the effect of extraneous variates in survey analysis.

2.5.4.1 Is the S.M.R. significantly different from 100?

Whenever the S.M.R. for a specific subgroup of the population has been calculated there is interest in determining whether it differs sufficiently from 100 for this to be unlikely to be a chance effect. The answer will be directly influenced by the number of deaths upon which the S.M.R. is based; this seems intuitively plausible, as if based on relatively few deaths, one or two more or less might have occurred within the data period and would have an appreciable impact on the results. The actual play of chance can be fairly readily estimated by a simple calculation as follows:

$$\text{indicator of chance effect} = \frac{(O - E)^2}{E}$$

where O is the number of observed deaths and E the number of expected deaths.

If, in a particular occupational group, the S.M.R. for leukaemia was 150 and this was based upon 24 observed deaths, then

$$\text{indicator} = \frac{(24 - 16)^2}{16} \qquad E = \frac{O}{\text{S.M.R.}} \times 100$$
$$= 4$$

but if this is based upon only 21 observed deaths, then

$$\text{indicator} = \frac{(21 - 14)^2}{14}$$

$$= 3$$

The indicator being used is in fact χ^2 (chi squared), and what is technically known as based on one degree of freedom in this comparison. The above fictitious examples have been chosen for ease of calculation and also because they span an important value of χ^2, i.e. 3.84. This is the figure for one degree of freedom, which, if exceeded for the specific set of data, indicates that the difference between the observed and the expected values has a probability < 0.05. This is the level usually used to reject the suggestion that the results are chance findings, in which case they are referred to as 'statistically significant'. (Some of the more general aspects of significance testing using chi-squared are covered in subsection 4.5.2.)

2.5.5 Future years of life lost

One alternative way of presenting data on mortality in a population involves consideration of the 'future years of life lost' for each particular death. For example, for a boy aged 15 to be killed in a road accident one can postulate that such a death involves the loss of a considerable number of 'expected years of life lost'. This introduces the concept of expectation of life; using age- and sex-specific mortality-rates for the latest available period, O.P.C.S. publish annually a life table and the associated expectation of life. The latest available material (O.P.C.S., 1982b) gives the expectation of life of a male at age 15 as 56.6 years; thus instead of counting a single death from road accident, the death of the 15-year-old can be considered to contribute 56.6 'future years of life lost'. With a relatively limited calculation the mortality for different causes can be converted to future years of life lost. There are two technical changes that can be introduced: (1) instead of counting the complete expectation, the years of productive life lost may be used (assuming for deaths under the age of 15 that 50 years of productive life are lost, and for any age over 15, the individual would have otherwise worked to 65); (2) an upper age-limit of 85 may be used to avoid some of the problems of including deaths for which the cause is uncertain and mortality beyond the span of the general deaths included in the calculation.

Table 2.3 sets out a sample of recent results for England and Wales. For a selection of sixteen causes, the number of deaths for (1) males and (2) females have been ranked; the table also gives the rank for each cause based upon the calculated future years of working life lost (F.Y.W.L.L.). To stress that the main use of this approach is to examine the relative toll from different diseases, only the ranks are quoted rather than the estimated figures for future years of life lost. Examining the ranks for males, shows that cerebrovascular disease, pneumonia and bronchitis decrease in importance; congenital malformations, perinatal deaths and accidents increase in impor-

Table 2.3 Relative mortality from various conditions when ranked by numbers of deaths and future years of working life lost (F.Y.W.L.L.), for persons aged 15–64 in England and Wales, 1979

| | Rank of mortality | | | |
| | Males | | Females | |
	Number of deaths	F.Y.W.L.L.	Number of deaths	F.Y.W.L.L.
All neoplasms*	3	2	3	1
Lung cancer	6	9	8	12
Breast cancer†	—	—	7	5
Leukaemia	14	15	14	16
Circulatory disease*	1	1	1	2
Ischaemic heart disease	2	3	2	8
Cerebrovascular disease	5	11	4	9
Respiratory disease*	4	7	5	6
Pneumonia	7	12	6	11
Bronchitis	8	14	9	15
Congenital malformations	13	8	12	4
Perinatal deaths	12	6	15	3
Sudden infant deaths	15	13	16	14
Accidents*	9	4	10	7
Motor vehicle accidents	10	5	11	10
Suicides	11	10	13	13

Source: *Mortality Statistics, England and Wales, 1979.* DH1 No. 8, O.P.S.C. (1982)

Note: The causes of death have been ranked by the absolute numbers of deaths at all ages in 1979, and the estimated contribution to future years of working life lost. As this is an alternative method of indicating the toll from the cause, the rank is quoted, rather than the estimated figures for years of life lost.

*These conditions are ranked as well as some selected causes within these broader headings.

†Not calculated for male breast cancer.

tance. The changes for females are broadly similar, though ischaemic heart disease has also dropped in rank when future working years are considered.

The regular presentation of such material for England and Wales began in the 1950s, though Logan and Benjamin (1953) who introduced the series pointed out that the concept had existed for over a hundred years as an extension of the use of life tables. Blyth Brooke (1954) exphasised its appeal in presenting a picture of the mortality for a particular locality. More recently Murray and Axtell (1974) indicated how the method could be used to indicate the impact of different cancers; Romeder and McWhinnie (1977) advocated its use for health planning, suggesting that it helped define priorities.

The calculation of expectation of life is one of the statistics that flows from calculating a life table (some aspects of life-table calculations are given in subsection 6.5.2). The extension of this to produce 'future years of life lost' requires limited manipulation of the relevant data; for the reader not averse to a little algebra, the calculation involves the following.

Calculation for all cases of death:

$$\text{total years lost} = (84.5 - y_i)d_i$$
$$\text{working years lost} = (64.5 - y_i)d_i + 50d_{0-14}$$

where y = single year of age, d = deaths at age i, and i = specific age.

This is provided for those who wish to carry out calculations themselves. The formula can be simplified by using five-year age-groups, especially for data on specific causes of death; at the same time the 84.5 and 64.5 can be replaced by 85 and 65, while y will represent the mid-point of the five-year age-group.

2.5.6 Multivariate analyses

In a classic experiment in which the two groups of individuals are alike except for one specific factor being investigated (see chapter 7), the main analysis may be very simple—a tabulation of the mortality of those exposed and those not exposed to factor X. However, the examination of national mortality data can involve the study of a whole complex of interrelated factors. If each of these factors can only have two states (for example, sex can be male or female, and marital status can be either married or other), the data can be looked at for each subgroup. With two factors there are four subgroups, while with ten factors there are 1024 subgroups. Such an approach has obvious problems, since it becomes increasingly difficult to present the material in a tabular form, and the numbers of subjects in each subgroup is very small. There are a number of statistical techniques that are suitable for the investigation of this class of problem.

Reference has already been made, in subsection 2.4.2 on collation studies, to the fact that a correlation coefficient may be calculated as a test of the association between mortality and some environmental factor. An associated technique is regression analysis, which quantifies the change in one measurement for unit change in an associated factor. Both these approaches can be extended to the simultaneous examination of several factors. When looking at mortality rates for different towns, Gardner (1973) had immediately available data on cause of death, age, sex, calendar period and place of residence. For individual towns he studied nine socio-economic indices, which he converted into a social-factor score, and he used an index of domestic air pollution, latitude, hardness of water and rainfall. The relationship of these factors was then examined by a multiple regression analysis that permitted scrutiny of the association between the factors and specific causes of death. This enabled the contribution of each of the various factors to different causes of death to be assessed and the size of their effects to be quantified. In addition, data on the factors for other towns were used to predict mortality rates and these were compared with actual and other theoretical results.

In discussion on variation of mortality in different localities, Pocock et al. (1981) pointed out that the areas involved may vary considerably in size of population and in the number of deaths involved. There may be an order-of-magnitude difference and the rates (or S.M.R.s) for larger populations should be given greater weight than the smaller ones. These authors point out that it is possible to take account of: (1) sampling errors, (2) the explanatory variables and (3) unexplained differences between the areas. Their method resulted in a weighting intermediate between none and one proportional to the population size.

As already indicated, another common focus of interest is variation of mortality over time. Bowie and Prothero (1981) point out that the methods often used to examine the association between a seasonally fluctuating factor (such as temperature) and mortality from a diverse disease such as ischaemic heart disease may provide spuriously high correlations. They demonstrate the application of a time-series analysis (which removes the autocorrelations of the two seasonal trends before testing the direct association).

The mathematical techniques that may be used for such work are beyond the scope of this book. Mention is made of such work to indicate the growing frontiers of analysis of such material and to emphasise the need for collaboration between the epidemiologist and the statistician.

References

Recommended reading

Alderson, M. R. (1974). *Central Government Routine Health Statistics.* Vol. 2, *Review of U.K. Statistical Sources* (W. F. Maunder, ed.), Heinemann, London

Other references

Aird, I., and Bentall, H. H. (1953). *Br. med. J.*, **1**, 799–801
Alderson, M. R. (1965). M.D. thesis. London University
Alderson, M. R. (1981). *International Mortality Statistics.* Macmillan, London
Alderson, M. R. (1983). U.K.—health and social factors. In *Textbook of Public Health* (W. W. Holland and G. Knox, eds), Oxford University Press, London
Barrett, J. C. (1973). *J. Hyg., Camb.*, **71**, 253–9
Blyth Brooke, C. O. S. (1954). *Med. Offr.*, **91**, 251–2
Bowie, C., and Prothero, D. (1981). *Int. J. Epidem.*, **10**, 87–92
Cameron, H. M., and McGoogan, E. (1981). *J. Path.*, **133**, 273–300
Case, R. A. M. (1956a). *Br. J. prev. soc. Med.*, **10**, 159–71
Case, R. A. M. (1956b). *Br. J. prev. soc. Med.*, **10**, 172–9
Chalmers, I., Newcombe, R., West, R., *et al.* (1978). *Hlth Trends*, **10**, 24–9
Chamblee, R. F., and Evans, M. C. (1982). *Am. J. publ. Hlth.*, **72**, 1265–70
Clarke, C., and Whitfield, A. G. W. (1978). *Br. med. J.*, **2**, 1063–5
Crawford, T., and Crawford, M. D. (1967). *Lancet*, **2**, 229–32
Crawford, M. D., Gardner, M. J., and Morris, J. N. (1968). *Lancet*, **2**, 827–32
Crawford, M. D., Gardner, M. J., and Morris, J. N. (1971). *Lancet*, **2**, 327–9
Dean, G. (1959). *Br. med. J.*, **2**, 852–7
Diehl, A. K., and Gau, D. W. (1982). *J. Epidem. Comm. Hlth.*, **36**, 146–9

Farr, W. (1840). Letter to the Registrar General. In *First Annual Report of the Registrar General*, H.M.S.O., London

Fox, A. J., and Goldblatt, P. O. (1982). *Longitudinal Study: Socio-economic Mortality Differentials 1971–5, England and Wales*, O.P.C.S., London

Fraser, P., and Doll, R. (1971). *Br. J. prev. soc. Med.*, **25**, 34–6

Frost, W. H. (1939). *Am. J. Hyg., Sect. A*, **30**, 90–1

Gardner, M. J. (1973). *J. R. statist. Soc. A*, **136**, 421–40

Greenberg, M. J. (1965). *Lancet*, **2**, 442–3

Greenwood, M. (1948). *Medical Statistics from Graunt to Farr.* Cambridge University Press, Cambridge

Haenszel, W. (1961). *J. natn. Cancer. Inst.*, **26**, 37–132

Hakama, M. (1980). *Wld. Hlth. Statist. Q.*, **33**, 228–40

Hakulinen, T., and Pukkala, E. (1982). In *Trends in Cancer Incidence* (K. Magnus, ed.), Hemisphere, Washington, pp. 111–23

Heady, J. A., and Kennaway, E. L. (1949). *Br. J. Cancer*, **3**, 311–20

Heasman, M. A., and Lipworth, L. (1966). *Accuracy of Certification of Cause of Death*, H.M.S.O., London

Hems, G. (1980). *Br. J. Cancer*, **41**, 429–37

Hill, A. B. (1955). *Proc. R. Soc. Med.*, **48**, 1008–12

Inman, W. H. W., and Adelstein, A. M. (1969). *Lancet*, **2**, 279–85

Kalton, G. (1968). *Appl. Statist.*, **17**, 118–36

Kallner, G., and Groen, J. J. (1968). *J. chron. Dis.*, **21**, 25–35

Kilpatrick, S. J. (1962). *Popul. Stud.*, **16**, 175–87

Knox, E. G. (1977). *Br. J. prev. Med.*, **31**, 71–80

Krueger, D. E., and Moriyama, I. M. (1967). *Am. J. publ. Hlth*, **57**, 496–503

Logan, W. P. D., and Benjamin, B. (1953). *Mon. Bull. Minist. Hlth*, **12**, 244–52

MacFarlane, A., Chalmers, I., and Adelstein, A. M. (1980). *Hlth Trends*, **12**, 45–50

McManis, A. G. (1964). *Med. J. Aust.*, **2**, 76

Manton, K. G., and Stallard, E. (1982). *Demography*, **19**, 223–40

Morris, J. N., Crawford, M. D., and Heady, J. A. (1961). *Lancet*, **1**, 860–2

Morris, J. N., Crawford, M. D., and Heady, J. A. (1962). *Lancet*, **2**, 506–7

Moriyama, I. M. (1982). *Potential of Records and Statistics from Civil Registration Systems*. Int. Inst. for Vital Registration and Statistics, Bethesda

Murray, J. L., and Axtell, L. M. (1974). *J. natn. Cancer Inst.*, **52**, 3–7

Office of Population Censuses and Surveys (1980). *Mortality Surveillance 1968–78, England and Wales*. O.P.C.S., London

Office of Population Censuses and Surveys. (1982a). *Infant and Perinatal Mortality, 1980, Monitor DH3 82/3*. O.P.C.S., London

Office of Population Censuses and Surveys. (1982b). *Mortality Statistics, D.H.1, No.8*. H.M.S.O., London

Osmond, C., and Gardner, M. J. (1982). *Statistics in Med.*, **1**, 245–59

Osmond, C., Gardner, M. J., and Acheson, E. D. (1982). *Br. med. J.*, **248**, 1005–8

Pocock, S. J., Cook, D. G., and Beresford, S. A. A. (1981). *Appl. Statist.*, **30**, 286–95

Polissar, L. (1980). *Am. J. Epidem.*, **111**, 175–82

Ramazzini, B. (1713). *De morbis artificium diatriba*, Geneva

Registrar General (1971). *The Registrar General's Decennial Supplement England and Wales, 1961. Occupational Mortality Tables*. H.M.S.O., London

Registrar General for Scotland. (1982). *Annual Report for 1981*. H.M.S.O., Edinburgh

Reid, D. D., and Rose, G. A. (1964). *Br. Med. J.*, **2**, 1437–9

Research Working Group (1980). *Inequalities in Health*. D.H.S.S., London

Romeder, J. M., and McWhinnie, J. R. (1977). *Int. J. Epidem.*, **6**, 143–51

Rosenbaum, S. (1963). *Br. med. J.*, **1**, 169–70

Shaper, A. G. (1981). *Lancet*, **1,** 1318

Stenhouse, N. S., and McCall, M. G. (1970). *J. chron. Dis.*, **23,** 423–31

Stevenson, T. H. C. (1923). *Biometrika XV*, 382–400

Stitt, F. W., Clayton, D. C., Crawford, M. D., and Morris, J. N. (1973). *Lancet*, **2,** 122–6

Stocks, P. (1952). *Br. J. Cancer*, **6,** 99–111

Stolley, P. D. (1972). *Am. Rev. resp. Dis.*, **105,** 883–90

Waller, R. E. (1981). *Environ. Intern.*, **5,** 479–83

Wingrave, S. J., Beral, V., Adelstein, A. M., and Kay, C. R. (1981). *J. epidem. Comm. Hlth*, **35,** 51–8

3 Routine Sources of Morbidity and Other Statistics

This chapter presents a brief description of the various sources of routine data that exist in the majority of developing countries. The first example relates to hospital discharge data; the other sources are presented in alphabetical order in subsections 3.1.1–3.1.8. There is then a brief comment on (1) population estimates and (2) statistics on some of the determinants of disease. In the standard format of all chapters, there then follow sections on principles of the use of routine data, ways of extending such use, and notes of some of the relevant statistical techniques.

This chapter covers a wide range of sources of routine statistics in a relatively short text. These have been described in greater detail in reviews by Benjamin (1968) and Alderson (1983).

3.1 Use of Hospital Discharge Statistics

The hospital inpatient enquiry (H.I.P.E.), which is processed by the O.P.C.S. on behalf of the D.H.S.S., accepts data for every tenth patient discharged from a general hospital in England and Wales. The particulars collected are limited to

(1) characteristics of the patient (sex, date of birth, marital status and address);
(2) administrative particulars (hospital, patient's record number, consultant, date of admission and discharge, source of admission, date on waiting list, type of bed, whether the patient was transferred to another ward or hospital, number of visits to theatre, and type of discharge);
(3) medical particulars (diagnoses and operations—if any performed).

Using the appropriate diagnostic codes to cover 'self-poisoning', Alderson (1974a) examined the age- and sex-specific admission rates for self-poisoning. These rates are shown in figure 3.1. There is a higher rate for females than males at every age recorded, and a peak for both sexes is at about twenty years. It was possible to obtain data that had been collected over a twenty-year period, and within the limits of the data, some examination could be made of the trend in admission rates over this period. The rates of self-poisoning for either sex and for ten-year age-groups from 15–24 through to 65–74 all showed a steady rise over these twenty years. This dramatic rise suggests that the sharp age-peak in figure 3.1 may be an artefact created by rates that are rapidly changing from year to year. The appropriate technique for examining such material has already been mentioned (see subsection 2.5.1). The data have only been available since 1953, but the data do enable the examination of three points on the cohort lines for

45

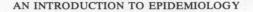

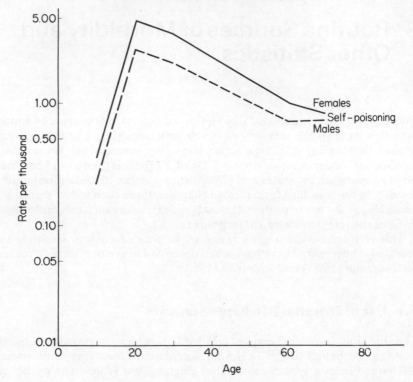

Figure 3.1   Suicide rates in 1971 and admission rates for self-poisoning for males
              and females by age, England and Wales (1972).
              Source: Alderson (1974a)

ten-year birth-cohorts. This material is plotted in figure 3.2 in which the age
peak has disappeared and for each cohort the admission rate rises with
advancing age, the age-specific rates for later cohorts being higher than for
earlier cohorts.

The above example indicates the way in which the routine material may be
handled in order to throw light on an important medical problem. Currently,
self-poisoning is the commonest cause of emergency admission to a medical
ward and creates a considerable problem as far as workload for the medical
staff is concerned. The prevalence of the condition is now sufficiently high to
create concern about the general health of such individuals and their peers.
It can be deduced from figure 3.1 that in the age period 15–24, approximately five admissions to hospital for self-poisoning will occur for every 100
women attaining the age of twenty-four (five per 1000 *per annum* over a
ten-year period).

It is important to point out that the basic data being examined are counts
of 'events' and the material does not directly identify the number of people
who poison themselves. It may well be that a few individuals entering
hospital a number of times have created the rise in the statistics. In order to
examine this subsidiary issue, Alderson (1974a) prepared a linked file for

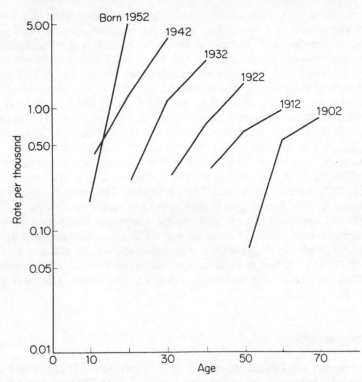

Figure 3.2 Admission rates by age for self-poisoning for cohorts of females born this century, England and Wales.
Source: Alderson (1974a)

such events in the Southampton area and examined this material to see whether the readmission rate was higher in the late adolescent males and females. There was no evidence for this hypothesis, thus suggesting that the rise in the admission rate since 1953 was due to an increased incidence of self-poisoning in succeeding generations and not because a few individuals had made repeated suicide attempts.

It must be pointed out that the examination of such routine data does not in any way provide a definite answer to a particular problem. The material can only provide some background information on the problem, and in certain circumstances can provide pointers to causation. Even if pointers can be deduced from the data, a special study will be required to provide a definitive answer.

The extent of the detail provided about any individual's admission to hospital is relatively limited and the statistical system for handling these data is chiefly geared to the preparation of background statistics that indicate the workload carried by the health service. This material has been predominantly used in the past as a source of information for management of the health service, including planning. This comes under the general topic of medical-care studies, and will be dealt with in greater detail in chapter 8. The material can also be used for aetiological studies and provided that the basic particulars are stored in a retrievable form, the material can be used as a starting point for detailed studies on individuals suffering from specific conditions. This use of the routine data will be discussed in subsections that deal with case–control and prospective studies (see 5.2.1.1 and 6.4.1).

Computer-held hospital-discharge diagnoses, and X-ray and operating theatre books, were used to identify all children in the North East of Scotland with acute intersusception in 1967–76. Compared with an earlier survey for 1950–9, there had been a decline in the age-specific incidence, which was greater in rural areas and for girls (Pollet and Hems, 1980).

Consideration in various countries has emphasised the importance of statistics of hospital activities and moved towards defining a minimum basic data set for all patients discharged from hospital. This was clarified at a meeting in the United States (National Centre for Health Statistics, 1972). Wagner (1976) reviewed the use of hospital discharge summary forms in Europe; more recently an E.E.C. working party has specified thirteen items that should be available to generate comparable and useful national statistics (Roger, 1981). A recent conference discussed the value of hospital statistics, and the availability and comparibility of such data (Lambert and Roger, 1982).

3.1.1 Abortion statistics

The Abortion Act 1967 came into effect on 27 April 1968. It permitted the termination of pregnancy by registered medical practitioners subject to certain conditions. Abortions may be carried out in N.H.S. hospitals, or in other approved institutions; only a very small proportion are carried out elsewhere, such as in service hospitals. Prior to the introduction of the Act there had been relatively few therapeutic abortions carried out in the N.H.S.

Table 3.1 just produces a simple example of the data available; these differences in the abortion-rates for single and 'other' women (i.e. married, separated, divorced, or widowed), and variation by age. The quarterly and annual publications can be used to examine variation in abortion-rates by characteristics of the women (age, marital status, parity, region of residence in England, nationality) or medical aspects (reason for termination, procedure, complications, associated sterilisation). Weatherall (1982) has used

Table 3.1 Legal abortion rates per thousand women, by marital status and age, for residents in England and Wales, 1980

Marital status	15–	20–	25–	35–	45+
single	17.9	26.4	24.4	7.0	0.2
other	12.5	10.9	10.3	6.2	0.4
all	17.6	18.7	12.0	6.2	0.4

Source: *Abortion Statistics for England and Wales, 1980,*
series AB no. 7, O.P.C.S. (1982)

information about reason for termination to align with trends in various congenital malformations—Down's syndrome, and major C.N.S. abnormalities.

The situation varies in different countries, depending on the legislation, and the attitudes of women and gynaecologists. Huldt (1968) presented data on deliveries, legal abortions (spontaneous and criminal) and other relevant operations (for ectopics, hydatidiform moles and missed abortions) in Stockholm for 1940–65. He suggested that from 1950 to 1961 the variation in the incidence of legal abortions distinctly affected the frequency of deliveries, but not that of criminal abortions. Between 1962 and 1965 the incidence of legal abortions in Stockholm increased substantially and there was a suggestion that criminal abortions might have then declined. There were no official statistics on criminal abortion, but the pointers available from cautious interpretation of available statistics were supplemented by a detailed prospective study of early pregnancy wastage in Uppsala county (Pettersson, 1968). He followed 1258 early pregnancies confirmed by laboratory tests and 463 women who applied for legal abortion. The spontaneous-abortion rates were 14 per cent and 12 per cent, respectively. It was suggested that 2–4 per cent of all pregnancies were being terminated by criminal abortion. This figure was partly derived from an analysis of the social class and marital status of women admitted with an incomplete abortion and pyrexia.

3.1.2 Cancer registration

On the basis of epidemiological, clinical and pathological features of Hodgkin's disease, MacMahon (1966) suggested that this disease may consist of several separate entities, one variety of which may be triggered off by infection. Fraumeni and Li (1969) and Cridland (1961) showed that an excess of cases presented are in the winter months. In earlier work in Denmark, Clemmesen et al. (1952) used a crude mapping technique that indicated microclusters of the disease.

Using the routine records of patients notified to the Manchester cancer register, Alderson and Nayak (1971, 1972) examined the data available for 737 patients for whom histological confirmation of the diagnosis was available. As figure 3.3 shows, there was a bimodal distribution of the incidence, with a pronounced trough in the incidence curves around early middle age. The bimodal swing in incidence according to age occurred in both males and females, but the percentage of the combined incidence that was due to males varied with age. A variation in the preponderance of males at different ages has been reported by other authors. Examination of the month of first attendance at hospital for each patient showed that an excess attended in May and June, and a deficiency at the end of the year. This spring peak was particularly apparent in patients aged fifty and over, and in males, findings that were very unlikely to be due to chance. Seasonal swings in the incidence of, and mortality from, other malignant diseases have been reported and a comparison was made with data for other malignant lesions

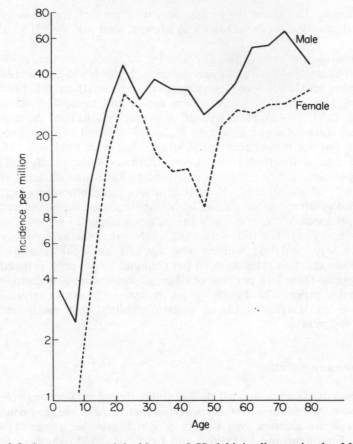

Figure 3.3 Average annual incidence of Hodgkin's disease in the Manchester region, by sex and age, 1962–8.
Source: Alderson and Nayak (1971)

registered in Manchester; comparable seasonal swings were observed.

Knox (1963) discussed the examination of low-intensity epidemicity and introduced a test for space–time clustering (see subsection 3.5.3). Applying Knox's technique to the data for 1962–5 indicated a significant space–time cluster of Hodgkin's disease. However, when seven years' data were used there was no statistically significant excess of cases occurring in a short space of time and living within a short distance of each other. With a short time interval between the initiation and development of disease, the technique used might be expected to pick up any clustering.

There are, however, two separate problems associated with the extremely crude routine data used in the study on Hodgkin's disease. The time of onset of that disease was identified by the date of the first hospital attendance and this might have been a long time after the initiating step. If there was considerable variation in the mean latent period, clustering would be extremely difficult to identify. The identification of location was the home address, plotted to the nearest tenth of a kilometre. If, however, the 'environmental' agent was acting away from the home environment it would be unlikely to pick up spatial clustering using the home address.

Smith *et al.* (1977) developed a technique to compare the network of contacts of Hodgkin's patients with that of controls; this overcomes the major disadvantage of a statistical clustering approach (see 3.5.3).

The analyses carried out by Alderson and Nayak (1971, 1972) did not provide any definitive answer on the possibility that an infective agent plays a part in initiating or promoting the development of Hodgkin's disease. The data used were collected as part of the national scheme of cancer registration and indicate the way in which the material can be tabulated, at very little extra expense or effort, in order to provide preliminary analyses of specific issues. By examining a variety of malignant diseases in this way it is possible that the results may indicate one or two specific forms of malignant disease that warrant more detailed investigation. Detailed case-control studies may be required to support the hypothesis that an infective agent is responsible, followed by a search for the agent. The use of other sources of routine data to study the relationship between exposure to infection and the onset of malignant disease is discussed in subsections 3.4.1 and 3.4.2.

Many countries have established national cancer registries, since Denmark set an example in 1942 (Clemmesen, 1965). The method of population-based cancer registration has been set out in MacLennan *et al.* (1978), while a more recent review (Magnus, 1982) covers both method and use, with particular emphasis on the activity in Nordic countries. An alternative to population-based registries are ones located at hospitals; their role has been set out in a handbook from the W.H.O. (1976). The W.H.O. *World Health Statistics Quarterly* contains articles on various topics, including ones based on international statistics of cancer registration. Statistics from seventy-eight populations registries in twenty-eight countries have been published by Waterhouse *et al.* (1976).

3.1.3 Congenital malformations

In 1961 the teratogenic action of Thalidomide was clearly enough established to justify the drug being promptly withdrawn from the market in the United Kingdom. This drug had been used for about three years in England and Wales, and it has since been estimated that during this period approximately 900 babies with gross limb malformations were born, owing to the ingestion of the drug by their mothers during early pregnancy. This tragedy acted as a stimulus for the development of a national scheme for the notification of congenital malformations in new-born babies in England and Wales.

Now each birth has to be notified by the attendant midwife or doctor to the district medical officer, and in 1964 the attendant at the birth was invited at the same time to provide information about the presence of congenital abnormalities. This is a voluntary scheme and the basic data may be collected in a variety of ways in different areas, but the bulk of notifications are made by midwives. A standard form is provided by O.P.C.S. on which the area authority is responsible for transcribing information about the place and date of birth, the mother's age, parity and place of residence, the sex of the child, and whether the child was born alive or dead and as a single or a multiple birth. The abnormalities present are indicated on a self-coding check list of sixty-six abnormalities, predominantly those that are easily recognisable at birth, together with a few that are unlikely to be discovered until later in life or at post-mortem. This material is processed by the O.P.C.S., with the aim of identifying local or national trends, in order to give as early a warning as possible of environmental factors that might contribute to a tragedy, such as that resulting from the use of thalidomide.

Hill and his colleagues (1968) discussed the problem of surveillance of the notification of data on congenital malformation. There are major methodological difficulties in repeatedly examining information relating to the sixty-six types of malformation for each health authority in England and Wales. Initially 17 300 frequencies had to be examined at monthly intervals and a technique for identifying nonrandom variation in these frequencies had not been fully developed. Hill *et al.* (1968) discussed two methods of computer analysis for surveillance of this material.

The first method involved comparing the observed number for a given malformation in an area with the number that would have been expected had the average rate of occurrence throughout the whole country been applied to that area. This method showed the areas in which the incidence of a given malformation deviated from the average rate for the country as a whole. It did not, however, indicate a change that uniformly affected the whole country and caused a variation in the mean rate of occurrence of that malformation.

The second method involved comparing the observed number of a particular malformation in each area with the previous monthly observations of the malformation in that area. If there was a significant upward trend compared with the previous average monthly incidence, the name of the area, the malformation in question and the results of the last six months were printed out by the computer. Hill and his colleagues provided an example of the computer output, indicating how this 'exception reporting' could attract attention to specific variations in the material, and relieve the statistician from perusing a tremendous mass of material at regular intervals.

In addition to computer analysis of the material, two further approaches can be used to monitor the occurrence of congenital abnormalities (Weatherall, 1974). A clerical file is kept of those authorities identified as having significant changes from month to month in their notifications of a particular abnormality. Also the material is examined to search for clustering of excess notifications, either in space or in time. For instance, high values for three adjacent authorities would be looked at much more closely than would such reports from three authorities scattered throughout England and Wales. Since 1967 the Medical Officer of Health has been informed of any significant increase of a particular malformation occurring in his area. It was hoped that the Medical Officer of Health would look into local conditions that might account for the increased incidence; increases may quite commonly have some administrative explanation, or be merely a sporadic increase and not indicative of the action of an aetiological agent.

The system for examining the congenital malformation data was set up as a result of a particularly disturbing problem. The number of new drugs coming onto the market each month is appreciable and the possibility of one of these drugs being used by a pregnant woman must always be borne in mind. It is not only therapeutic agents that can introduce a teratogenic factor: irradiation and infectious diseases have also been postulated as harmful agents in the past. In a prospective study of influenza infections in pregnancy, women so infected delivered more babies with congenital abnormalities than the controls (Griffiths *et al.*, 1980).

Statistics may be provided from: clinics with a particular responsibility for certain abnormalities, notification within seven days of birth as in the English system, and registration of malformations detected in birth cohorts at any age. The development of such systems has been described by Weatherall (1982), while Flynt and Hay (1979) reported on the variation of approach in thirteen locations participating in international exchange of statistics.

3.1.4 Health interview surveys

Table 3.2 shows the percentage of males and females aged 45–64 who reported limiting long-standing illness, by socio-economic group, from the national household survey in Great Britain. This indicates little difference between the sexes, but appreciable variation in the percentage from the professional to the unskilled manual group. The identification of such variation does not answer questions—but may guide thought and further enquiry towards consideration of differences in exposure to aetiological agents, in response to such agents, or in access, uptake or response to health care.

The data used in table 3.2 are from the 1980 General Household Survey; this survey was initiated in Great Britain in 1971. The intention was to create a survey that was developed in close collaboration with a number of

Table 3.2   Percentage of males and females aged 45–64 reporting limiting long-standing illness, by socio-economic group, England and Wales, 1980

Socio-economic group	Males %	Females %
professional	21	21
employers and managers	20	21
intermediate and junior nonmanual	29	25
skilled manual and own-account nonprofessional	29	26
semiskilled manual and personal service	31	32
unskilled manual	36	28

Source: *General Household Survey, 1980.* O.P.C.S. (1982)

government departments, such that the material collected was closely linked to their needs for information on housing, employment, education, health and social services, transport, population and social security. There had been a national 'Survey of Sickness' in England and Wales in the period 1944–52. The development of national health surveys in the European Economic Community is reviewed in Armitage (1977), while the role of such surveys in gauging population health needs are discussed by Alderson and Dowie (1979). The next chapter deals with the method of such surveys.

3.1.5 Hospital statistics

The lead example for this chapter presented data derived from discharges from general hospitals. The points made there are now amplified by consideration of data for patients treated in psychiatric hospitals. Figure 3.4 shows the admission rates in England and Wales for psychiatric patients per 100 000 population, by age and sex for the years 1954 and 1971. Admission rates have been plotted on a log scale, because of the wide variation in these data for different age-groups. A general trend is seen in all the curves, with a low rate of admission in young persons, rising to a level that remains fairly steady from about thirty years of age onwards. This is in contrast to admissions to acute hospitals, where admissions rise sharply with advancing age. It can be seen from the pairs of curves for both 1954 and 1971 that female admission-rates are higher throughout adult life. Also, both male and female rates were considerably higher in 1971—the increase being tenfold for the youngest, fourfold for the young adult and twofold for the elderly.

This is only one facet of the change that has occurred in the care of patients with mental illnesses. The admission-rates have risen at a time when there has been considerable development of community services for the care of the mentally ill; this may seem strange. However, analysis of other material shows that the proportion of patients whose duration of stay is over two years has also dropped over the past twenty years. These changes have been accompanied by a steady decrease in the average length of stay (a few months or even weeks) and a higher re-admission rate.

The documentation of these changes is not merely a dry exercise in the examination of 'historical statistics'. The mentally ill occupy just over a third of all health-service beds. It is important, therefore, to have a clear picture of the current use of such beds together with an indication of the trends. The information mentioned above may be combined to provide a projection of the facilities required over the coming years. For the past twenty-five years, this is an issue that has been hotly debated, and there is still disagreement about the appropriate number of beds to be provided in any given locality. This is partly because of over-optimism in the 1950s when the number of very long-stay patients in psychiatric hospitals began to fall. Some planners have been carried away by their enthusiasm for community care, and have perhaps overestimated the impact that this will make on the requirements for admission. The basic data collected in the Mental Health Enquiry

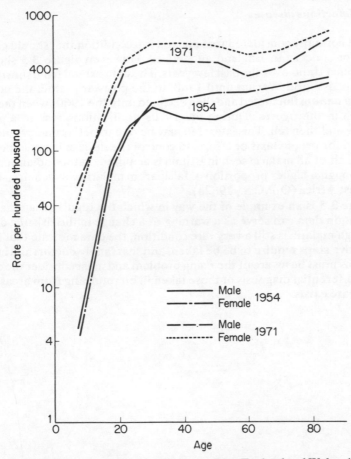

Figure 3.4 Psychiatric admission rates by age and sex, England and Wales, 1954 and
1971.
Source: *Statistical Report Series*, No. 12. D.H.S.S., H.M.S.O. (1971);
Statistical and Research Report Series, No. 6, D.H.S.S., H.M.S.O. (1974)

provides a background to a consideration of this important issue. (It will be
discussed further in section 3.4.3, in relation to psychiatric registers, which
have provided more precise guidance.) The important point to stress at this
stage is that routine material can make a contribution, but must be interpreted with caution and supplemented with studies in depth.

The basic data for the Mental Health Enquiry are initiated at hospital
level, where a form is completed shortly after admission of each patient, one
copy of which is then submitted to the D.H.S.S. for data processing. On
discharge of that patient a further form is submitted, which includes some of
the particulars that were included on the first form; these suffice for a
manual or computer linkage of the two sets of data. Material can be
generated about the characteristics of the patient, the reasons for admission,
the duration of stay, and the disposal.

3.1.6 Infectious diseases

It is not normally considered that malaria is a condition that should give any cause for concern in England and Wales. However, figure 3.5 shows an unexpected trend over the past few years. The data extend from shortly after the Second World War up until 1980. In the postwar period, the notifications *per annum* fluctuated and then declined until the 1960s when there was a trough in the figures. During the 1970s notifications rose to a peak in 1978–9 and then fell. This latest fall may be due to better understanding of the need for prophylaxis or efforts to control the disease in endemic areas. About half of all malaria seen in Britain is acquired on the Indian subcontinent, though a higher proportion of falciparum malaria was acquired in East and West Africa (O.P.C.S., 1982a).

Figure 3.5 is an example of the way in which the regular examination of notification data can serve as a warning of a change in the risk of a disease. Although malaria is still a very rare condition, the data indicate that further preventive steps require to be be taken, and that family doctors and hospital clinicians must be aware of the rising problem and must consider the disease in the differential diagnosis of those taken ill on returning from areas where the disease exists.

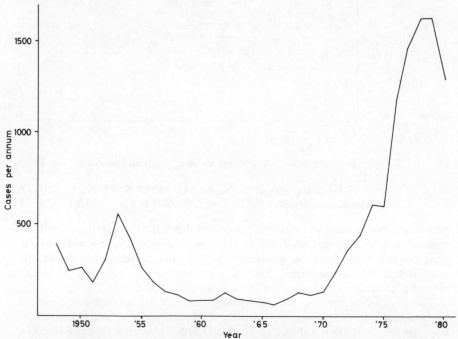

Figure 3.5 Annual number of cases of malaria notified in England and Wales, 1948–80.

Source: *Annual Report of the Chief Medical Officer to the Ministry of Health (1949–73); Communicable Disease Statistics, England and Wales*, MB2 No. 7 (1980)

Notification of infectious disease has been compulsory for the whole of the present century. It is usually suggested that the purposes of these notifications are as follows: to facilitate local administrative action when an epidemic occurs; to provide background information for epidemic control; for the measurement of morbidity; for administrative action that relates to the care of individuals; and for medical intelligence required in the management of epidemics at national or regional level. The data would also be of value in the planning of long-term provision of facilities, and could be used in mounting epidemiological research. Compared with some of the other sets of routine data discussed in this section, statistics for infectious diseases are of limited value as the importance of infectious disease is declining in this country. In fact, infectious diseases are now responsible for only a very small proportion of deaths in the United Kingdom and only limited morbidity.

Notifications of infectious disease are processed by O.P.C.S., and statistics appear in their weekly, quarterly and annual publications. In addition, confidential information received from public health and hospital laboratories in the United Kingdom and Republic of Ireland is collated by the Public Health Laboratory Service and published in their regular *Communicable Disease Reports*. These provide descriptions of significant outbreaks, giving epidemiological, clinical and laboratory details. Also, statistical data and brief descriptions are provided for other reported infections. This material is of particular interest to those involved in the diagnosis and treatment of infectious disease, and the series provides a classic example of epidemiology monitoring the distribution of infectious diseases.

Considerable use has also been made for research purposes of basic data flowing through the notification system for infectious diseases. The material has contributed to studies on the relationship of infectious disease to congenital abnormality (see subsection 6.4.6) and the development of malignant disease (see subsection 3.4.1).

One volume of the W.H.O. *World Health Statistics Annual* publishes statistics on notifications of infectious disease, while issues of the *World Health Statistics Quarterly* contain articles with detailed analysis of data on particular infections.

A different system exists for handling returns for sexually transmitted disease, with returns from venereologists being collated by the British Co-operative Clinical Group (for example, see the report on homosexuality and venereal disease, 1980). Limited data have also been reported by the Communicable Disease Surveillance Centre (1982). The need to monitor such statistics is shown by McCutchan *et al.* (1982), who reported an alarming increase in the indigenous (as compared with the earlier rise in directly or indirectly acquired abroad) cases of penicillinase-producing gonorrhoea in Great Britain in 1977–81.

3.1.7 Morbidity statistics from general practice

For a number of years, hospital discharge data have suggested that there is a considerably higher referral rate and subsequent discharge rate from hospital, for patients who reside in urban areas compared with those living in rural areas. It has never been clear just by examining the hospital data whether there is in urban areas a higher incidence or prevalence of morbidity, a differentially higher referral rate, or a greater provision of hospital facilities.

In the 1950s a study was carried out for one year in which records were completed in 106 family practices distributed throughout the country. This showed a higher consultation rate in rural practices (Logan and Cushion, 1958). A second national study on morbidity in general practice began in 1970, and results from this have been published (O.P.C.S., 1974). This study was based on 53 practices involving 115 principals and just under 300 000 patients. Table 3.3, which has been abstracted from this report, shows the general practitioner referral rates per 1000 population to different agencies involved in health care according to place of residence. It can be seen for each of the referral rates provided that there is a higher figure for those living in rural areas, although for some of the items the percentage difference is slight. The excess of referrals to outpatients and of emergency admission from rural areas, however, sharply contradicts published data on discharge from acute hospitals. The explanation of such differences is not obvious, but the data are not compatible with the earlier suggestion that morbidity is more prevalent in the urban areas, which thus require more hospital care.

Table 3.3   General practitioner referral rates per 1000 population, by type of referral and place of residence

	Type of referral						
Place of residence	Emergency admission	Out-patients	Investigation	Local authority	Multiple	Other*	All
urban	15.8	83.6	100.6	5.2	2.3	5.5	213.1
rural	24.8	92.6	135.9	8.5	4.3	11.2	277.3
all areas	18.3	86.0	110.1	6.1	2.9	7.0	230.4

* Other = optician, chiropodist, dentist, etc.

Source: *Morbidity Statistics from General Practice.* O.P.C.S. (1974)

The incidence of the morbidity in persons living in urban and rural areas is not just an academic problem. It is important to have a clear idea of the health problems of people living in different parts of the country, in order to estimate the appropriate balance of facilities required to meet their needs. The reported higher consultation rate in family practice and higher referral rate for persons resident in rural areas requires careful consideration in relation to the higher hospital discharge rate for persons resident in urban areas.

Lambert (1974) pointed out that the national morbidity study depended on a small selection of practices, and actual practice behaviour might be different in the survey practices compared to that throughout the country. The report also discussed the validity of the items recorded, including the referral rates—although there was no suggestion of major errors in these. For a number of years, it has been known that practice lists tend to be inflated; this is due to the delay in deleting records of patients who have moved away or have died. This would affect the denominator in the calculation of the rates, although particular care was taken to determine accurately the list sizes prior to the study. There might have been some slight bias in inflation between urban and rural practices. The definition of what constitutes an urban or a rural location is arbitrary, and this in itself might have created confusion, particularly when comparing different sets of data using different classifications. Also, some patients might have received care from ancillary staff in the practice, and thus would not figure in the data on contact or referral rate although they had received appropriate treatment. In other circumstances, patients might have gone directly to a hospital accident or emergency department for minor treatment without first contacting their general practitioner.

3.1.8 Sickness-absence statistics

One of the aspirations at the time of the introduction of the N.H.S. was that the provision of available care to all segments of the population would, in due course, improve the general health, thus cutting down the need for additional facilities. This would reduce the overall morbidity and sickness absence. Bevan, supported by Beveridge and his colleagues, suggested in the 1940s that the N.H.S. might be a self-limited expense. This was later described by Powell (1962) as a 'miscalculation of sublime proportions'.

Morris (1965), in a perceptive examination of published statistics on sickness absence, commented on the steady rise in the number of new claims for sickness benefit during the summer period (May–August) from 1949 to 1964. Further data on this issue are shown in figure 3.6. Two curves are plotted, one based on the average new claims for sickness benefit per week in January–March each year, the other on the average weekly figures for May–August each year. The 'winter' curve tends to vary from year to year owing to the variation in epidemics of influenza and prevalence of upper respiratory tract infections. A three-year moving average was therefore calculated, and superimposed on the original curve. This technique tends to eliminate the fluctuations and enables any trend to be more readily identified and compared with the 'summer' curve. The graph has been plotted on a log scale so that the relative change in the two curves can be directly compared. Morris drew attention to the abrupt change that occurred in 1953, with a steadily rising number of claims after that time. The rise in new claims was greatest for short-term absence, which comprises the majority of spells of incapacity. He commented that 'influenza' was the predominant diagnosis in the growing number of claims, but that sickness absence had to be labelled as something, and if influenza was responsible then it was an 'epidemic summer distemper'!

The above example indicates the way in which the routine material may be used. The National Insurance Act 1946 provided for the compulsory

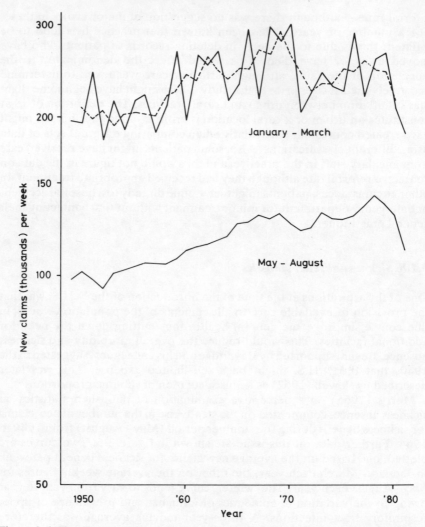

Figure 3.6 Trends in average new claims for sickness benefit per week in the United Kingdom, 1949–81 (continuous lines); three-year moving average for January–March (broken line).
Source: *Digest of Statistics Relating to Incapacity for Work*, circulated by Ministry of Pensions/D.H.S.S., *Social Security Statistics*, D.H.S.S., and for 1980–81 *Monthly Digest of Statistics*, Central Statistical Office

insurance of everybody between leaving school and retirement, with the exception of married women not in paid employment and one or two specific occupational categories. For the first time this made possible the collection of national data on sickness absence. Since 1950 the annual reports of the Ministry of Pensions and National Insurance (now a part of D.H.S.S.) have given some information about sickness absence in England, Wales and

Scotland. This material is derived from the initial, intermediate and final certificates issued to a 2½ per cent sample of individuals who have been certified as being unfit for work. This material provides tabulations of the numbers of spells of incapacity and the duration of incapacity, in relation to such factors as age, sex and cause of incapacity. The material provides general background information about the morbidity affecting the working population.

When using the routine data as an index of the incidence of morbidity in the community it must be stressed that the examination of such relatively crude data can only permit very cautious interpretation. Alderson (1967) suggested that, apart from any direct effect of occupation on health, incapacity rates in the current British situation might be influenced by a number of overlapping factors.

(1) The place of residence of the worker, including the influence of environmental factors and the availability of medical care.
(2) The multiple processes of selection of an individual 'into' and 'out of' a particular occupation, which are in part related to physical, mental and physiological demands of the job.
(3) The financial and social consequences of declared illness, including membership of a sick-pay scheme.
(4) The completeness of notification of incapacity (for example, certain professional workers may not be required to produce certificates unless incapacity is prolonged).
(5) The general and particular unemployment situation.
(6) The morale within an industry.
(7) Other, little understood, subcultural factors.

Taylor (1971) observed that personal and group attitudes are far more important in determining actual levels of sickness absence than are objective medical and demographic features.

In addition to providing background information, there are some specific uses of the data. For example, each local office handling new claims checks the trend for these during the winter and when there is a 150 per cent rise from one week to the next in new claims a warning is circulated to various authorities, this information being useful as a guide to pressure on the health services. Such a dramatic rise is usually caused by the spread of influenza, which can result in a dramatic increase in the number of patients referred for emergency admission to hospital and at the same time can reduce availability of nursing and other hospital staff. Such a warning may therefore be used to control the admission of nonurgent cases in order to leave sufficient resources available to cope with the medical emergencies.

In addition the basic data has been applied in specific research studies. A combination of sickness-absence and maternity-benefit records has been used to identify pregnant women who had had infectious diseases and who were at risk of delivering a child with congenital abnormality (see section 6.4). Another application has been in linked studies examining the factors that contribute to variation in the length of sickness absence (see subsection 8.1.4).

3.1.9 Population estimates

The previous and the present chapter have referred to the use of various rates, or age-standardised statistics; both these will require population estimates for their production. These estimates will usually be national or small-area statistics and this section discusses their source. Rather different is the need for denominator data for 'non-population based' event statistics, such as contact data from general practice; there are quite different sources of figures for persons served by the practice, which are briefly discussed in subsection 3.2.3.

A national census has been held in Great Britain every ten years since 1801, with the exception of 1941. The vast majority of the population are counted at the census in their own homes (or someone else's)—usually on a Sunday in April. There are also arrangements for enumeration of those present in institutions. The range of topics on which information is collected has extended from the beginning of the century, reaching a peak of thirty questions in 1971. From the point of providing a denominator for calculating rates, the main demographic items are sex, date of birth and marital status. More extended epidemiological analysis can be performed using the other material; this is discussed in the next subsection.

The development of censuses and comparisons with other countries have been reviewed by Redfern (1981). The United States has had a decennial census since 1790; legislation was passed in 1976 permitting a mid-term census from 1985. Australia and Canada take quinquennial censuses, while France has held them at irregular intervals (from six to eight years). Each of these countries uses self-enumeration. In Scandinavia the population registers are maintained with up-to-date addresses; these registers serve as alternative sources of statistics and affect the need for and design of population censuses. The main census schedules used in Australia, Canada, France and the United States are all considerably longer than that employed in Great Britain. This permits questioning about (1) a wider range of topics, such as: fertility, nationality and ethnicity, former economic activity, income, rental, heating and fuel, (2) more detailed questioning on education, and employment.

The census provides the main source of detailed statistics; annual estimates are produced which take account of (1) the increment in the age of the population, (2) the occurrence of births and deaths, and (3) estimates of migration into and out of the country and locally. The difference between the population estimates which have been carried forward from the 1971 census and the estimates derived from the 1981 census have been calculated for England and Wales and each of the local-government areas. These differences have been published for seven age-groups (O.P.C.S., 1982b); though there was only a 0.2 per cent difference for the total population, there were larger discrepancies for various age groups.

3.1.10 The determinants of disease

In studying the health of the community it is important to have access to data on various factors that are thought to be associated with variation in risk of disease. The following brief notes indicate the various sources of such material, though the grounds on which some of the factors are thought to be related to health or disease are beyond the scope of this section.

The census provides information on household composition, household amenities, education, occupation and migration. This is complemented by the material from the General Household Survey (see subsection 3.1.4), which covers demographic particulars, housing, employment, education, family formation, smoking and alcohol consumption.

The National Food Survey quantifies the food entering a sample of households, but excludes meals bought and consumed outside the home, and some items such as alcohol or confectionery. The published data cover nineteen items of food intake, giving nutrient values for various classifying characteristics of the population such as age of housewife. This material is supplemented by that obtained from the Family Expenditure Survey, including expenditure on food and alcohol. Other data on agriculture, fisheries and food production appear in the *Annual Abstract of Statistics*.

Occupational data are collected in the census and the G.H.S. and also in the biennial Labour Force Survey, though this only produces counts at the level of 27 industry orders and 16 occupational groups.

Over the past few years there has been an annual publication, *Digest of Environment and Water Pollution Statistics*, produced by the Department of the Environment. This covers data on smoke emissions, sulphur dioxide by source, radioactivity, noise, waste and water supply, heavy metal and organochloride concentrations in fish and shellfish.

Rather indirect measures of environmental pollution are indices of industrial productivity. The *Annual Abstract of Statistics* provides data on: consumption of coal, coke, gas, petroleum and oils; production of iron, steel, and other metals, and a range of items such as cotton, man-made fibre, jute, paper, timber, fertilisers, various chemicals, rubber and various manufactured goods.

3.2 Principles of the Use of Routine Data

Chapter 2 discussed the principles of the use of mortality data. Equally applicable to the use of morbidity data are the points made there on: descriptive studies (examination of variation by person, place and time), generation of hunches, testing hypotheses and monitoring the public health. Obviously, there will be some variation in the detail of the approach, depending on the particular topic being studied and aspects of the data available for study. Examples of use of material have already been given in the preceeding sections 3.1—3.1.10; particular emphasis is now placed on the way of monitoring of the public health. As with any source of data, the validity requires careful consideration prior to interpretation; this is discussed in 3.2.2. Because of the wide variety of sources of morbidity statistics, some guide is given on this in subsection 3.2.3. A brief comment is made on confidentiality.

There are four different approaches to the use of such material:

(1) Examination of the published tables.
(2) The central-government departments processing such data usually produce, in addition to the published tables, a range of more detailed tabulations, which may be available on special request.
(3) The basic items entered into these national systems will permit an extensive range of analyses well beyond the range of that routinely published and it is possible to request a special tabulation from the D.H.S.S. or O.P.C.S.
(4) The basic items entered into the systems may be handled in ways other than by tabulation, particularly by the use of linkage between two or more routine input systems.

In addition to the use of data input into these routine systems (either in its raw state or in published form), there is an immense amount of valuable material in routine records, which is retrievable by special search. The use of such data greatly extends the range of topics that can be studied because the number of items that are 'hidden' in local record systems is inevitably so much greater than the restricted range of detail covered by the national data-collection systems. Many of the principles involved in scanning and analysis of such retrievable data are identical to the other activities discussed in this chapter. A discussion of this type of study is therefore included (subsection 3.4.5), even though it does not involve the use of data available in a national system. Some authors refer to this collection of retrievable data as a 'survey', but the issues involved are more comparable with those involved in using routine data rather than in organising and carrying out a survey.

3.2.1 Monitoring the public health

It has already been explained (3.1.3) how the notification system for congenital malformations is used to check each month for variation in the number of notifications for a particular malformation in each district in England and Wales. This is an example of a very specific monitoring system, which requires speedy notification of malformations detected around the time of birth, and a computer-generated statistic to identify local variation in reporting. Now that a number of countries are running local, regional, or national schemes there is the facility to exchange information on particular suspect hazards (e.g. recent concerted action over an anticonvulsant drug following initial reports in one region of France; Bjerkedal et al., 1982).

Influenza can produce major disruption during a severe epidemic, due to the large proportion of key staff in various organisations who may be suddenly incapacitated. Tillett and Spencer (1982) have described how various sets of data may be used to detect the onset of an epidemic: weekly number of deaths; weekly deaths from respiratory disease; morbidity recorded in forty-one sentinel practices; laboratory isolates of the appropriate virus; number of new claims for sickness benefit. The best predictor is the crude statistics of total deaths, rather than the other morbidity data, which all suffer from various biases as indicators. Spicer (1979) has described a mathematical approach to the early detection of influenza epidemics, using the Kermack–McKendrick model fitted to data on weekly deaths for all influenza epidemics in England and Wales in the period 1958–73 (excluding those with bimodal curves).

Some aspects of monitoring the public health overlap with medical-care issues, where variation in delivery of care may be associated with alteration in various indices of outcome. This is discussed further in subsection 8.1.6.

Apart from these clearly defined topics where there is regular activity on examining time trends, some of the other sources of morbidity data can also be used in this way. The incidence of malignant disease does not change rapidly, but regular scrutiny of trends by site may provide warning of health problems (see Alderson, 1982). A tabulation of trends in hospital discharge has now been produced using statistical 'surveillance' techniques to identify those conditions for which the age-specific discharge rates or mean duration of stay had altered significantly in the period 1968–78 (D.H.S.S. *et al.*, 1981).

3.2.2 Validity of morbidity and other routine data

The validity of each of the various categories of data needs to be very carefully assessed, both when considering the use of the data to study a particular topic and when drawing conclusions. A number of studies have been carried out on each of the categories of data; there is not the space to describe each of the studies, though the following provides a précis of the main points.

Abortion statistics. The Chief Medical Officer to the Ministry of Health (1972) made some reference to incompleteness of notification.

Cancer registration. Nwene and Smith (1982) used five independent sources of information about patients with cancer, these were lists of patients under follow-up at some hospitals where meticulous care was taken to maintain contact with such patients, or region-wide lists of subjects with (1) children's tumours and (2) ovarian tumours which were being studied for other reasons. For eleven stites there was thought to be 94 per cent registration, but this varied with site and source of information. Benn *et al.* (1982) discussed other ways of checking completeness.

Congenital malformation. In 1966 a memorandum on screening for dislocation of the hip in new-born infants was issued to general practitioners, hospitals and local health authorities. The annual report of the Chief Medical Officer to the Ministry of Health (1967) pointed out that if there was a substantial increase in screening for this condition, a rise in the number of notifications of congenital dislocation of the hip would be expected; such an increase was in fact observed in 1967. Weatherall (1970) pointed out that it was reassuring that the computer surveillance methods were sufficiently sensitive to identify these increased rates. Other work by Weatherall (1969) indicated considerable variation in the efficiency in reporting congenital malformations, which means that the observed rates must be interpreted with caution.

In Exeter and Devon, a more thorough investigation of the child population has indicated that the proportion of malformations found and reported in the national scheme varies with the type of malformation. The levels detected for all but a few internal malformations were thought to be sufficient to expose any increase in incidence (Vowles *et al.*, 1975). In a case–control study (Greenburg *et al.*, 1977) out of 2867 notifications that were originally sampled, further enquiry by the local health authority indicated that 77 were normal babies who should not have been notified. Nevin *et al.*, (1978) used data from various sources to indicate the limited deficiences from notification.

General household surveys. The general issue of validity in surveys is dealt with in some detail in the next chapter (4.2.6). A particularly apposite study in Sweden (Brorsson and Smedby, 1982) showed false-positive reporting of 12.8 per cent and false-negative reporting of 13.4 per cent when comparing subjects' recall with doctors' records. The misclassification of reported visits varied with age and self-reported state of health.

Hospital discharge statistics. Alderson and Meade (1967) compared the accuracy of hospital discharge data with mortality statistics for patients who had died in hospital—they suggested there were appreciable errors in the principle condition treated for about 13 per cent of completed forms. Before studying the seasonal variation in admission to Scottish hospitals, Dunnigan *et al.* (1970) examined 1093 records where the discharge diagnosis had been coded to 'heart disease specified as involving coronary arteries'; 65 per cent were judged to be unequivocal myocardial infarction and 27 per cent myocardial ischaemia. In the majority of patients their diagnoses had been the primary reason for admission. More recently Lockwood (1971) demonstrated that there was a high degree of accuracy of such data; others have produced a range of opinions (see McNeilly and Moore, 1975; Patel *et al.*, 1976; Martini *et al.*, 1976; Cameron *et al.*, 1977; Rees, 1982; Whates *et al.*, 1982). Goldacre (1981) provided some general warnings about the interpretation of hospital discharge statistics.

Forster and Mahadevan (1981) provided some data on the validity of the information from the mental-health enquiry, based on an examination of 824 records in one locality in northern England. The error rates were high for source of referral (20.5 per cent wrong), diagnosis (14.8 per cent wrong) and outcome (10.8 per cent wrong).

Infectious-disease notifications. Stocks (1949) and Taylor (1965) emphasised that the completeness of notifications varied from one disease to another, being poor for the milder conditions. Lambert (1973) and Goldacre and Miller (1976) suggested that about half the patients with meningococcal meningitis were notified. There is strong circumstantial evidence to

question the validity of whooping-cough notification, partly due to confusion with infection from various respiratory viruses (Stewart, 1980).

Davies *et al.* (1981) identified a number of problems with notification of
tuberculosis, including duplicate notifications, changes in diagnoses, post-
humous registration, and definition of respiratory disease. The impact of this
on the statistics and possible solutions were discussed. Adler (1980) noted
appreciable variation in the method of diagnosis of sexually transmitted
diseases and use of treatment before diagnosis. He suggested that an
uniform approach was required to improve the usefulness of the notification statistics.

Morbidity statistics from general practice. A vital element in such studies is
the estimation of the number of patients, by sex and age, served by the
general practices in any study. Lees and Cooper (1963) identified problems
of definition, inflation and net change in practice list. The first national
morbidity survey had an inflation of 1.1 per cent, though this was reduced to
0.7 per cent on investigation. Other studies have identified variation of 20
per cent (Backett *et al.*, 1954), and 14 per cent (Morrell *et al.*, 1970). Less
extreme variation was found by Fraser (1978) and Fraser and Clayton
(1981).

Another issue is, to what extent does contact with a G.P. indicate
population morbidity? A number of studies have indicated that there is a
varying degree of self-care and undetected disease (Horder and Horder,
1954; Last, 1963; Kessel and Shepherd, 1965; Cartwright, 1967; Wadsworth *et al.*, 1971).

Equally important is the validity of data recording. The accuracy of the
analyses depends on the errors in capture, coding and processing of the
material. This has been discussed by many authors (see Dawes, 1972;
Munro and Ratoff, 1973; Morrell and Nicholson (1974). Other aspects of
data validity and coding accuracy have been investigated by Hannay (1972)
and Kay (1968).

In the second national morbidity study, the validity of the practice
registers was checked, indicating a true inflation of about 1.1 per cent (Royal
College of General Practitioners *et al.*, 1974). An attempt was made to
check the morbidity data, which indicated some diagnostic problems and
variation between the practices; coding errors resulted in only marginal
variation in the morbidity recorded. It appeared that about 3.5 per cent of
consultations and 2.4 per cent of episodes recorded on practice records were
not on the computer records, while 0.35 per cent of the events on the
computer file could not be identified in the practice notes.

Studies of this nature involve volunteer G.P.s and it is not known how
typical these are, but Crombie (1975) has suggested that a family doctor can
have some influence on the diagnostic patterns and differences in case-mix
that he draws towards himself. A report (Royal College of General Practitioners *et al.*, 1979) examines some of the characteristics of the practices
and concludes that morbidity rates were likely to vary in relation to the
location of the practices, size of partnership, doctors' age, and availability of
ancillary staff.

Sickness absence. The many aspects bearing on claims for sickness absence have already been listed (see 3.1.8). Semmence (1973) has carried out a direct check on 74 men having a hernia repair—in only 4 did the final certificate (the one used for statistical purposes) identify the operation.

Population estimates. In 1981 it was estimated that 0.63 per cent of people had been missed in the census, but about 0.17 per cent had been double-counted (i.e. a net underenumeration of less than 0.5 per cent). In parallel with checks of enumeration, a post-enumeration survey has followed each census since 1961 to assess the validity of the answers. Gray and Gee (1972) provide the latest results of such a check.

Conclusion. An extensive review of the validity of the various sets of morbidity data (Alderson, 1983) suggested that with care the material can be of value, but that variation by place or time can readily be biased by the error rates of the primary data.

3.2.3 Sources of data

The potential user of routine data must accumulate knowledge of what is available and where it can be found, including an idea of the unpublished material that can be obtained by a direct approach to the departments responsible. It must be borne in mind that only a restricted set of tables will have been provided in the published reports. Often by requesting unpublished analyses, or by obtaining a special computer analysis, the material can be set out in ways that are more relevant to the specific issue that the user wishes to explore. A charge is sometimes levied for special computer analyses, but even so this charge is small compared with the cost of *ad hoc* collection of comparable data. The Central Statistical Office provides a free booklet, *A Brief Guide to Sources of Government Statistics.* This, together with two pamphlets produced by the Stationery Office on the publications from the D.H.S.S. and O.P.C.S., provides an introduction to the range of material that is available. More comprehensive reviews of this material are provided by Benjamin (1968) and Alderson (1974b).

In subsection 2.2.1.2 mention was made of the role of the W.H.O. in collating and publishing mortality statistics from member countries. W.H.O. also plays an important role in making available a range of morbidity and other health statistics for countries able to contribute relevant data. One volume of the *World Health Statistics Annual* provides data on notifications including the age, sex and seasonal distribution of new cases for about forty different infectious diseases; other tables cover the prophylactic vaccinations given against thirteen infectious diseases. In addition to this annual publication, the brief weekly report published by W.H.O. is an important monitor of the spread of major epidemics of infectious disease and of the outbreaks of rare, but highly fatal diseases, such as Lassa fever.

The W.H.O. *World Health Statistics Quarterly* has current statistics on mortality and morbidity, together with a section dealing with a specific subject. These subjects provide a more detailed review of a selected topic that may relate to a specific cause of death, the incidence of a particular disease, such as cancer, hospital-treated morbidity, provision of health-care facilities, medical or health-service manpower and trends in population/ morbidity/mortality. These special reports provide a digest of statistics together with a commentary, which identifies pitfalls in the interpretation of the material. The one difficulty about using the material is that the topics covered follow no set pattern and a cumulative index is not provided.

3.2.4 Confidentiality

An extremely important aspect of all epidemiological work is the preservation of confidentiality. This issue raises problems in the collection, transmission, storage and use of all information relating to identifiable individuals. The particular aspects will depend on the conditions under which information was originally obtained. Inclusion in cancer registration at national level of named data permits identification of duplicate registration, but stringent control must be maintained of this information which has been provided without the patients' knowledge (particularly because some patients may not know that they actually have cancer). The Medical Research Council (1973) have set out guidelines for the use of medical information for research.

Particular issues to consider are whether: (1) an assurance (even implied) has been given to the provider of information not to use or divulge this except for stated purposes, (2) information can be transferred from the initial custodian to some other user, (3) linkage of two sets of data creates additional concern about breach of confidence, (4) publication can result indirectly in identification of individuals, such as by tabulation of data by several classifying variates so that counts in some cells are based on one or two events or individuals.

Security can be enhanced where those handling the data have signed the Official Secrets Act, or some other statement giving an assurance not to divulge information. For computer-held material, there are also technical devices to scramble material so that interpretation by others is difficult.

3.3 Advantages and Disadvantages of Routine Data

The main advantage of routine data is that the material is published and available on a bookshelf, while being updated with regular publications. There is, however, some delay between the actual event, capture of the relevant data, processing and publication. In certain circumstances, delay can be reduced by obtaining unpublished analyses direct from the central office some time before publication of the relevant volumes. To have material such as described in section 3.1 regularly produced is a tremendous advantage, especially when the alternative is an *ad hoc* study to collect the relevant data. Compared with mortality data the range of issues covered by the routine data is extremely wide. Subjects covered include socio-demographic characteristics of the general population, contact with family doctors and details about inpatient care in general and psychiatric hospitals. Additional particulars are collected about special problems, such as abortion, cancer, congenital abnormality and infectious diseases. Compared with the complexity of many of the issues that require to be studied, either in examining the causes of the disease or the response to care, the data are, however, still extremely limited. Potential users should develop an awareness of the ways in which the routine data may be used to throw light on specific issues, as a preliminary to detailed study. Sometimes the careful examination of routine data can even answer questions, but this is rare, and as a general rule any study carried out using such material will only be a preliminary to a definitive study. By use of the routine data that is immediately available guidance can be given in the planning of many detailed studies, so that these are efficient and directed most appropriately at the specific issues in question. Often a careful review of the routine material will enable the research worker to design his special enquiry so that it is more satisfactory and produces the answers required in a more economical fashion.

The chapter on mortality data mentions some of the standard problems associated with such routine data: these include difficulties over completeness, delay, accuracy, coding, retrievability, applicability, flexibility, acceptance and confidentiality. All these difficulties also occur in the handling of routine morbidity data. It is important to be aware of the problems of completeness and accuracy of the material, not as a barrier to the use of data, but as a guide to the cautious but correct interpretation of the material.

The delay between an event and publication in a series is irritating rather than a major fault with the material; there are relatively few issues that are changing so rapidly that the lack of the latest annual publication proves a disaster.

The additional information that can be provided by morbidity data was indicated by a study carried out in Nova Scotia by Deutscher *et al.* (1971). They compared the age and sex trends for ischaemic heart disease, cerebrovascular disease, hypertension and diabetes, using mortality and hospital discharge data. Compared with mortality statistics for ischaemic heart disease, the morbidity among younger subjects and females was greater than expected. This suggested that the case fatality increased with advancing age and was higher in men than women. Inpatient morbidity for hypertension and diabetes was more prevalent among women; but the opposite was true of cerebrovascular disease. It was postulated that premature death from ischaemic heart disease might selectively remove men with hypertension and diabetes.

A specific issue that can create difficulty in the examination of routine data is the change in the coding or classification system used for one set of data, or variations in classification between two or more sets of data. For example, when examining the discharge rates in patients with heart disease over a twenty-five-year period, difficulty is created by the change in coding of disease, which occurs about every ten years with the International Classification (this has already been discussed in subsection 2.2.6). However, difficulties can be created by change in classifying any of the variates used in the handling of data. Tabulation of first admissions to psychiatric hospitals, as a percentage of total admissions, from 1952 onwards showed a steady rise until 1970, when there was a sudden fall. The reason for this was that the wording of the question used to elicit whether an admission was a first one or a readmission was changed in that year, with a dramatic impact on the figures. The new wording might have provided more valid data, but it created difficulty in examination of a trend.

Other problems occur when trying to compare data from two or more statistical systems, for instance when examining the geographical variation in sickness absence by diagnosis and in hospital discharge rates. Difficulty occurs because different geographical areas are used to provide basic aggregation of the material.

A more specific point relates to the use of material for specific age-groups. It is sometimes found that denominators for calculating rates, such as in the published results of a census, provide age and sex breakdowns that differ from the basic aggregation of morbidity data, or two sets of morbidity data may use different cutting points when identifying age-specific figures. These difficulties occur because the prime user of one set of material may have had different interests and approaches to the use of the material, and these may have had a powerful influence on the method of processing. In the accumulation and processing of routine data, the basic material should always be retained in the system, even if published material is aggregated; various combinations and permutations of the data may then be produced on special request.

As in the case of mortality data, the strength of the analyses is enhanced by examining the routine data in relation to other material; this is discussed in subsection 3.4.1. Apart from a simple combination of two sets of data there may be the actual linkage of specific items of information derived from two or more sets of data. This use of linked data has already been mentioned under mortality data and will be discussed further in sections 3.4.2 to 3.4.4.

3.4 Extensions of the Use of Routine Data

Previous sections have discussed the basic ways in which routine data may be examined. The first step beyond direct analysis of such material is the simultaneous examination of data from two or more sources. This analysis may be merely by tabular or geographical presentation, or accompanied by statistical analysis of varying complexity. An example of this approach is given in subsection 3.4.1.

A more powerful approach to the use of routine data can be obtained by special linkage of the elements of data from two or more routine systems. This may be done (1) as an *ad hoc* exercise for a specific research project, (2) as a routine for collection of data concerning a specific medical problem, such as mental illness, or (3) by the systematic ongoing linkage of different categories of records for a defined population. These three quite different approaches are described in subsequent subsections. The section ends with a discussion of the use of retrievable data.

3.4.1 *Collation studies*

The first report of the Oxford Survey of Childhood Cancers (Stewart *et al.*, 1958) showed an excess of mothers of children with cancer reporting a viral infection during pregnancy, compared with control mothers. In order to explore this issue further, Fedrick and Alberman (1972) used death-rates of children under five dying of cancer from the Registrar General's reports, adjusted to identify estimated year of birth. This material was then compared with estimates of the prevalence of influenza during the preceding winter, based on sickness-absence statistics. The data were examined graphically for the period 1955–64; figure 3.7 shows the relationship. There are two peaks in the rate of incapacity due to influenza per 100 000 working women. The first of these peaks coincided visually with a rise in the death rate from leukaemia, with a less pronounced rise for the second peak incidence in influenza. The association was less clear for the death-rates for all neoplasms, or death-rates for all neoplasms less the leukaemias. In addition to a graphical presentation, a statistical analysis was used in which allowance was made for overall trend in the cancer death-rate over a period and then correlation coefficients were calculated between the sickness-absence statistics and the death-rates. There was a highly significant correlation with deaths attributed to the leukaemias, including reticuloses.

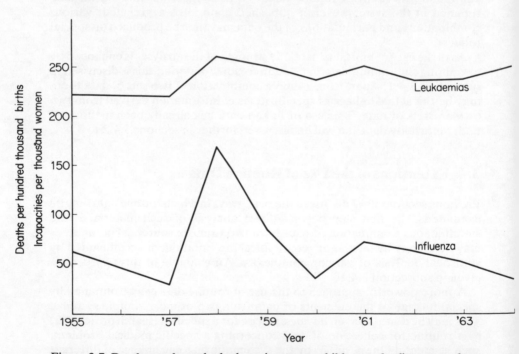

Figure 3.7 Death-rate from the leukaemias among children under five years of age according to estimated year of birth compared with the prevalence of influenza during the previous ten winters.
Source: Fedrick and Alberman (1972)

This report stimulated Leck and Steward (1972) to examine material in the Manchester hospital region. They used a slightly different technique to identify the occurrence of an epidemic of influenza, defining this as a rise of 50 per cent from one week to another in new claims for sickness benefit. Also, they were able to use the actual date of birth of children who had been registered as developing cancer. Their material was examined in tabular and statistical form, but the incidence among children born after six influenza epidemics in the period 1951–68 was no higher than among children born at other times.

A number of other studies that have examined this issue have been discussed in a review of the epidemiology of leukaemia (Alderson, 1980).

Rather different from collation of event data with environmental data is the alignment of data from different sources in order to extend the power of the descriptive material. Ashton (1981) indicated how routine data could be used to monitor the 'control of fertility' at local level. He advocated alignment of: population data by age group, G.P. payments for family planning, prescription data for oral contraceptives, family-planning clinic returns, hospital statistics on sterilisation and vasectomy, statistics of legal abortions, and birth statistics. He emphasised that material on adoption, spontaneous abortion and purchase of contraception were difficult to obtain, and advocated surveys to collect data on sexual activity and sex education.

3.4.2 Ad hoc *linkage of routine data*

The use of routine data for a preliminary exploration of the hypothesis that Hodgkin's disease may be partially determined by infection has already been discussed (see subsection 3.1.2). A more specific examination of this issue has been possible through a study of linked data, which brought together a list of individuals who had suffered from mononucleosis and collated this against all registrations for Hodgkin's disease.

Rosdahl *et al.* (1974) used the records of the State Serum Institute in Copenhagen to identify all individuals who had had a positive Paul–Bunnell test from 1940 to 1969. Over this period there were 17 000 subjects whose reaction was identified as positive. The identification particulars of all these individuals were then compared against the registration particulars for all patients in Denmark with Hodgkin's disease. The names of seventeen individuals appeared in both sets of data. The case records of most of these individuals were traced and it was possible to confirm that there was clinical as well as serological evidence for the mononucleosis.

The expected number of cases of Hodgkin's disease was calculated by applying the national sex, age and calendar-period incidence figures to the numbers of man years at risk, again tabulated by age, sex and period (see subsection 3.5.2 for a discussion of the method). The expected number of cases was found to be significantly lower than the number actually identified among males, but not for females. The authors were careful to point out that the data did not prove that there was a causal relationship between infectious mononucleosis and Hodgkin's disease; it could be that those diseases were both more prevalent in a certain section of the population. It was also possible that patients in the presymptomatic stage of Hodgkin's disease were susceptible to infection, although special studies have not confirmed this. Despite the fact that the number of cases developing Hodgkin's disease was significantly in excess of the expected figure, the proportion affected was very small compared with the total number of positive cases of infectious mononucleosis.

The names of individuals notified in Leicestershire in 1975 as suffering from tuberculosis were used to classify the patients into those who were and were not Asians; census, birth and migration records were used to estimate the age/sex distribution of the Asian population. Using these data, Clarke *et al.* (1979) estimated that this ethnic minority group had a notification rate seventy times that of the general population.

3.4.3 Registers

Baldwin and Hall (1971) provided a very detailed analysis of the attrition of the long-stay mental-hospital population and the associated recruitment rate to this category of patients. This was based upon data collected in the North-east Scottish Psychiatric Register. They described various models that indicated the functioning of mental hospitals, in an approach to assist in the evaluation of psychiatric hospitals and planning. The attrition of the long-standing population can be examined by calculating direct estimates of the probability of leaving hospital, taking into account age, sex and length of stay of the patients. Using this approach the data showed a nonlinear outcome with a relatively short period required to halve the number of long-stay patients, but a very long period before all such patients would have left hospital. As might be expected, marked differences were shown for subjects of different age and sex, although there was little variation through-out the period examined (1956–70). These authors contrasted the difference in the projected rundown of the patients using their technique to that obtained by Tooth and Brooke (1961) using a much simpler approach.

The North-east Scottish Psychiatric Register is one of several similar registers that have collected particulars about individuals and the care they have received from the psychiatric services; these have usually included admissions and also attendance as outpatients, domiciliary visits and even contact with other agencies. The registers have been restricted to patients in a defined geographical area and have been maintained so that recontact with the psychiatric services provides information for a cumulative patient file. Studies have been carried out using material from such registers, which provide leads to the aetiology and natural history of mental illness, including the genetic influence. A quite separate series of analyses has been carried out on the current workload and trends in workload, to provide a more sophisticated planning tool than that available from the national data.

Registers basically consist of lists of individuals whose eligibility for registration depends on a particular attribute. A considerable number of different registers exists in the medical field; the function of these varies widely, and as a consequence, the recorded information other than full identification particulars also varies. It is essential that the information stored in a register is accurate and retrievable. Only then may it assist (1) with the care of an individual, and (2) with the administration of the service, either by helping local management and planning, or national planning. Depending on the prime aim of the register, the information stored may vary from a single entry to a cumulative file for a chronic disease, such as psychiatric problems. In the latter, each contact with the services is documented and information sent through to the register. Research may be facilitated by the presence of a register either by a direct analysis of the material held (an example has been provided in subsection 3.1.2), or more indirectly by assisting as a starting point in retrospective or as an end-point in prospective studies.

Consideration of registers is simplified by bearing in mind a classification of the different types of register existing in this country. The main division is between those registers that play a part in the delivery of health care to individuals and those storing information for planning and research purposes.

Action registers

(1) Individuals requiring some preventive action, such as children due for immunisation and vaccination, or women due for cervical cytology are identified.
(2) Genetic registers have now been developed, with computer-held data used to recall at appropriate intervals members of affected families for investigation or advice. These are particularly likely to be of benefit for the study of dominant disease of adult onset (see *The Lancet*, 1979).
(3) Those individuals, who are at special risk of the onset of disease and for whom regular check up has been shown to be beneficial can be kept under surveillance. Many local health authorities have run 'at risk' registers for children. Despite the clear lead given by Sheridan (1962), these registers have had a troubled history owing to imprecise definition of objectives, reasons for entry onto the register and methods of surveillance (Oppé, 1967; Grundy, 1973). Other categories of individuals at risk may be: persons exposed to occupational hazard, such as dye, rubber and cable workers (Parkes, 1967); middle-aged males with precursors of coronary artery disease (Morris *et al.*, 1967); those having had medical treatment with known side-effects, such as ^{131}I treatment (Barker and Bishop, 1969); and the elderly (Alderson, 1974c).
(4) Certain categories of patient may require recall for supervision of maintenance therapy, such as persons with pernicious anaemia.
(5) Registers are now being compiled by departments of social service, for those with a wide range of physical, mental and social handicaps requiring after-care (Hutton *et al.*, 1974).
(6) The entire population are identified on the N.H.S. Central Register, which exists to facilitate the work of family practitioner committees, and in particular arranges for the transfer of patients' records on moving and registration with a new general practitioner.

Information registers

(1) Disease groups have already been discussed under cancer registration, (see subsection 3.1.2) and in the initial example on psychiatric registers in this section. Other conditions now being registered are children with phenylketonuria, diabetes, or Burkitt's lymphoma.
(2) Doctors and many ancillary staff have registered qualifications. Although basically designed to control 'fitness to practise', these registers may assist in manpower planning.
(3) The foundation of the vital statistics system is the registers of births, marriages and deaths.

Some of the general problems of the assembly of routine mortality and morbidity data apply to the compilation of registers. However, it is generally felt that the more closely linked the register is to the delivery of medical care, the more accurate the material can become; actual use in patient care should identify discrepancies, duplications and other deficiencies in the material. Where population-based registers have been set up for administrative and research purposes, the drive and enthusiasm of the individual responsible for the registers play a large part in determining the accuracy and efficiency of the process. At a recent conference on psychiatric registers some of the problems of maintaining them were discussed (Hall *et al.*, 1974). Tunstall Pedoe (1978) has discussed the purpose of heart-attack registers and the difficulties inherent in using such registers.

Brennan and Knox (1973) examined the blind register in England. After a detailed analysis of the variation in registration rate by local authorities, they concluded that despite variation from the small size of certain of the local authorities, differing age structures, and differing true incidence and prevalence of blindness, there remained variation in the registration rates, which was unexplained. It was felt that the most probable reason for this was the attitudes of patients, doctors and social workers. In particular, they suggested that the threshold effect plays a part (a phenomenon parallel to that already mentioned under morbidity in general practice—subsection 3.1.7). It was proposed that the blind register was not sufficiently accurate for medical research purposes; this seems a slightly over-pessimistic point of view. Alderson (1972) discussed the general problem of maintaining and using a cancer register. The subsection on cancer morbidity (3.1.2) has briefly indicated some of the aspects of cancer registration, both hospital- and population-based. Weddell (1973) reviewed the registers in use throughout the health service.

Irgens and Bjerkedal (1973) described the history and contribution of the Norwegian leprosy register, which was established in 1856. At that time, leprosy was a major health problem in the country and the registry played a significant part in the control of the disease in rural districts. In addition, it assisted in the planning of medical facilities by quantifying the trend in prevalence of leprosy, and clearly demonstrated the usefulness of central patient registries in the solution of a range of public-health problems. Over 100 years later, the initial concepts are being adapted to the solution of present issues—supported by advances in technology which greatly influenced the mechanics of the systems.

Bodenham and Wellman (1972) reviewed the requirements for a health information system. Among other issues, they examined the current use of the multiple discrete registers in the health service. They advocated that a basic register of the people in each area should be automated and have linked to it, as interrelated functions, all subsidiary registers. This is a concept with a number of major issues still to be resolved—would such a master register be cost-effective and acceptable on the grounds of confidentiality?

Some of the difficulties of maintaining a register were described by Jones *et al.* (1981). They used the Scottish Automated Follow-up Register of patients with thyroid disease to check on the reasons for discontinuance of surveillance. From 5.4 to 8.4 per cent of patients from four teaching hospitals were lost to follow-up over an eight-year period. The main reasons for this were: patient movement, patient non-compliance, general practitioner withdrawal of the patient, and retention at specialist clinics.

3.4.4 Record linkage

Quite different from the *ad hoc* linkage of two sets of routine data is the establishment of ongoing linkage of such material in order to provide cumulative records of events occurring to individuals in a defined population. This is not a new concept, having been described in considerable detail in the last century by Farr (1861), who identified as a long-term aim the recording of all cases of sickness in the population, in order to study the effect of therapeutic methods on the duration and fatality of all forms of disease. Although his ideas were sound, the opportunity to translate them into practice did not arise until the middle of the present century.

Stocks (1944) again advanced the argument in favour of continuous health histories of a large number of individuals of all occupations and classes, involving the morbidity recording of incapacity, attendances at hospital and details of deaths. A pilot scheme for the linkage of elementary data concerning each birth (whether at home or in hospital), each discharge from hospital and each death in the population of the city of Oxford and of Oxfordshire was started in 1962 (Acheson, 1967). The aim of the record linkage was to provide, as an ongoing operation, selected medical data from a defined population arranged prospectively by persons, family and community in order to provide a facility for epidemiological research, and information of value for management and planning in the health service.

Acheson (1968) described a number of operational and service applications of the material. These included identification of obstetric risk in relation to place of delivery, identification of deaths occurring after hospital discharge with notification of the hospital concerned, and identification of babies at risk and the provision of lists to the medical officer of health. Other applications included the identification of women developing carcinoma of the cervix and the notification of these to the cytology laboratory, identification of patients treated in hospital with nonpulmonary tuberculosis and notification of these to the medical officer of health (who had previously been receiving incomplete formal notification of these patients), and an examination of the relationship between admission and readmission, so that hospital statistics could be analysed, taking into account readmission in persons with chronic disease. This has been discussed in some detail by Hobbs *et al.* (1976).

A practical issue of importance to obstetricians, paediatricians and pregnant women is the risk of a mother having a premature baby if her previous baby was premature. The Oxford record linkage study was used by Hobbs (1968) to study the risk of repeated prematurity. Using the data for the period 1962–5, out of 22 000 women who were delivered in the population, 3439 had babies delivered after two or more pregnancies. It was possible to relate the birth weight of the earlier-born child to that of the later-born child and table 3.4 shows the findings. Just over one-fifth (44/207) of the mothers who had had one premature baby (defined by birth weight) were likely to have another in their next pregnancy. Another way of expressing this, is that 30 per cent (44/149) of mothers who had a later-born premature child would have previously had a premature baby. The implications of such an issue for the management are that if all women who have had a premature baby are booked for delivery in fully equipped hospitals, one can be sure that at least a third of those who have had premature babies in subsequent deliveries will be delivered in the most appropriate place.

The medical record facility developed in Scotland has been described by Heasman and Clarke (1979). The objects are: (1) to provide economical collation of events occurring to an individual to permit statistical analysis, (2) to enable individuals to be followed up, and (3) to produce person-based statistics. The Scottish system uses records on: general hospital discharges, obstetric discharges, mental and mental deficiency admissions and discharges, cancer registration, school medical examinations, handicapped children register, and death and stillbirth registrations. An important point is that for each project a linked file created *ad hoc* is used. The system has been used for epidemiological and health services research, and to follow up specific groups of individuals.

Table 3.4   Number of babies weighing up to 5¼lb and over 5¼lb born to mothers having two singleton babies in the Oxford Record Linkage Study area in 1962–5

Earlier-born birth weight	Later-born birth weight		All
	< 5¼lb	> 5¼lb	
< 5¼lb	44	163	207
> 5¼lb	105	2767	2872
all	149	2930	3079

Source: Hobbs (1968)

Linkage of basic demographic particulars for over forty thousand subjects to details of prescriptions, and records of hospital admissions, obstetric deliveries, and deaths suggested that such information would be of value for both generating and testing hypotheses about adverse drug-effects. Skegg and Doll (1981) indicated that this would be particularly so for: (1) delayed effects, (2) sudden deaths outside hospital and (3) effects on the foetus.

3.4.5 Use of retrievable data

At the time of diagnosis of thyrotoxicosis, many patients give a history of recent emotional disturbance. This has resulted in the popular belief that stress is in some way implicated in the pathogenesis of this disease. Hadden and McDevitt (1974) tested this hypothesis by examining retrievable data on the level of treatment for thyrotoxicosis before and during the disturbances in Northern Ireland. The civil disturbances began at the end of 1968; the data were therefore examined for the three-year periods 1966–8 and 1969–71. Three different methods were employed for identifying new treatment for thyrotoxicosis. Records were examined for the main hospitals in which surgery was carried out in order to identify the number of thyroidectomies performed during the relevant period. Radioactive iodine treatment is carried out at only two centres in Northern Ireland, and it was possible to obtain the total number of patients treated with a first dose of ^{131}I during the two three-year periods; care was taken to eliminate second or subsequent doses given to the same individual. In Northern Ireland, all prescriptions issued by family doctors and dispensed by pharmacists are processed by computer for the Northern Ireland Central Services Agency for Health and Social Services. It was possible to determine the total number of carbimazole (5 mg) tablets prescribed each year during these periods, and assuming that on average a patient receives 30 mg per day, the total number of patients treated was estimated. Table 3.5 shows the findings of the study. The variation in the numbers of patients treated by carbimazole and radioactive iodine was very small, and there was a decline in the number of patients undergoing thyroidectomy. Over all there appears to be very little change in the treatments carried out in the control and study periods, and there is no evidence that environmental stress has added to the number of cases requiring treatment.

Table 3.5   Numbers of patients receiving treatment for thyrotoxicosis since the civil disturbances in Northern Ireland and in the preceding three years

| | Number of treatments | |
| | Control period | Stress period |
Treatment	1966–8	1969–71
30 mg carbimazole/day	1556.2	1571.6
first dose of ^{131}I	319	312
thyroidectomy	173	122

Source: Hadden and McDevitt (1974)

This study is an excellent example of the way in which retrievable data can be handled to provide a quick examination of a specific issue. There was no routine data available in published form that could immediately answer the question, but by retrieving data already recorded it was possible to compare the three-year control period and the subsequent three years. By using three sources of data, there was a greater chance of excluding bias and of producing a more refined probe of the situation; with careful interpretation conclusions could then be derived. An estimate had to be made of the validity of the data and the likelihood of bias in the recording which might have altered the accuracy between the two periods. Other changes likely to affect the incidence of the disease or the treatments were also to be taken into account. However, as indicated by Susser (1974), caution was required because (1) there were many different forms of stress and response to stress varied, and (2) the data did not rule out cessation, with the onset of the troubles, of a falling number of treatments prior to 1966.

The approach of delving into medical and other records to retrieve data for examination of particular issues deserves careful thought before mounting a more complex study. It is usually considerably cheaper than a special survey—even a limited cross-sectional one—and provided that the 'retrievable' data extend over a number of years this can provide an answer much more quickly than by collecting fresh material. An important general issue that warrants consideration is how far the routine data-collection systems discussed in earlier sections of this chapter require amplification so that they can automatically tackle some of the problems that in the past have been looked at by surveys and other special studies. This general issue of feasibility of extending routine information systems to the level at which they are comprehensive and can tackle any fresh problem will be discussed further in section 8.1.6.

3.5 Statistical Techniques

Three different techniques that may be applied in the analysis of routine morbidity data will now be considered. The first is a graphical approach to the examination of regularly acquired counts, such as new spells of sickness absence, to identify a change in trend in the figures. The second technique is used to convert a series of pairs of dates, for example, for irradiation and subsequent death to an estimate of years lived and thus expected numbers of deaths by cause. The final technique to be discussed enables a search to be made of incidence date for evidence of low-grade epidemicity.

3.5.1 Cusums

An example in subsection 3.1.8 on the trend in sickness-absence certification was accompanied by figure 3.6 which showed the notifications in the winter and summer periods for 1949–81. The conversion of such data to a cusum is a technique for producing a continuous series by a method that tends to remove the irregular fluctuations in the data and accentuate any short-term change in trends. The calculation of a cusum is quite simple. A reference figure has to be selected, which may, for example, be the expected average reading. For each new reading, the reference figure is subtracted from this value and a cumulative total of the result produced by adding each successive difference. This cumulative figure is the cusum. The data from figure 3.6 have been converted into cusums and are presented in figure 3.8; the reference figure was the mean of the first three readings, rounded to a convenient whole number. Comparison of figures 3.6 and 3.8 shows that the technique has accentuated the point at which the notification changed; from the mid-1950s onwards a steadily rising curve has occurred. There is no indication that the steady increment in new spells of sickness absence has diminished.

Woodward and Goldsmith (1964) prepared a monograph that brought together a collection of techniques based on cumulative sums which should be widely applicable. They discussed the basic method and a range of specific applications, including a statistical technique for assessing change in a plotted curve. Hill *et al.* (1968) used this approach to monitor the notification of congenital abnormalities for the United Kingdom. The derived cusum was not plotted graphically, but was tested using a computer;

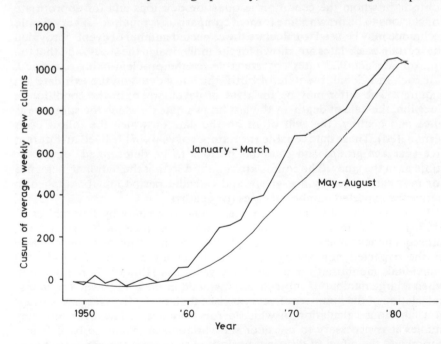

Figure 3.8 Cusum of average weekly claims for sickness benefit for (a) January–March and (b) May–August, 1949–81.
Source: *Digest of Statistics Relating to Incapacity for Work*, circulated by Ministry of Pensions/D.H.S.S., *Social Security Statistics*, D.H.S.S., and for 1980–81 *Monthly Digest of Statistics*, Central Statistical Office

the output highlighted any significant monthly changes in the values. In addition to applying formal tests of significance, it was possible to use a graphical approach by placing a 'V'-shaped mask over the plotted cusum (see discussion in Woodward and Goldsmith, 1964). Healy (1968) discussed some of the uses of cusums in the medical field. He emphasised that the procedure has the effect of magnifying small, abrupt changes, which are themselves too small to be visible in the surrounding 'noise' of a fluctuating series. Later, Chaput de Saintonge and Vere (1974) questioned why doctors didn't use cusums. In their paper they provided examples of this technique's use in the clinical field to determine any change in clinical measurements in patients undergoing therapy. Robinson and Williamson (1974) pointed out that cusums could be used to monitor measurement errors; introduction of a systematic error is quickly reflected by a change in slope of the graph.

3.5.2 Person-years at risk

Frequently in epidemiological studies, data are collected about subjects who have been exposed to aetiological risk at different times, and who are then followed up over a period. During this time they may develop the particular condition that is being studied. A count is then made of the number of subjects in whom the condition in question develops and for appropriate conclusions to be drawn some form of comparison is required. A very simple technique may be used to calculate the expected number of events, provided that certain basic dates are known for the individual in the study, and that the appropriate national rates are available for the problem being examined. For each individual, the date of birth, the entry date and the exit date are required. The latter may be the date of development of the condition in question, the date of death, or the last known date on which the subject was alive and healthy (this will often be the date on which the follow up is terminated). These dates enable the number of years of life lived in different five-year age-groups and calendar periods to be determined for all the subjects in the study. The counts are required so that the national incidence (or mortality) rates by age-group and calendar period may be applied to derive the expected number of cases (or deaths).

In subsection 3.4.2, reference was made to a study by Rosdahl *et al.* (1974) on the relationship between infectious mononucleosis and the subsequent development of Hodgkin's disease. This required the calculation of the expected number of cases of Hodgkin's disease among 17 000 individuals monitored for up to thirty years. As Hill (1972) pointed out, when a large number of subjects are included in the study, even the simple calculation of the numbers of years at risk tabulated by five-year age-groups is a laborious calculation in which errors may occur. However, in many studies it is necessary to consider the variation in incidence by calendar period and the effect of different periods of time since the exposure to the aetiological agents. (For example, radiation is thought to have a peak effect on the development of malignant disease about ten years after exposure.) Hill (1972) described a computer program that he had devised which facilitated the handling of such material.

The calculation of person-years at risk is in itself only a preliminary to the application of national or other standard rates of incidence (or mortality). Case and Lea (1955) discussed the statistical technique involved in comparing the mortality of a 'closed population' with the expected mortality. This work has been greatly facilitated by the activities of Case and his colleagues (1957). These workers prepared an impressive range of serial mortality-rates for the calculation of the expected number of deaths in a wide range of specific conditions. Apart from malignant diseases, for which there have been appropriate publications for England and Wales over the past twenty years, there are no other morbidity data. Thus, expected figures for myocardial infarction cannot be calculated using national incidence rates; instead one would have to rely on statistics derived from the published results of appropriate prospective studies.

Cramer and Crombie (1981) drew attention to the effect of using five-year age-specific rates to calculate expected incidence or deaths. They pointed out that only if the single-year age structure of the study population contained several age-groups with large changes in size would five-year rates introduce large errors. In this case, they advocated interpolation to produce single-year rates.

The technique for testing whether the number of observed deaths is significantly greater than expected is discussed in subsection 10.5.2.

3.5.3 Space–time clustering

Knox (1963) in discussing the problem of detecting low-intensity epidemicity pointed out that where the occurrences were few in number, and sparsely scattered in time, there was difficulty in identifying an epidemic. He also drew attention to the fact that an epidemic is often 'recognised' on a time basis, but that distribution of the cases in space must also be taken into account. He suggested a method of analysing such data in a more discriminating manner than had been employed in the past. Instead of the conventional analysis by examining the distribution of events by location or by time of occurrence (which results in a series of small subdivisions), he substituted an analysis that took into account three components: (1) the time distribution of cases; (2) the space distribution; and (3) a measure of the space–time interaction. The analysis used the simultaneous measurement and classification of the time and distance intervals between all possible pairs of cases. An appropriate test of the distribution so obtained was suggested, and tested against a specific example (the distribution of children born with clefts of the lip and palate, in Northumberland and County Durham).

Other more sophisticated mathematical approaches to this issue have subsequently been devised, but a discussion of these is beyond the scope of this text. However, it is still agreed that Knox's approach provides an appropriate examination of the basic issue. It has been pointed out by Pike and Smith (1968) that if the disease being studied has a long latent interval, examination of space–time interaction is not appropriate. Under these circumstances there is a need to test the link between each patient and others from whom he could have caught the disease. Pike and Smith described an extension of Knox's test which enabled this issue to be examined and provided a method of testing the distribution so observed for significance.

An early warning of the fallibility of using place of residence to study clustering of disease was given by Maxcy (1926); he showed no aggregation when mapping endemic typhus by place of residence, but clear clustering when using place of employment. It was the rats near the place of work which acted as the reservoir of disease, with rat fleas being the insect vector. More recently Smith *et al.* (1977) have used a case–control technique to examine person-to-person contact in preference to statistical testing of space–time clustering. These limitations have not prevented the mathematical techniques from showing positives with: meningococcal disease (Goldacre, 1977), Burkitt's lymphoma in East Africa (Williams *et al.*, 1978), and juvenile diabetes in Oxfordshire (Mann *et al.*, 1978).

References

Recommended reading

Benjamin, B. (1968). *Health and Vital Statistics*. Allen and Unwin, London

Other references

Acheson, E. D. (1967). *Medical Record Linkage*. Oxford University Press, London
Acheson, E. D. (1968). *Record Linkage in Medicine*. Livingstone, Edinburgh
Adler, M. W. (1980). *Comm. Med.*, **2**, 109–19
Alderson, M. R. (1967). *Br. J. prev. soc. Med.*, **21**, 1–6
Alderson, M. R. (1972). In *Cancer Priorities* (G. Bennette, ed.), British Cancer Council, London, pp. 101–7
Alderson, M. R. (1974a). *Lancet*, **1**, 1040–3
Alderson, M. R. (1974b). *Med. Geriat.*, **4**, 156–63
Alderson, M. R. (1974c). *British Central Government Health Statistics*. Heinemann, London
Alderson, M. R. (1980). *Adv. Cancer Res.*, **31**, 2–76
Alderson, M. R. (1982). *The Prevention of Cancer*. Arnold, London
Alderson, M. R. (1983). U.K.—Health and social factors. In *Textbook of Public Health*. (W. W. Holland, R. Detels, and G. Knox, eds.), Oxford University Press, Oxford
Alderson, M. R., and Dowie, R. (1979). *Health Surveys and Related Studies*. Pergamon, Oxford
Alderson, M. R., and Meade, T. W. (1967). *Br. J. prev. soc. Med.*, **21**, 22–9
Alderson, M. R., and Nayak, R. (1971). *Br. J. prev. soc. Med.*, **25**, 168–73
Armitage, P. (1977). *National Health Survey Systems in the European Economic Community*. Commission of the European Communities, Luxembourg
Ashton, J. R. (1981). *Comm. Med.*, **3**, 44–54
Backett, E. M., Heady, J. A., and Evans, J. C. G. (1954). *Br. med. J.*, **1**, 109–15
Baldwin, J. A., and Hall, D. J. (1971). In *The Mental Hospital in the Psychiatric*

Service (J. A. Baldwin, J. H. Evans, and D. J. Hall, eds.), Oxford University Press, London, pp. 151–90

Barker, D. J. P., and Bishop, J. M. (1969). *Lancet.*, **2**, 835–8

Benjamin, B. (1968). *Health and Vital Statistics*. Allen and Unwin, London

Benn, R. T., Leck, I., and Nwene, U. P. (1982). *Int. J. Epidem.*, **11**, 362–7

Bjerkedal, T., Czeizel, A., Goujard, J., *et al.* (1982). *Lancet*, **2**, 1172

Bodenham, K. E., and Wellman, S. (1972). *Foundations for Health Service Management*. Oxford University Press, London

Brennan, M. E., and Knox, E. G. (1973). *Br. J. prev. soc. Med.*, **27**, 154–9

British Co-operative Clinical Group (1980). *Brit. J. vener. Dis.*, **56**, 6–11

Brorrson, B., and Smedby, B. (1982). *Statist. Tidsskr.* **20**, 31–40

Cameron, H. M., Clarke, J., and Melville, A. (1977). *Hlth Bull.* **35**, 113–4

Cartwright, A. (1967). *Patients and Their Doctors*. Routledge Kegan Paul, London

Case, R. A. M., and Lea, A. J. (1955). *Br. J. prev. soc. Med.*, **9**, 66–72

Case, R. A. M., and Pearson, J. T. (1957). In *Studies on Medical and Population Subjects No. 13*. H.M.S.O., London, pp. 30–99

Chaput de Saintonge, E. M., and Vere, D. W. (1974). *Lancet*, **2**, 120–1

Chief Medical Officer to the Ministry of Health (1967). *On the State of the Public Health for the Year 1966*. H.M.S.O., London

Chief Medical Officer to the Ministry of Health (1972). *On the State of the Public Health for the Year 1971*. H.M.S.O., London

Clarke, M., Samani, N., and Diamond, P. (1979). *Comm. Hlth*, **2**, 23–8

Clemmesen, J. (1965). *Statistical Studies in Malignant Disease*. Vol. 1, Munksgard, Copenhagen

Clemmesen, J., Busk, T., and Nielsen, A. (1952). *Acta radiol.*, **37**, 223–30

Communicable Disease Surveillance Centre (1982). *Br. med. J.*, **284**, 124

Cramer, N., and Crombie, I. K. (1981). *J. Epidem. Comm. Hlth*, **35**, 146–9

Cridland, M. D. (1961). *Br. med. J.*, **2**, 621–3

Crombie, D. L. (1975). Personal communication

Davies, P. D. O., Darbyshire, J., Nunn, A. J. *et al.* (1981). *Comm. Med.*, **3**, 108–18

Dawes, K. S. (1972). *Br. med. J.*, **3**, 219

Department of Health and Social Security, Office of Population Censuses and Surveys, and the Welsh Office (1981). *Trends in Morbidity 1968–78 Applying Surveillance Techniques to the Hospital In-Patient Enquiry, England and Wales*. O.P.C.S., London

Deutscher, S., Robertson, W. B. C., and Smith, A. P. (1971). *Br. J. prev. soc. Med.*, **25**, 84–93

Dunnigan, M. G., Harland, W. A., and Fyfe, T. (1970). *Lancet*, **2**, 793–7

Farr, W. (1861). *Report of the Committee on the Preparation of Army Medical Statistics*. Br. Parl. Papers, 1861, xxxvii

Fedrick, J., and Alberman, E. (1972). *Br. Med. J.*, **2**, 485–8

Flynt, J. W., and Hay, S. (1979). Report of variation in approach in 13 programmes visited in 1975. In *Epidemiologic Methods for Detection of Teratogens* (M. A. Klingberg and J. A. C. Weatherall, eds), Karger, Basal

Forster, D. E., and Mahadevan, S. (1981). *Comm. Med.*, **3**, 160–8

Fraser, R. C. (1978). *J. R. Coll. gen. Pract.*, **28**, 283–6

Fraser, R. C. and Clayton, D. G. (1981). *J. R. Coll. gen. Pract.*, **31**, 410–9

Fraumeni, J. F., and Li, F. P. (1969). *J. nat. Cancer Inst.*, **42**, 681–91

Goldacre, M. J. (1977). *Int. J. Epidem.*, **6**, 101–5

Goldacre, M. J. (1981). *Comm. Med.*, **3**, 60–8

Goldacre, M. J., and Miller, D. L. (1976). *Br. med. J.*, **2**, 501–3

Gray, P., and Gee, F. A. (1972). *A Quality Check on the 1966 Ten Per Cent Sample Census of England and Wales*. H.M.S.O., London

Greenberg, G., Inman, W.H.W., Weatherall, J. A. C., Adelstein, A. M., and Haskey, J. C. (1977). *Br. med. J.*, **2**, 853–6

Griffiths, P. D., Ronalds, C. J., and Heath, R. B. (1980). *J. Epidem. Comm. Hlth*, **34**, 124–8

Grundy, P. F. (1973). *Lancet*, **2**, 1489

Hadden, D. R., and McDevitt, E. G. (1974). *Lancet*, **2**, 577–8

Hall, D. J., Robertson, N. C., and Eason, R. J. (1974). *Proceedings of the Conference on Psychiatric Case Registers.* H.M.S.O., London

Hannay, D. R. (1972). *Lancet*, **2**, 371–3

Healy, M. J. R. (1968). *Br. med. Bull.*, **24**, 210–4

Heasman, M. A., and Clarke, J. A. (1979). Hlth Bull. **37**, 97–103

Hill, I. D. (1972). *Br. J. prev. soc. Med.*, **26**, 132–4

Hill, G. B., Spicer, C. C., and Weatherall, J. A. C. (1968). *Br. med. Bull.*, **24**, 215–8

Hobbs, M. S. T. (1968). A study of birthweight and other factors in sibship. In *Record Linkage in Medicine* (E. D. Acheson, ed.), Livingstone, Edinburgh

Hobbs, M. S. T., Fairbairn, A. S., Acheson, E. D., and Baldwin, J. A. (1976). *Br. J. prev. soc. Med.*, **30**, 141–50

Horder, J., and Horder, E. (1954). *Practit.*, **173**, 177–85

Huldt, L. (1968). *Lancet*, **1**, 467–8

Hutton, D. S. S., Imber, V., and Mitchell, H. D. (1974). *J. R. statist. Soc.*, **137**, 483–512

Irgens, L. M., and Bjerkedal, T. (1973). *Int. J. Epidem.*, **2**, 81–9

Jones, S. J., Hedley, A. J., Young, R. E., Dinwoodie, D. L., and Bewsher, P. D. (1981). *Comm. Med.*, **3**, 25–30

Kay, C. R. (1968). *J. R. Coll. gen. Pract.*, **16**, 162–6

Kessel, W. I. N., and Shepherd, M. (1965). *Med. Care*, **3**, 6

Knox, E. G. (1963). *Br. J. prev. soc. Med.*, **17**, 121–7

Lambert, P. M. (1973). *Comm. Med.*, **129**, 279–81

Lambert, P. M. (1974). *Personal communication*

Lambert, P. M., and Roger, F. H. (1982). *Hospital Statistics in Europe.* North-Holland, Amsterdam

Lancet. (1979). *Lancet*, **1**, 253

Last, J. M. (1963). *Lancet*, **2**, 28–31

Leck, I., and Steward, J. K. (1972). *Br. med. J.*, **4**, 631–4

Lees, D. S., and Cooper, M. H. (1963). *J. Coll. gen. Pract.*, **6**, 408–35

Lockwood, E. (1971). *Br. J. prev. soc. Med.*, **25**, 76–83

Logan, W. P. D., and Cushion, A. A. (1958). *Morbidity Statistics from General Practice.* Vol. 1, H.M.S.O., London

McCutchan, J. A., Adler, M. W., and Berrie, J. R. H. (1982). *Br. med. J.*, **285**, 337–40

MacLennan, R., Muir, C., Steinitz, R., and Winkler, A. (1978). *Cancer Registration and Its Techniques.* International Agency For Research in Cancer, Lyon

MacMahon, B. (1966). *Cancer Res.*, **26**, 1189–200

McNeilly, R. H., and Moore, F. (1975). *Hosp. Hlth Serv. Rev.*, **71**, 93–5

Magnus, K. (1982). *Trends in Cancer Incidence.* Hemisphere, Washington

Mann, J. I., Thorogood, M., and Smith, P. G. (1978). *Lancet*, **1**, 1369–70

Martini, C. J. M., Hughes, A. O., and Patton, V. A. (1976). *Br. J. prev. soc. Med.*, **30**, 180–6

Maxcy, K. F. (1926). *Pub. Hlth Reps.*, **41**, 2967–95

Medical Research Council. (1973). *Br. med. J.*, **1**, 213–6

Morrell, D. C., Gage, H. G., and Robinson, N. A. (1970). *J. R. Coll. gen. Pract.*, **19**, 331–42

Morrell, D. C., and Nicholson, S. (1974). *J. R. Coll. gen. pract.*, **24**, 111

Morris, J. N. (1965). *Proc. R. Soc. Med.*, **58**, 821–9

Morris, J. N., Kagan, A., Pattison, D. C., Gardner, M. J., and Raffle, P. A. B. (1967). *Lancet*, **2**, 553–9

Munro, J. E., and Ratoff, L. (1973). *J. R. Coll. gen. Pract.*, **23**, 821–6

National Centre for Health Statistics (1972). *Uniform Hospital Abstract: Minimum Basic Data Set.* D.H.E.W. Publ. No. 73–1451, Washington

Nevin, N. C., McDonald, J. R., and Walby, A. L. (1978). *Int. J. Epidem.*, **7**, 319–21

Nwene, U., and Smith, A. (1982). *Br. J. Cancer*, **46**, 635–9

Office of Population Censuses and Surveys (1974). *Morbidity statistics from general practice, second national study 1970–1. Studies on Medical and Population Subjects*, No. 26, H.M.S.O., London

Office of Population Censuses and Surveys (1982a). *Communicable Disease Statistics, 1980.* H.M.S.O., London

Office of Population Censuses and Surveys (1982b). *A comparison of the Registrar General's Annual Population Estimates for England and Wales compared with the results of the 1981 census.* O.P.C.S., London

Oppé, T. E. (1967). *Cerebr. Palsy Bull.*, **9**, 13–21

Parkes, H. G. (1967). Industrial aspects of prevention of cancer of the bladder, in *The Prevention of Cancer* (R. W. Raven and F. J. C. Roe, eds.), Butterworths, London

Patel, A. R., Gray, G., Lane, G. D., Baillie, F. G. H., Fleming, L., and Wilson, G. M. (1976). *Hlth Bull.*, **34**, 215–20

Pettersson, F. (1968). *Epidemiology of Early Pregnancy Wastage.* Svenska Bokforlaget, Stockholm

Pike, M. C., and Smith, P. G. (1968). *Biometrics*, **24**, 541–56

Pollet, J. E., and Hems, G. (1980). *J. Epidem. Comm. Hlth*, **34**, 42–4

Powell, J. E. (1962). *Proc. R. Soc. Med.*, **55**, 1–6

Redfern, P. (1981). *Population Trends*, **25**, 3–15

Rees, J. L. (1982). *Br. med. J.*, **284**, 1856–7

Robinson, D., and Williamson, J. D. (1974). *Lancet*, **1**, 317

Roger, F. H. (1981). *The Minimum Basic Data Set for Hospital Statistics in the EEC*, Commission of the European Communities, Luxembourg

Rosdahl, N., Larsen, S. O., and Clemmesen, J. (1974). *Br. med. J.*, **2**, 253–6

Royal College of General Practitioners, Office of Population Censuses and Surveys, and Department of Health and Social Security (1974). *Morbidity Statistics from General Practice, 1970–71.* H.M.S.O., London

Royal College of General Practitioners, Office of Population Censuses and Surveys, Department of Health and Social Security (1979). *Morbidity Statistics from General Practice, 1971–72.* H.M.S.O., London

Semmence, A. (1973). *J. Soc. occup. Med.*, **23**, 36–48

Sheridan, M. D. (1962). *Mon. Bull. Minist. Hlth*, **21**, 238–45

Skegg, D. C., and Doll, R. (1981). *J. Epid. Comm. Hlth*, **35**, 21–31

Smith, P. G., Pike, M. C., Kinlen, L. J., Jones, A., and Harris, R. (1977). *Lancet*, 59–62

Spicer, C. C. (1979). *Br. med. Bull.*, **35**, i, 23–8

Stewart, G. T. (1980). *Br. med. J.*, **2**, 451–2

Stewart, A., Webb, J., and Hewitt, D. (1958). *Br. med. J.*, **1**, 1495–1508

Stocks, P. (1944). *Proc. R. Soc. Med.*, **37**, 593–608

Stocks, P. (1949). *Sickness in the Population of England and Wales, 1944–47.* H.M.S.O., London

Susser, M. (1974). *Lancet*, **2**, 951

Taylor, I. (1965). The notification of infectious diseases in various countries. In *Trends in the Study of Mortality and Morbidity*, W.H.O., Geneva

Taylor, P. J. (1971). *Publ. Hlth Lond.*, **85,** 298–302

Tillett, H. E., and Spencer, I.–L. (1982). *J. Hyg. Camb.*, **88,** 83–94

Tooth, G. C., and Brooke, E. M. (1961). *Lancet*, **1,** 710–3

Tunstall Pedoe, H. (1978). *Br. Heart J.*, **40,** 510–15

Vowles, M., Pethybridge, R. J., and Brimblecombe, F. S. W. (1975). Congenital malformations in Devon, their incidence, age and primary source of detection. In *Bridging in Health* (G. McLachlan, ed.), Oxford University Press, London

Wadswoth, M. E. J., Butterfield, W. J. H., and Blaney, R. (1971). *Health and Sickness: the Choice of Treatment.* Tavistock, London

Wagner, G. (1976). *Uses of Hospital Discharge Summary Forms in the European Region.* W.H.O. European Office, Copenhagen

Waterhouse, J., Muir, C., Correa, P., and Powell, J. (1976). *Cancer Incidence in Five Continents.* Vol. III, International Agency for Research in Cancer, Lyon

Weatherall, J. A. C. (1969). *Med. Offr*, **121,** 65

Weatherall, J. A. C. (1970). *Proc. R. Soc. Med.*, **63,** 1251–2

Weatherall, J. A. C. (1974). *Personal communication*

Weatherall, J. A. C. (1978). *Population Trends*, **11,** 27–9

Weatherall, J. A. C. (1982a). *Hlth Trends*, **14,** 85–8

Weatherall, J. A. C. (1982b). Epidemiology of congenital malformations in Europe. Paper given to *National Conference on Congenital Malformations*, Ferrara, 24 September, 1982

Weddell, J. N. (1973). *Int. J. Epidem.*, **2,** 221–8

Whates, P. D., Birzgalis, A. R., and Irving, M. (1982). *Br. med. J.*, **284,** 1857–8

Williams, E. H., Smith, P. G., Day, N. E., Geser, A., Ellice, J., and Tukei, P. (1978). *Br. J. Cancer*, **37,** 109–19

Woodward, R. H., and Goldsmith, P. L. (1964). *Cumulative Sum Techniques*, Oliver and Boyd, Edinburgh

World Health Organisation (1976). *Handbook for Standardised Cancer Registries*, W.H.O., Geneva

4 Surveys

This chapter discusses the simplest class of *ad hoc* study that can be mounted to complement the examination of routine mortality and morbidity data. Section 4.2 covers the principle of survey design, including subsections on response and issues involved in collecting accurate data. These two subsections provide considerable detail on these topics, as many of the points made are applicable to other types of study dealt with in the following chapters. The final section on statistical methods mentions the use of a few standard tests of significance, the intention being to indicate the types of situation in which such tests can or should be applied. Subsections deal with quantification of the validity of survey data and some ways of estimating the sample size required for a particular study; these two issues often receive relatively limited attention in standard statistical texts.

A survey may be defined as a special inquiry which collects planned information from individuals (usually a sample) about their history, habits, knowledge, attitudes or behaviour. In addition to asking questions, the respondents may be examined or various investigations carried out (such as collection of sera for laboratory analyses). An extension of the general technique may involve the abstraction of particulars from retrievable records (rather than the direct inquiry from individuals).

4.1 Basic Example of a Survey

A survey on drinking in England and Wales was carried out in 1978; out of the representative sample of 2000 persons aged 18 or over on the electoral

Table 4.1 Alcohol consumption by marital status and sex in England and Wales, 1978

Weekly consumption*	Single male %	Single female %	Married male %	Married female %	Divorced or separated male %	Divorced or separated female %	Widowed male %	Widowed female %
None	4	9	6	9	0	11	15	25
Occasional	9	20	19	31	14	23	37	40
1–20 units	44	61	52	58	54	59	30	34
21–35 units	20	7	12	2	18	4	7	1
36–50 units	11	3	7	1	11	4	9	
51 + units	12		5		4		2	

Source: Wilson (1980)

*A unit is equivalent to half a pint of beer, a single measure of spirits, a glass of wine, or a small glass of fortified wine.

89

register, 96 per cent were contacted and 86 per cent were interviewed using a structured questionnaire (Wilson, 1980). There was some suggestion that nonparticipants contained a higher-than-average proportion of heavy drinkers. Table 4.1 presents one aspect of the findings.

The study was commissioned by the D.H.S.S. in order to identify patterns of alcohol consumption—this was required as there had been reports of an increase in the number of persons affected by various problems stemming from 'heavy drinking'. The survey accounts for about half of the estimated consumption from Customs and Exicse returns, which is about the usual coverage from such surveys. This shortfall is estimated to be due to under-reporting and loss of heavy drinkers in the respondents. The report discusses the study design, comparison with Customs figures and the General House-hold Survey, and presents data on: patterns of consumption, demographic and occupational variation, leisure, drinking before driving, influence of work, development of drinking habits, and opinions on drinking problems.

4.2 Principles Involved in Surveys

The most important aspect in planning any study is to define the aim. Only when this has been done is it possible to consider the type of study that would meet this aim. No simple guidance can be given to ensure that this vital aspect of any study is adequately dealt with, but many of the general points considered in this and the next three chapters are relevant to this issue. In addition to clarifying the aim of the study, one must know the resources available, the time by which an answer is required, and the degree of resolution of the problem which is appropriate. The type and complexity of the survey will depend on these factors. It is assumed that as a preliminary to the planning of a new study, the scientific literature has been reviewed and an examination made of any relevant routine data.

4.2.1 Choice of study population

Having clarified the aim of the study, the research worker must then identify a suitable study population and specify the categories of data that are to be collected. The choice of a study population depends on a subtle balance of a number of issues (suitability, feasibility and availability). One approach is to select a representative sample of the country's population (see subsection 4.2.2 for a discussion of the techniques and problems of sampling). Provided that the sample is representative and of adequate size and that valid data have been collected, the findings should be of general application. Often logistic and cost considerations will lead to the selection of other study populations.

Many valuable studies have been carried out on specific groups of subjects, such as persons working in a particular factory, living in one locality, or attending specific schools. In cross-sectional studies of defined groups, such as those working in a particular occupation, one must always consider how representative the study population is of the general population. Most adult groups will in fact be a 'survivor' population, and the bias from internal migration was clearly demonstrated by Hill (1925). For example, if the occupation being studied is one that requires physical activity, those working in the occupation will be men (1) who have felt inclined to undertake such work and (2) who have not left the work because they found the environment or circumstances disagreeable. A proportion of the subjects will have left after initial experience, and these may be an extremely biased group. The remainder are, therefore, those who have self-selected themselves for the occupation and having tried it out have remained.

One source of a list of individuals is the electoral roll. West (1977) drew attention to other errors in the electoral register and emphasised that the public had very limited time in which to check particulars and notify corrections. Philipp *et al.* (1982) discuss the biases of use of the electoral register, such as a deficiency of 3–6 per cent of residents, a specific lack of new residents, the loss of individuals from recently demolished housing, and the lack of individuals from multi-tenancy dwellings. In a check carried out in 1981, 6.5 per cent of those eligible for entry were not included on the register of electors for their qualifying address on the qualifying date of 10 October 1980, while it was estimated that between 6 and 9 per cent were incorrectly included on the registers (Todd and Butcher, 1982).

4.2.2 Sampling

In the majority of special enquiries, one issue that should be considered early in the planning stage is the need to conduct the survey on a sample basis. The following points should be considered:

(1) A sample survey may be the only feasible way of collecting the relevant data.
(2) Financial and personal resources may be such that a sample survey is all that is possible.
(3) A sample survey produces the goods quickly.
(4) Accuracy can be increased in a restricted survey.
(5) The response rate may be higher.

However, use of a sample may not be appropriate for the following reasons:

(1) Data may have to be collected for other reasons from the entire population.
(2) Rare events may warrant a complete coverage.
(3) Sampling may create a feeling of discrimination.
(4) If theory suggests a sample of 75 per cent is required, it is preferable to cover the whole population.

A properly drawn random sample will enable the results in the survey to be considered and conclusions to be made about the population as a whole. This will be so only if the sample is a truly random one and if no factor, other than chance, determines if an individual is included in the sample. Technically each individual should have the same probability of being selected and every possible combination of samples of a given size should be equally likely to be selected.

In order to draw a sample, a nominal role of all the members of the population eligible for the study is required, from which a restricted number of individuals can then be selected. The sample should be drawn at random, either by shuffling and dealing cards representing the total population or by using random-number tables to identify the selection from within the nominal role. Random selection of individuals has a very definite meaning and is far removed from purposeful selection of individuals who are available or who are likely to help. An alternative form of sample, which is usually acceptable, is systematic sampling. In this approach the units selected in any one sample occupy related positions in the sampling frame and only the first to be selected is chosen at random. For example, having chosen the number 3 at random out of numbers from 0 to 9, a 10 per cent systematic sample may then be drawn by using subjects number 3, 13, 23, 33 and so on.

There are various special techniques that may be introduced to increase the efficiency of the study. One technique is known as multistage sampling; this is used to concentrate the resources of a large survey, such as a national one, on a limited number of areas. For example, instead of selecting a random sample from the entire population of England and Wales, a restricted list may be drawn up by selecting a sample of local authorities. Then within these selected authorities a sample of streets may be chosen; finally individuals are selected for interview. In certain circumstances, it is worth considering balancing the characteristics of the sample with regard to particular attributes. For example, in drawing up a sample of individuals to question about the health service, it may be considered important to get an equal number of males and females in the sample, and to exclude children. This merely necessitates the drawing up of two separate nominal rolls, one for men and another for women, both excluding children. From each of these lists an equal number of subjects are taken at random.

This technique of stratified sampling may be extended. Separate sampling frames, for example, could be identified for different areas of residence, for either sex, and for individuals in particular occupational strata. By identifying these separate facets of the sample frame, random selection would then result in the appropriate balance of individuals in each of the chosen groups. Variable-sampling fractions may be used to increase the information available for groups of special interest or for those categories with relatively few individuals represented. It is intuitively plausible that the weight that can be placed on the observation depends partly on the number of subjects studied. The variable-sampling fraction is used to ensure that minority groups of special interest are adequately represented in the sample. Stuart (1968) discussed the ideas underlying the theory of sampling and the effect of various sampling strategies on the interpretation of the collected data.

4.2.3 The problem of nonresponse

It seems intuitively likely that low response in a survey may be accompanied by difficulty in interpreting the results obtained. This subsection discusses the factors associated with poor response in surveys, and then the bias that can result from this; finally some suggestions are made about the ways in which subjects can be motivated in order to obtain an adequate response-rate with a minimum of bias.

Much of the original literature on response in surveys has little to do with medical studies and it is not clear to what extent it is therefore relevant to studies on cause of disease. Where there seem to be general principles involved these have been quoted, even if not documented by any definitive study in the medical field. Because the issue of bias in response rate is crucial to the interpretation of survey data, it seems somewhat surprising that so little in the way of adequate method studies to quantify the effects has been reported.

There are three different aspects that need to be considered: (1) the topic of the study, (2) the study design and (3) attributes of the target population.

4.2.3.1 The effect of the topic

It is suggested that the topic of the enquiry has an overall effect upon the response rate. It is particularly because of this that examination of response rates in nonmedical studies may bear little upon the issues of epidemiological work. The influence of the topic was demonstrated by Scott (1961) and Clausen and Ford (1947); they showed that the addition of questions of broader interest to a questionnaire reduced the nonresponse rate. This suggests that it may be possible to introduce such a minor modification into any specific study in order to boost the response.

Linked to the issue of the topic is the organisation responsible for the study. Scott (1961) suggested that enquiries identified as originating from the government had a better response, while Cartwright and Ward (1968) found a positive influence when questionnaires were sent from a local department, in this case Sheffield University, as compared with a London-based research unit.

4.2.3.2 The effect of study design

There are two approaches to collecting data from individuals in a survey, namely personal interviews and self-completion questionnaires. Commercial experience has suggested that the response rate from postal questionnaires is lower than that obtainable by personal interviews. Mork (1970) commented that the experience from epidemiological studies conducted in different countries does not support this contention. Scott (1961) reviewed fifteen surveys where the response rate was over ninety per cent, which is the target figure usually set. Epidemiologists are increasingly coming to rely on postal questionnaires and work has been done on the various factors associated with such questionnaires that can influence response rate. This is, however, not a new topic; in the middle of the nineteenth century, Babbage (see Morrison and Morrison, 1961) studied factors affecting survey response. Cartwright (1978) obtained a higher response from interviews than from postal surveys in a number of studies, but the difference in response was not statistically significant. She argued that the relatively minor improvement in response did not in itself justify the additional cost of interviewing.

A postal questionnaire may be addressed to each individual in the sample, or merely to 'The Occupier'. A covering letter may be used either as part of, or separate from, the questionnaire. This letter may be duplicated or printed, and signed or stamped with the name of the sender. There is no clear evidence that any of these variations influence the response rate. Kaplan and Cole (1970) looked at the impact of the covering letter being signed by a name considered to be Jewish, one considered to be Irish and one name not associated with any particular ethnic group. There was no evidence that any such variation in the questionnaire or covering letter materially influenced the response rate. A similar result was achieved by Kelsey and Acheson (1971), who found that the difference in the covering letters (typed, duplicated or signed) made no impact on the proportion of useable responses.

In a survey of physicians' attitudes to postgraduate education in Georgia, the format of the questionnaire (both its design and method of production) and the class of postage used were examined. An 'attractive business letter format' sent by first-class mail had a response of fifty-seven per cent, while mimeographed postcards sent by bulk mail had one of only thirty-four per cent (Gullen and Garrison, 1973).

Scott (1961) noted that, although common sense suggested there should be a limit to the length of a questionnaire that could be expected to obtain a satisfactory response, evidence gave surprisingly little support to this view. In a study on various aspects of obstetric care, Douglas (1948) found no appreciable difference in response from mothers sent a short or long questionnaire (with the latter including somewhat specific details about expenditure). Markush (1966) found no appreciable difference in the overall response-rate for two questionnaires of different lengths, although doubling the number of questions did create variation in the response from the three subgroups in the study. Relatives of British and Norwegian migrants dying in the United States gave a lower response to the long form and relatives of United States native decedents gave a slightly better response. The family expenditure surveys of the government social survey provided evidence (Kemsley and Nicholson, 1960) that indicated that the actual length was immaterial, but more important were the experience and training of the interviewers—part of whose job was to persuade people that co-operation is vital and worthwhile. Kaplan and Cole (1970) also observed little or no adverse effect from increasing the length of the questionnaire. To confuse the issue slightly, there was an English study by Cartwright and Ward (1968), which obtained a lower response with the much longer of two questionnaires. However, these questionnaires differed appreciably in content and the amount of detail required. It appears, therefore that there is no clear evidence that length affects the response rate. In general, once the respondent has decided that the study deserves his attention, he is not directly influenced by the length of the questionnaire.

Various approaches for the distribution and collection of questionnaires have been tried. Direct postal return is the most usual method. Scott suggested that a stamped return envelope produces a higher response than a prepaid one. With surveys of occupational groups, internal mail systems or direct delivery can be used. Another approach is the 'group' interview, at which the respondents are directly instructed on the purpose of the survey and on how to complete the form, and are then left to complete the questionnaires themselves (often in a large room holding up to a hundred people). In the case of completion of the form at home, Kemsley and Nicholson (1960) found a higher response rate when the research worker distributed and collected the forms. In a postal survey on headache sent to a sample of the electoral roll in Southampton, Newland *et al.* (1977) used first- and second-class stamps and prepaid/business reply for mail-out and return of the questionnaires. White and brown envelopes were also used. No difference was found in response from cheaper postage or brown envelopes. In a survey of health-care institutions it appeared that the order of the questions and the perceived length affected response, while the drafting of the covering letter and the promise to share results did not (Mullner *et al.*, 1982).

4.2.3.3 The effect of attributes of the target population

A number of studies have examined the impact of various aspects of the target population upon response rate. These can be considered first in general terms, as the major demographic factors, and then some of the more specific facets of the population studied. The following notes deal with: age, sex, social class, urban/rural residence, household composition, aspects of the health of the respondents, and general attitudes to surveys.

(1) Age. Hill (1951a) clearly showed the influence of age. In a postal survey of doctors, the proportion of nonresponders rose from two per cent in doctors under thirty-five, to nearly ten per cent in those who were aged sixty-five and over. Cochrane (1954), Kemsley and Nicholson (1960), and Kaplan and Cole (1970) found a similar deficit of response by the elderly in surveys of the population as a whole. It appears to be a general rule that the elderly are less inclined to participate in studies; the main exception to this would presumably be those studies that have a specific appeal to that section of the population.

Confidential linkage of information obtained at the 1971 census with particulars of responders and nonresponders in (a) the United Kingdom Expenditure Survey (Kemsley, 1975) and (b) the National Food Survey (Kemsley, 1976) showed a close relationship between decrease in response and increase in age.

(2) Sex. The influence of sex does not appear to be clearly defined. Cochrane (1954) reported a lower response in females in some of his population studies in South Wales, while an American population study (Gordon and Kannel, 1968) had a lower response in males. There is also no indication in the literature that marital status is an important component on nonresponse. For example, in a careful study of the reluctant participants in a breast cancer screening programme, Fink *et al.* (1968) showed no influence of marital status. (This is a particular example in which one might have expected to observe such an effect owing to the personal nature of the investigation.)

(3) Social class. One finding from the literature on general surveys is the effect of education and occupational status of the respondent on the response. In a prospective heart study in Los Angeles using a postal questionnaire, there was lower response in blacks, those of socio-economic status 5, and the older age groups (Reader, 1960). Both Gordon and Kannel (1968) and Kaplan and Cole (1970) reported a lower response-rate among those residing in an area with a high proportion in the lower social classes. Kemsley (1975, 1976) found a lower response with social class IV and V respondents or those who had had no formal educational attainment. The relationship was not straightforward, as there was also a lower response in those who were self-employed. Similarly, Tiblin (1965) found an excess from low-income groups among nonrespondents in a Swedish population survey.

In the National Child Development Study (Goldstein, 1976) children who refused to co-operate at sixteen had reading, mathematics, and I.Q. scores that were four to six months in advance at eleven years of those who continued to collaborate. In contrast, those who could not be traced at sixteen were nearly one year behind at eleven. It was felt that the bias in the mental measurement of responders was greater than that for measures of physical growth.

(4) Urban/rural location. There is conflicting evidence of the effect of place of residence with variation in response from urban/rural areas and small/large towns. Gray (1957) found a response bias in favour of urban residence. In a study of breast screening in Norway, there was a higher response in those living in the rural areas; in general, the response improved as the distance to the nearest town increased.

(5) Household composition. The analyses on the two national surveys carried out in Britain (Kemsley, 1975, 1976) showed that there was an appreciably lower response where the household: consisted of an individual living alone; did not contain any children; had a head of the household who was single, widowed or divorced; consisted of unrelated individuals living in the same household; had one or more other households living in the same dwelling.

(6) Health of the respondents. It seems likely that if the individual ap-

proached is seriously ill, he may be much more likely not to participate in any survey. This will also be aggravated by the obvious inability of someone ill in hospital to respond in surveys of those living at home. In the follow up of doctors originally sent questionnaires in 1953, Doll and Peto (1976) suggested that the effect of nonresponse due to ill health at the time of the initial questionnaire mail out had disappeared by the fourth year of follow up.

Apart from major incapacitating illness having an effect, it is important to consider if other disease prevalent at the time of a survey has an important effect. Harris *et al.* (1971) examined the prevalence of physical abnormalities in those responding quickly and slowly to a survey of handicap in England and Wales. There was no alteration in the prevalence of abnormality in those who responded after considerable delay. Rather different was the finding in a study of peptic ulcer, when information was collected from control families. When this was classified according to degree of cooperation during the survey, a considerably higher proportion of the 'uncooperative' families were found to have evidence of major social and psychological problems (Morris, 1975).

(7) General attitudes to surveys. Obviously it is difficult to study a rather vague concept. In a review of nineteen studies carried out by her unit, Cartwright (1978) noted that there had been a decrease in participation rate of general practitioners between two surveys carried out on the same topic in 1964 and 1977. This drop had occurred despite the support of the professional representative body for the study in 1977 (this had not been sought at the time of the earlier survey).

(8) Conclusions. The point of agreement is that the topic of the study is of overriding importance, while some of the characteristics of the population approached also have a powerful influence upon response. In particular, the age and social class have been reported as being closely linked to participation. The mechanics of the survey do not seem important (e.g. the method of mail out or return of postal questionnaires); the difference between the respective responses from interview and postal studies seems small compared with the cost of the two methods.

4.2.3.4. Bias introduced by nonresponse

The preceding subsections have indicated that respondents in any survey are likely to differ in some of their characteristics frm those who do not respond. The important issue is whether this will introduce a bias into the study that cannot be overcome by appropriate analysis; if such a bias exists, how large is its effect? One of the major factors identified above was a relationship with age; it is also a fact that many conditions will increase in incidence or mortality with advancing age. This could be allowed for in the analysis of a survey, but more difficult to adjust for is interaction between exposure to an aetiological agent and response rate (bearing in mind that in many surveys of the general population there will be a tendency to fail to get replies from those who are seriously ill).

The bias introduced into surveys by nonrespondents was clearly reviewed by Cochrane (1954). In presenting results from surveys carried out in South Wales, he showed a rather complex bias. Prevalence of pneumoconiosis was higher in those who came most readily for examination while the prevalence of tuberculosis was higher in those reluctant to participate in the survey. Cochrane commented on the general phenomenon, which holds for many diseases, that those most likely to be affected come forward less willingly for investigation. This phenomenon has been reported in relation to a number of other population studies and screening investigations, such as for malignant, chronic respiratory and coronary artery diseases, developmental abnormality of children, and hearing defects in children. A specific example is the examination of 'well women' for early carcinoma of the cervix. A number of authors (MacGregor et al., 1966; Osborn and Leyshon, 1966; Sansom et al., 1970) reported that the response rate was lowest in social classes IV and V, and these are groups in which there is a high prevalence of positive cervical smears. Fink et al. (1972), in a screening programme for breast cancer, studied the prevalence of lesions and the stage of disease in the ready and in the reluctant participants. They found no appreciable difference between these two groups. However, the breast cancer lesions that were subsequently brought to the attention of medical care by the nonparticipants in the study were at a more advanced stage than those detected in the screening examinations. Pedersen (1966) drew attention to the self-selection that takes place with many screening programmes and the bias that this can create.

In order to assess the bias introduced into any large-scale study by nonresponse, it is essential to try to obtain some information about the individuals who initially refused to participate. Lambert (1972) arranged for a sample of nonrespondents in a large-scale postal enquiry on cardiorespiratory disease to be approached and interviewed. An attempt was made to find out about their characteristics, smoking habits and prevalence of symptoms. There was the expected variation in demographic characteristics, with overrepresentation of rural residents and those in social classes IV and V. The smoking habits and prevalence of symptoms in the nonrespondents did not differ to an appreciable extent from the original respondents. Oakes et al. (1973) contacted members of the Kaiser-Permanente (one of the largest health insurance foundations in the USA) in Oakland and Berkeley, asking questions about smoking, disability, and 'feeling well at present'. Five waves of questionnaires were mailed at three-week intervals to those not responding; after this 66.8 per cent had answered. A personal letter from the chief physician was then sent, followed by attempts to interview over the telephone, or contact at home by personal visit. Finally, 91.4 per cent of subjects provided information (excluding those whose address had changed). Smokers tended to respond more slowly than nonsmokers. This tendency was reversed in men and women stating they were limited in activity or did not feel well. The initial responders would have produced biased results by containing a disproportionate number of sick and disabled smokers.

Harris et al. (1971) found that there was no alteration in the prevalence of abnormality in those who only responded after considerable delay; this was used as indirect evidence that the nonresponders were unlikely to be a biased subgroup of the total study population.

Tiblin (1965) had an 88 per cent response in a population survey on fifty-year-old males in a large town in Sweden. Some information on all subjects was directly available to the investigator. Details included income, civil status, place of birth, reported sickness absence, the proportion with a disability pension, and those on the register of the temperance board (that is those who had been reported to the board because of excessive alcohol consumption). In the nonrespondent group there was an excess of individuals who had been drawing sickness benefit for long periods of time, who had disability pensions or who were known to the temperance board. A further sample of about 10 000 men born in 1915–25 living in the same city (Göteborg) in 1970–73 were invited to complete a questionnaire on heart disease and then attend a screening examination. Comparison of the participants with the 25.2 per cent of nonparticipants showed that the latter had evidence of higher prevalence of chronic diseases and alcoholic problems with higher mortality by 4 July 1973 (Wilhelmsen *et al.*, 1976).

Mention has already been made (4.2.3.3, paragraph 6) of the finding, among the controls in a study of peptic ulcer, of evidence of major social and psychological problems in a high proportion of 'unco-operative' families.

Kemsley (1976) compared the characteristics of the nonresponders in two national surveys. Overall, the response to the Food Survey was considerably lower (50–55 per cent) than to the Family Expenditure Survey (70 per cent); there was appreciable difference in the responses associated with differences in household attributes. It was thought that this differential response was compatible with bias in association with low response.

Cartwright (1978), in some of her unit's medical-care studies, had arranged interviews of patients and doctors in the same localities. She was thus able to contrast the patients' comments about doctors who did and did not respond. In a study of prescribing, patients were more likely to state their doctor had enough time to listen if their doctor had responded, but there was no difference in contact rate with the two categories of doctor. In another study of terminal illness, noncollaborating doctors were less frequent in their visiting of patients, less likely to have arranged a district nurse, and less likely to have spent time discussing the illness with relatives. However, she concluded that the differences detected did not indicate a large bias between responders and nonresponders.

In certain prospective studies, it has been possible to examine the mortality of the respondents in relation to that of the nonrespondents. Gordon and Kannell (1968), Doll and Hill (1964), and Horowitz and Wilbeck (1971) found that the mortality rate among nonrespondents was higher shortly after the initial survey (as one would expect if nonparticipation was caused by a severe illness at the time). However, the excess mortality did not disappear after a number of years of follow up in any of these three studies. Doll and Hill suggested that this was an indication that there was a general association between mortality and the tendency not to reply to an inquiry, whether the tendency was due to a deliberate refusal (which was rare) or to a mere neglect of these things (which was frequent). Doll and Peto (1976) subsequently suggested that the effect of nonresponse due to ill health at the time of the initial questionnaire mail out had disappeared by the fourth year of follow up.

Sheik and Mattingly (1981) found more nonresponders to a mail survey of disabled persons were biased with respect to results of rehabilitation, return to work, or use of vocational training. Rather different were the findings in a study to screen for hypertension in which ninety-two per cent of the potentially eligible were eventually examined. There was no difference in the diastolic blood-pressure in those who came readily or only after intensive persuasion (Silman and Locke, 1982).

4.2.3.5 Motivation of subjects

It is generally suggested that, for any survey, the response rate will be related to the degree of motivation of the subject. There is, however, no definite evidence from surveys that indicates the best approach to motivation. Research workers have considered the specific problem and have then decided what steps they thought were most appropriate to boosting motivation. There do not appear to have been any controlled studies, in which different approaches have been assessed in a scientific fashion. The general literature suggests that painstaking follow up of nonrespondents is the most rewarding approach to boosting response (Scott, 1961).

Many research workers have documented the effect of care and persistence; the number responding gradually rises with each subsequent approach. Cochrane (1954) suggested that it takes as much effort to increase the response rate from 75 to 90 per cent, as the effort required to obtain the initial response of 75 per cent. In a number of early studies in South Wales, considerable effort was made to warn the population of the impending study by the use of the press and radio. However, the research workers in South Wales were convinced that local contact (door-to-door visiting) was the essential prerequisite for an adequate response rate. After trying a number of different approaches, they used a home visit to inform individuals about the impending survey, and to try to persuade reluctant particpants to take part in the study. There is no clear guidance as to the optimum number of follow up attempts; for example, do too many approaches harden attitudes to refusal? Nor is there any indication as to the appropriate interval between attempts.

Kemsley and Nicholson (1960) reported a series of trials in which various levels of payment were used. For a one-week survey on household expenditure, the response rose from 33 per cent with no payment, to 49.4 per cent when the payment was 10s 0d (£0.50p) for each person within the household completing the form. (This material was collected in the late 1950s when obviously the value of money was different. Over the past few years, the response rate in this ongoing survey has improved considerably compared with these earlier figures.)

Earlier it was suggested that the length of interview or questionnaire and the number of times an individual is asked to participate do not radically alter the response rate. Once an individual has agreed to take part in a study, he will apparently do so with relatively little default as the complexity of the study grows. However, one should bear in mind the warning of Hill (1951b) who suggested that for every question inserted in a questionnaire, the research workers should put at least three questions to themselves—Why should a survey be carried out, by what means and when? In addition, there must be a detailed consideration of every question to be included in the survey. Although questionnaire design may play a part, the important element appears to be the general message initially conveyed to the subject and the impact that this makes in stimulating him to respond. The proportion of outright refusals to participate is generally extremely low, thus re-emphasising the relevance of Cochrane's approach which was persistent encouragement to sway those who were just hesitant.

4.2.4 Categories of data

A wide range of information may be used in epidemiological studies. The simplest data relate to the characteristics of individuals or households, such as the sex of subjects, their age, marital status, number of children born alive and currently living, literacy or degree of education, and ethnic group. This may often be supplemented by information about the occupation, industry and employment status of those at work; such information can provide an indirect indication of the economic status of individuals. In addition, information may be sought on the environment (biological, physical and chemical) of the home and workplace; other environmental data, such as quality of housing and population density, may also be obtained. A further category of information is the individual's attitudes, particularly those regarding health and the use of the health services. In certain circumstances it is relevant to quantify personal behaviour—for instance, diet and smoking and drinking habits.

All this information may then be related to a 'measure of health', or more usually disease state. Identification of biochemical, physiological or psychological abnormalities that have not been recognised by the individuals may be involved. Confirmation of the presence of early or established disease may occur. One of the most important aspects of data collection is the steps that have to be taken to ensure the quality of data is satisfactory. This issue is discussed at considerable length in subsection 4.2.6.

4.2.5 Methods of data collection

After the extent of the information required for the study is decided on, the method of collecting it should then be considered. Whenever possible a standardised record-sheet should be used in order to increase the accuracy of data recording and to facilitate processing. Where questions have only a few possible answers, it is a good idea to specify these on the record sheet; the appropriate answer can then be clearly marked on the form, either by the individual concerned or by the interviewer. Consider, for example, a question about the respondent's marital status. Answers will usually fall into one of the following categories: single/married/widowed/separated/divorced; some people's marital status may not conform to any of these standard categories and it is always useful to have as one of the answers 'other'. As a general rule the form should allow for 'not known', 'not asked', 'not answered', 'not recorded' and 'not applicable' Specification of the range of anticipated answers requires confirmation using pilot questionnaires. Also, there must always be room to record comments, particularly where an individual's answer will be coded 'other'. Other questions will result in quantitative answers, and these can be handled by providing boxes in which the appropriate figures may be written. For example, with the question 'How many children have you?' two boxes would allow for the relatively rare cases of more than nine.

Responses may be collected from individuals either by asking them questions or sending postal questionnaires for completion at home. There are minor variations in these two different approaches, such as handing out the questionnaire to a group gathered into a (large) room, in order to go over the reason for the study or the points that the respondent should consider before completing a complex set of questions. A member of the survey team may then quickly check over the answers given in returned form. Also, though the above referred to 'postal' questionnaires, there are a variety of ways in which the forms may be distributed and collected—such as via the internal mail for individuals in some large organisations.

4.2.6 Accuracy of data

This subsection first discusses the importance of accurate data in general terms and then considers the three categories of survey data: (1) subjects' responses, (2) clinical examination findings and (3) results from special investigations.

4.2.6.1 The importance of accurate data

In all studies it is important to be sure that the data collected are as accurate as possible. The common sources of error and bias, and the various ways in which they may be quantified, will be discussed. When commenting on the accuracy of any particular 'instrument', it is usual to distinguish the reliability of the data collected from the validity. Reliability is the extent of agreement between repeated measurements, and consists of the sum of variation in the item being assessed and the error introduced by the observer collecting and processing this information. Validity of the technique is the extent to which a method provides a true assessment of that which it purports to measure.

Wherever possible a research worker will use an 'instrument' that has already been standardised and validated. Even so, in any major study it is important to check the accuracy of the data collected by such means. In many projects, particularly those tackling new problems, specific methods for collecting relevant and accurate data need to be developed. This may necessitate lengthy method studies as a preliminary in order to develop suitable ways of collecting data—especially when the field survey involves large numbers of subjects and requires a simple technique for collecting data on attitudes, habits, symptoms, signs or results from investigations.

In order to indicate the range of 'instruments' that have been developed a few specific examples are given. Some of these studies are referred to in greater detail later in this section, while comment will be made at the appropriate place in later chapters where particular studies have involved detailed work in the development of methods of data collection.

Cochrane and his colleagues (1951), when studying the prevalence of respiratory disease, developed a standard questionnaire to elicit symptoms of respiratory disease, while Rose (1962) was responsible for developing and validating a questionnaire to detect the presence of cardiovascular symptoms. The situation is more complex when studying behaviour. Marr (1965) described a tested method of obtaining data on dietary intake, while Yasin et al. (1967) devised and validated a questionnaire to assess habitual leisure activity.

Many epidemiological surveys have involved the recording of physical signs and much work has been carried out perfecting the method of obtaining valid material from clinical examination. Rose and Blackburn (1968) described the steps they took to reduce the errors in the collection of data from cardiovascular surveys. As a specific example, Rose et al. (1964) described the work that led to the production and testing of a new machine for recording blood pressure. As an example of the improvement of the reliability and validity of data from investigation, Blackburn and his colleagues (1960) standardised the technique for recording and interpreting E.C.G. tracings obtained in surveys.

Some of the error introduced in data collection will be random and this can result in the incorrect classification of individuals, or the recording of too high to too low values for continuous variates. It is important to have some guide as to the degree of this random variation. Once this variation has been quantified, there are statistical techniques available for overcoming the influence of random variation in the interpretation of collected data. Another issue that has to be considered is the introduction of bias into data collection. Particular ways of phrasing questions, consistent faults in the technique of examining patients, or errors in the method of analysing investigations can introduce a bias into the results. Use of more than one observer often introduces differences in the bias of the results, while the degree of bias may vary between subgroups of the subjects in the study. This complicates the interpretation of the material much more than the presence of random error. In assessing the reliability, validity and bias in the data-collection system, it is usual to consider (1) the innate variability in the subjects being observed, (2) the error or biases introduced into the subjects' responses because of the experimental situation and (3) the contribution of observer error or bias. The interplay of these factors will be mentioned in subsection 4.5.3. Where a particular investigation is used to classify individuals into 'healthy' and 'diseased' subgroups, it is usual to consider the sensitivity and specificity of the test that is used. Sensitivity is a measure of the extent to which the method gives results free from false negatives (that is, it fails to pick up as diseased those individuals who suffer from the condition). Specificity is a measure of the extent to which a method gives results free from false positives (that is, the degree to which the technique falsely classifies as diseased subjects that are in fact healthy).

It is essential that the error rate of various 'instruments' used in epidemiology are known before the data collected by them is interpreted. This is a similar approach to any other scientific work—it is essential to calibrate a new instrument before it is put to use and to recalibrate the instrument at appropriate intervals. The term 'instrument' may be used in the epidemiological field to refer to the techniques for collecting (1) written or verbal information from subjects, (2) observations after examination of the subjects or (3) data from the investigation of the subjects. Only when one has a precise indication of the accuracy rate of the measurements to be made in a study is it possible to plan carefully and determine the size of the study; this will be dealt with in subsection 4.5.4. At this stage, it is sufficient to say that if an instrument used is of low accuracy, then the larger the number of observations, the easier the interpretation will be. Often there are various techniques for collecting the same item of information with varying levels of accuracy; the least accurate technique may be the easiest to apply. Thus, the main options will be either to study large numbers of subjects with a crude instrument, or to study a small number of subjects with a more accurate technique. Precise information about the error rate will be required in order to decide which is the more appropriate tactic. The other main reason for requiring information about the accuracy of data collection is the part this plays in the interpretation of data from surveys. Only when there is clear information about the validity of the techniques used is it possible to interpret results with certainty.

A full discussion of the acquisition of clinical data from history and physical examination is provided by Feinstein (1964), though no estimates of error rates and biases are provided.

4.2.6.2 Accuracy of subjects' responses

When questioning patients, information may be obtained about current symptoms, and about the habits and characteristics of the individuals, or about previous history. It is important to consider these three facets in a different light. Some of the early work carried out on the recording of symptoms in population surveys was in the study of respiratory diseases.

Cochrane and his colleagues (1951) noted a significant variation in the proportion of miners reporting various symptoms (cough, sputum, pain in the chest, dyspepsia) when interviewed by different observers. A planned study clearly showed the influence of a standardised questionnaire in improving the consistency in the answers. Fairbairn et al. (1959) showed that health visitors obtained as reliable results as doctors using the questionnaire. Further use of the questionnaire showed a relationship between positive responses and measured evidence of impaired respiratory function (Sharpe *et al.*, 1965; Fletcher and Tinker, 1961; College of General Practitioners, 1961).

Histories may be obtained by interview with or without a standard questionnaire, or by a questionnaire that may be completed by the respondent either under supervision or with the aid of written instructions. Each of these approaches has been carefully studied and the validity of the material collected assessed and related to the costs involved in obtaining it. There is evidence that the attitude and manner of the interviewer, and even the sex of the interviewer, can affect the respondents' answers (Kannell *et al.*, 1969; Columbotis *et al.*, 1968). Self-completion questionnaires, especially when these can be distributed to respondents and then returned by post, involve far less labour than interviews carried out on a one-to-one basis. This is a good example of a situation in which clear information about the relative accuracy of the different approaches is required, thus enabling one to assess whether the vast increase in the number that can be studied using self-completion of the questionnaire outweighs the diminution in the accuracy of the data collected. Milne and Williamson (1971) warned that automatic administration of a questionnaire can generate a 'response set' where a positive answer to a series of questions is the first alternative (after a correct answer of yes to the first one or two questions, this response may then be given incorrectly to subsequent questions).

Considerable work has been done on the collection of information about patients' current habits and characteristics. For example, much work has been involved in the collection of data on smoking habits. No direct validation study of such questionnaires has been carried out, although Doll and Hill (1950), and Todd (1966) have reported on the reliability of statements about smoking habits. Indirect validation of the questionnaires has been demonstrated by the relationship between reported smoking habits and assessment of respiratory functions (Bewlcy *et al.*, 1973; Holland and Elliott, 1968). Even for relatively simple matters, such as age, there is a tendency for the answers to be inaccurate. Firstly it is common to round age to certain terminal digits, with preference for recording ages with a terminal digit of 0, 5 and 8. This was observed by Farr (1841) when examining the tabulations by single year of age of the national mortality data, and was also noted in the 1961 census (General Register Office, 1968). In contrast, there is the tendency for certain sections of the population to introduce bias. For instance, women approaching middle age consistently understate their age, while the elderly and especially the very old subjects tend to exaggerate their age.

Stewart (1982) analysed the self-reported height and weight against measurements for 3373 subjects and concluded that the information is reliable and valid, even for groups in whom poorer quality data might be expected, such as the overweight. This was also quantified by Palta *et al.* (1982) who compared self-reported with measured height and weight in a survey in Minneapolis. Height was overstated by 1.3 per cent by men and 0.6 per cent by women, whilst weight was understated by 1.6 per cent by men and 3.1 per cent by women.

In a study of the epidemiology of cervical dysplasia, Armstrong (1980) noted that patients asked about age at first coitus did not show embarrassment and appeared certain of their answers. However, of women aged twenty and over at first marriage, first birth, or first abortion, about one-quarter reported first coitus under the age of seventeen. If these answers are valid, it suggests that the factual items on age at marriage and pregnancy are poor surrogates for the age of onset of sexual behaviour. In an attempt to check the validity of data on sexual intercourse, Kunin and Ames (1981) asked a small group of women to keep diaries. Some information was recorded on a diary of all daily activities using fifteen-minute intervals, and running for seven days. For the rest of the month the women were merely asked to record frequency of intercourse and menstruation. The study continued for six months. Considerably more frequent intercourse was recorded in the daily activities calendar than for the remaining twenty-one days of the month. The full weekly records were consistent from one month to the next, indicating that one week of recording should be adequate to classify each woman. There was appreciable variation with different days of the week, indicating that a full week was required.

One of the most difficult topics to study in large samples is diet; the following paragraphs indicate some results of checking the quality of data. Hankin *et al.* (1975) developed a questionnaire to estimate the current frequencies and quantative intakes of selected food items. Interviewers were asked to agree on sizes of small, medium and large servings of each item in the questionnaire. These servings were weighed and photographed in colour. The assessment consisted of an item-by-item recall about foods eaten yesterday. After the diet for the previous day had been recorded the entire list was reviewed to obtain estimates of frequency and amount consumed during the previous seven days. They examined the validity of the method in 1973–4 among fifty randomly selected subjects. The subject and his wife were visited at their home and provided with seven-day forms for recording frequencies and relative amounts, together with the pictures of serving items for thirty-three foods. The interviewer demonstrated the way of recording the information and asked the subject to bring the material back when coming for examination at the end of the week. When the subject presented himself for the examination, an interviewer then asked the respondent to record thirty-three food items consumed yesterday and the previous week; this recall had not been indicated in the preliminary contact with the subject. The analysis compared the daily diaries with the recall at the end of the week.

Comparison of the quantative intakes of the thirty-three food items showed appreciable variation for some of the foods. The major discrepancies—quoting the mean value in grams for diary and then recall—were: beef (57.3; 32.0), chicken (18.3; 11.6), luncheon meat (9.6; 4.5), Japanese soup (96.5; 44.6), green tea (45.1; 33.6), black tea (135.3; 79.2), coffee (291.1; 345.6), milk (74.4; 50.1), fruit drinks (92.4; 54.0). All the discrepancies of greater than 25 per cent provided a higher estimate of intake from the diary than the recall. The correlations between the two sources of data were higher for items that were eaten habitually (such as eggs, rice, lettuce, green and black tea, coffee and milk) or for items that were thought to be associated with specific events (such as consuming shrimp, dried fish, pickled Chinese cabbage). The technique for recording the data obtained frequency as well as serving size; the correlations between the two sources of data were slightly higher when serving size was taken into account than for the correlations between the frequencies alone. Comparable results have been obtained by Nomura *et al.* (1976) and Jain *et al.* (1980); these indicate the difficulty in assessing nutrient intake in healthy individuals (let alone in case–control studies).

Israel *et al.* (1979), in a laboratory study of psychology students, found that requests to self-monitor smoking behaviour produced reactive effects upon smoking itself. This occurred even though there was no suggestion that the investigation was in any way related to the frequency of smoking or attempting to influence such behaviour. This illustrates the general concern that the study group may be (perhaps subconsciously) influenced to alter their behaviour.

Todd (1978) drew attention to the discrepancy between surveys of cigarette consumption and estimated national consumption, demonstrating that this varied from country to country. He suggested that the wording of questions, whether they were asked in the context of health inquires, and anti-smoking propaganda could influence the validity of the answers. He noted the highest deficiency had occurred in the U.S.A. (in 1975, survey results had to be inflated by 56 per cent to agree with national data). One problem with inflating in this way was the assumption made on degree of under-reporting in men and women. Kozlowski *et al.* (1980) reviewed the degree of error in self-reporting of smoking habits, while McKennell (1980) reported up to fivefold differences in children's smoking statements depending on whether these were obtained at home or school.

Edwards *et al.* (1973) reinterviewed forty men and their wives after an interval of two to three months. About seventy per cent were consistent on number of days a week they drank, the expenditure on drinking, and the amount and frequency of drinking over the past year. Cross-check of methods of assessing drinking behaviour suggested that quantity–frequency questioning might underestimate certain patterns of alcohol consumption that are associated with health risk (Sobell *et al.*, 1982). Comparison of eight laboratory tests for detection of excess drinking and three brief, standard interviews suggested that the latter were more effective than the best laboratory test (γ-glutamyl transpeptidase). The questionnaires were thought suitable for detecting high-risk groups (Bernadt *et al.*, 1982).

When asking patients about their medical history (either their exposure to aetiological factors or their health in the past), due consideration has to be given to the influence of the current situation and of the recent past, both of which may stimulate or depress recall of past events. This point will be dealt with in greater detail in relation to case–control studies (see section 5.3). When questioning patients about their previous health, it has been shown that the validity of the answers deteriorates with the increase in the period over which attempts are made to collect information. In the survey of sickness carried out in this country over thirty years ago (Stocks, 1944 and

Stocks, 1949), subjects consistently reported a higher prevalence of illness in the four weeks preceding interview than in the period four to eight weeks before. This finding was observed whatever the month of interview. It was unlikely therefore that this was a genuine effect of secular variation in prevalence of disease, but was an effect of loss of data due to memory bias. The General Household Survey (O.P.C.S., 1973) provided some evidence that there was a drop in recall even when using a short reference period of only two weeks. The relationship between use of hospital services reported during an interview and the actual evidence from examination of hospital records showed discrepancies in recall. Some studies showed a modest tendency to under-report such events (National Centre for Health Statistics, 1965; Vessey *et al.*, 1974), while Palmer *et al.* (1969) suggested that a sample in North Lambeth tended in general to over-report.

Earlier in this section, attention was paid to the use of a questionnaire to obtain symptoms of respiratory disease. Another standard questionnaire used in many epidemiological studies is the London School of Hygiene's questionnaire on cardiovascular symptoms. Development of this question-naire was discussed by Rose (1962), and its validation reviewed by Rose and Blackburn (1968). Many other clinical fields of enquiry have been investi-gated in an attempt to obtain reliable and valid information, and each of these has required careful consideration of the phrasing of the questions used. In the General Household Survey an attempt was made to identify the prevalence of long-standing disability. The original question used in 1971 was split into two linked questions in 1972, with the result that there was an appreciable drop in the number of positive responses. The results shown in figure 4.1 serve as a warning of the effect that change in a question can have.

Detailed studies have been carried out in the psychiatric field, with the examination of the large and persistent differences in the admission statistics by diagnosis between American and British hospitals. Cooper *et al.* (1972) suggested that most of these differences were spurious and generated by variation in interpretation of symptoms and the use of different diagnostic labels. Further work in an international pilot study of schizophrenia has led to the development of standardised instruments and procedures for assess-ment of patients with mental disorders in different countries (W.H.O., 1973).

Kneale and Stewart (1980) compared the history of X-ray to mothers and fathers of children who had died from malignant disease in the period 1953–60 and parents of control (living) children. In general, the histories of paternal X-ray were obtained from the mothers. X-rays reported in preg-nancy have been checked against medical records. The relative risk of maternal and paternal X-ray to abdomen, chest or extremities was examined for preconception and postnatal periods. The preconception risks ranged from 1.06 to 1.33, while the postnatal risks were from 0.83 to 1.00.

For preconception abdominal X-rays (which might have affected the child), there was no significant difference between cases and controls. For X-rays which could not have affected the child (preconception to chest or extremities, or postnatal) mothers of dead children reported significantly more X-rays before conception and significantly fewer postnatally.

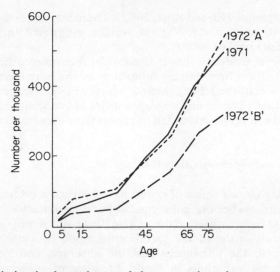

Figure 4.1 Variation in the estimate of the proportion of persons suffering from chronic illness by age, in relation to question used, United Kingdom, 1971–2

1971 Those answering 'Yes' to 'Do you suffer any long-standing illness, disability or infirmity which limits your activity compared with most people of your own age?'
1972'A' Those answering 'Yes' to 'Do you suffer from any long-standing illness, disability, or infirmity?'
1972'B' Those also answering 'Yes' to 'Does it limit your activities compared with most people of your own age?'

Source: *General Household Survey*, O.P.C.S., H.M.S.O. (1973)

This analysis indicates different facets of memory bias, but does not suggest that the estimates of risk from foetal irradiation were inappropriate.

The Nottingham Health Profile is a self-administered questionnaire designed to provide a measure of perceived health problems. Patients with osteoarthritis were given the questionnaire to complete on two occasions four weeks apart. Results showed a high level of reliability for reported number and types of health problems (Hunt *et al.*, 1981). Watkins *et al.* (1982) found a poor relationship between doctors' diagnoses of lower respiratory illness and maternal recall of these illnesses in their infants. However, the group of children reported by their mothers to have had bronchitis or pneumonia in the first year of life appear to suffer more respiratory illness than other children. Reinterview of over twelve thousand people in Finland after a three-year interval suggested that information about myocardial infarction was reliable. Responses on diabetes and stroke were subject to error, with the latter showing under-reporting (Tretli *et al.*, 1982). Comparison of data on drug usage from interviews, medical records and pharmacy records showed variation for different types of drugs—from 69 per cent agreement for barbiturates to 87 per cent for hypertensive treatment (Paganini-Hill and Ross, 1982). There was even closer agreement for reported diseases, and for height, weight, menstrual and reproductive variables (90 per cent or better).

Also, there is evidence that it is considerably more difficult to obtain correct information from certain subgroups of the population, such as the psychiatrically disturbed. For example, Murray (1973) suggested that those persons habitually consuming large quantities of analgesics are emotionally disturbed and are very likely to fail to report their excessive consumption of these drugs.

4.2.6.3 Accuracy of examination findings

When studying the influence of raised blood-pressure on health, a number of research workers became concerned about the accuracy with which blood pressure could be measured. Rose et al. (1964) and Armitage et al. (1966) showed, as well as the innate variation in blood pressure, that an error occurred due to the instrument and the observer. Gardner and Heady (1973) indicated variations in blood pressure of subjects in the same situation, but in the presence of different observers. Other studies of the relationship between body build and cardiovascular disease required the measurement of skin-fold thickness, which may be used as an estimate of obesity. An instrument was devised by Edwards et al. (1955) which was suitable for survey work and which provided consistent and valid measures of skin-fold thickness. Ruiz et al. (1971) showed how the selection of the specific site for measurement of skin-fold thickness affects the reading; even with a shift of only a few centimetres significantly different values were obtained.

In a study of women over forty attending for screening for breast cancer, Chamberlain et al. (1975) tabulated the independent opinions of clinical and radiological observers. Table 4.2 shows the agreement between nurses and clinic doctors. The 1215 women were followed up for six months and then re-examined. Table 4.3 compares the combined opinion on initial screening against the status of the women at six months.

Table 4.2   Agreement between nurses and clinic doctors on the need to refer subjects to a surgeon, after screening 999 'well women' for breast cancer

Action recommended by nurse	Action recommended by clinic doctor		
	Referral	No referral	Total
referral	43 (5)*	46 (1)	89
no referral	46 (3)	864 (3)	910
total	89	910	999

Source: Chamberlain (1982)

*Numbers in parentheses indicate cancers detected within six months

Table 4.3   Diagnosis reached by six-month review compared with conclusion on initial screening of 1215 'well women' by nurse, clinic doctor and mammography read by two radiologists

Screening conclusion	Diagnosis by six-month review				
	Cancer	Biopsy: non-malignant	Surgical assessment no biopsy required	No surgical assessment	Total
malignant	14	38	20	6	78
benign	3	64	77	9	153
not referred	2	—	—	982	984
total	19	102	97	997	1215

Source: Chamberlain (1982)

The Yorkshire Breast Cancer Group (1977) arranged for 242 patients with breast lesions examined by ten consultant surgeons to be also seen by a research registrar. The degree of observer variation differed from one clinical item to another; there was agreement on the presence of supraclavicular nodes in 96.9 per cent of the comparisons, but only 45.4 per cent for tumour size within 2 cm, or pectoral muscle fixation in 35.5 per cent of comparisons.

Other facets of clinical examination to be studied in this way have been: examination of the heart (Raftery and Holland, 1967); physical signs in airways obstruction (Godfrey et al. 1969); physical signs in ulcerative colitis (Graham et al., 1971); the detection of absent pulses in the peripheral limbs (Meade et al., 1968).

The problem of digit preference mentioned in the previous section can also cause problems with observer bias. In a population survey of blood pressure in Bergen, it was noted that there was a marked tendency to record values rounded to a value in mmHg ending '0', rather than in '5' (Bøe et al., 1957).

4.2.6.4 Accuracy of investigation results

With the increase in the investigation of patients for diagnostic purposes and in order to control therapy, a considerable amount of work has been carried out on the accuracy of such measures. The initial stimulus came from those working in laboratories responsible for investigating patients, and further interest was generated by the collection of large volumes of data in population surveys. The use of the E.C.G. was introduced into clinical practice at the beginning of this century. However, it was only after the collection of tracings from large numbers of individuals in population surveys that interest developed in assessing the validity of interpretation of such recordings. A number of studies have been mounted in which different techniques for recording the electrical changes were used, and the interpretation of individual records by a number of observers compared (Higgins *et al.*, 1963). In addition, the findings of different observers have been related to the prevalence of other indices of cardiovascular disease, and the development of disease and death on follow up. Rose and Blackburn (1968) described a technique for reducing the inter- and intra-observer variation in the interpretation of E.C.G.s.

The accuracy of certain biochemical determinations, such as serum cholesterol levels (and their relationship to the prevalence or subsequent development of cardiovascular disease) has been studied. There have also been a number of studies on the accuracy of haematological measurements, such as the haemoglobin levels, packed cell volume and serum iron estimations. Whitehead (1974) reviewed the development of quality-control techniques in the laboratory. It was suggested that by the adoption of standard methods and the monitoring of any variations, the precision of the results may be improved. An earlier study by Whitehead (1965) showed how different technicians could influence results independently of technique and subject variation. Of particular interest to epidemiologists has been the observer variation in the interpretation of X-rays (Yerushalmy, 1947) and the assessment of respiratory function (Wright and McKerrow, 1959). In a deliberate test of observer variation of reading mammograms a set of 100 films was read by 9 radiologists (Boyd, 1978). Using 4 categories of diagnosis, and 4 of recommendation, all 9 observers only agreed on 4 of the 100 films; 5 observers agreed for 73 of the diagnoses but only 30 of the recommendations. The films had been selected to contain 10 biopsy-proven cancers; one radiologist read 9 and another 57 as 'possibly or definitely malignant'. Biopsy or aspiration was recommended from 15 to 47 of the films.

With growing interest in the screening of 'well women' for *in situ* carcinoma of the cervix, studies have been carried out on the reliability and validity of cervical cytology (Yule, 1972). Husain *et al.* (1974) drew attention to the very wide range of error rates that had been reported (from 1.1 to 30 per cent). However, comparisons were difficult because of variation in the lesions assessed, different methods of sample collection, and use of a variety of methods to calculate the results. As far as sample collection was concerned, it could involve different sites (from cervical scrape, vaginal aspiration or vaginal irrigation); the sampling method may or may not directly access the squamo-columnar junction in the cervical canal (in older women this junction 'retreats' up the canal).

In an extension of the results from the Christie Hospital, Yule (1974) presented data on rescreening of 14 437 women after 3 months. Of 25 smears positive at the second screen, 9 on rereading should have been identified as positive on first screen, while 16 were sampling deficiency. These 25 positive smears were 14.9 per cent of the total positives at first plus second screening.

The reason for stressing the errors that may occur in patients' responses, observers' findings and results of investigation is to emphasise that attention to such detail can reduce the variation and improve the quality of survey data. The use of data in the clinical field is usually quite different. Large-scale epidemiological studies may have to classify individuals on the basis of one measurement of a particular variate. A discussion on the classification of individuals as 'at risk' from coronary artery disease from a single measurement of the blood cholesterol was presented (Heady, 1973). In a clinical situation on the other hand, information from history, examination and investigation is collated and reviewed, with subtle judgement being made about individual items out of line with the general profile of a disease. If doubt arises in interpretation, the patient may be observed over a period of time and repeat measurement made and assessed.

4.3 Advantages and Disadvantages of Surveys

A survey is the simplest type of study that can be carried out and is usually descriptive in nature. The approach may be used (1) to tackle a wide range of issues not covered by routine data, or (2) for the exploration in depth of an issue by collating detailed information.

The main advantages in surveys lie in their ability to cover gaps in the items in routine data-collection systems. A survey will often permit the collection of material that is not readily catered for in routine returns: the latter are usually quite good at recording the events that occur (e.g. has a patient been to hospital, or who referred them), but they are not so suitable for identifying the reasons for the various actions; this will often require specific questioning of a sample of subjects about the factors leading to their actions.

Rather different from the coverage of such issues of detail that are better collected in surveys, there is the fact that new situations may arise that require the analysis of quite fresh items of information. Obviously, a routine data collection system has a degree of built-in inertia. For example, over the past twenty years the pattern of food consumption has altered, with increasing use of 'fast foods' requiring the minimum of preparation and home cooking. Rather different questions may be required to identify the exact particulars of an individual's diet (e.g., it is no use just recording that soup has been eaten, as there are considerable differences between home-made soup, tinned soup, packet soup requiring twenty minutes to cook, and 'instant soup').

Having established that there is a gap in the routine data collection, there will be a modest delay in the planning and execution of the survey. This may not be a major delay, and the judicious balance of routine and survey systems should provide a full range of information and the best value for money.

4.4 Extension of the Method of Surveys

As far as a relatively rare disease is concerned, or one whose duration is limited, surveys prove an inadequate approach to studying the prevalence of the condition. (This does not apply to the investigation of very common conditions like upper respiratory tract infections, nor to very chronic conditions such as disabling rheumatoid arthritis.) Thus for cancer their use is really restricted to providing background information about the distribution of habits, attitudes, or symptoms that can occur with cancer.

For other diseases a survey that identifies subjects who do and do not have the disease can be linked to an examination of the factors associated with the distribution of the disease (e.g., is osteoarthritis more or less common in social classes I or II, or does it particularly occur in people with certain jobs?). This approach is not really suited to the study of malignant disease, though it may be used for investigating the factors associated with prevalence of precursor lesions. (For example, what is the reproductive history of women found, on mammographic survey, to have certain patterns of breast duct?)

The use of a survey of the population to identify cases and controls for a study of the aetiology of the disease is dealt with in the next chapter (see subsection 5.2.1.1).

Analysis of casualty records for 1557 burns and scalds in children under twelve treated in Bradford in 1969–73 suggested that children in overcrowded and New Commonwealth immigrant families were associated with increased risk. Interview of parents of seventy-eight children was used to cross-check this finding, but no clear explanation was obtained in the second survey (Learmonth, 1979).

4.4.1 Combination of two surveys

In 1966–8, questionnaires were mailed to the next of kin of 19 526 persons aged 35–84 dying in the United States; in 1967 a household survey was carried out which also collected information on smoking from over sixty thousand adults in the same age range. Results from these two cross-sectional surveys were combined by Enstrom and Godley (1981); they showed that the cancer mortality in male nonsmokers was 47 per cent of that in smokers, while in female nonsmokers it was 33 per cent. The largest cancer-rate reductions were concentrated in the respiratory system. This indicates how the results of two quite separate surveys may provide a more powerful probe of an issue.

4.4.2 Comparison of high- and low-prevalence localities

The International Agency for Research on Cancer (1977) investigated the diet in small samples of men living in Denmark and Finland, as part of a study of the aetiology of colo-rectal cancer. This is one variant of survey design which may be used to provide an analytical study, to probe aetiological relationships more fully than by the mere description of the characteristics of locations with differences in the incidence or mortality from cancer. Where there is known (major) difference in the incidence of a particular disease, probability samples of the population are selected and detailed information collected from the individuals about all potentially relevant factors.

In the Finnish study, it was decided to investigate residents from a rural location, while the Danish sample was drawn from persons living in an urban area. The main focus of enquiry was diet and a day's weighed dietary survey was carried out, which was supplemented by questioning about food habits, drinking and smoking. Other information was collected about: single stool transit time, faecal flora and faecal steroids.

Such a study has the advantage that it can probe for variation in various aspects of way of life and also quantify the local environment to a much greater extent than is possible in any descriptive study restricted to the use of routine data. The power of the study will depend in part upon the extent of the difference in incidence between the two study locations. If there are no clear leads to the aetiology of the disease being studied, then this approach can be used as a preliminary screen to search for variation in exposure to different environmental factors that might have a bearing on the aetiology of the disease.

Obviously, one would not expect such marked differences between the subjects in the different locations as between cases and controls (see next chapter); however, this type of survey does avoid the conceptual problems involved in choosing ideal controls. The inferences that may be drawn from any differences noted in the samples from the two populations is that they are associated with a difference in risk of the cancer of a stated order of magnitude. It cannot be directly argued that a high level of exposure to a specific factor leads to or causes the disease being studied (though the results may be compatible with this).

4.5 Analysis of Survey Data

A brief introduction to the techniques of checking, sifting, sorting, counting and tabulating data is provided. An indication is given of the ways in which survey material can be examined by the application of statistical tests prior to the derivation of inferences; one subsection deals with the testing of the validity of data. The final subsection provides a brief guide to the consideration of sample size required in a study.

4.5.1 Preliminary analysis of survey data

Proposals for analysing the material should always be considered in the planning phase of a study, and one important issue to clarify early is the system for data recording. The way in which the data is laid out on initial recording can often facilitate the maintenance of accurate records that are easy to analyse. Where very simple surveys have been carried out on less than 100 subjects, it is often possible to use the original data-recording sheets for analysis, since these may be manually sorted into piles and counted. For larger survey numbers, it may be possible to use edge-punched cards. These require standardisation of the answers to the individual questions, so that the material can be broken down into yes/no responses to specific questions; sex can be coded as yes or no to male, and punched accordingly. The completed cards can then be sorted using a thin rod, such as a knitting needle, which enables one to readily sort the material. There still remains the problem of counting to produce an analysis and the use of edge-punched cards is suitable only for approximately 100 to 1000 cards. Beyond this number the sorting and counting becomes tedious, even for the relatively restricted range of particulars that can be handled on such a card. Where a greater quantity of data has been collected, mechanical or electronic systems may be considered for processing the data. The applications of such techniques are beyond the scope of this book.

The first essential in survey analysis is that the research worker becomes completely familiar with the material that he has collected. This process can most easily be approached by simply sorting through all the data to find the mean value, the maximum, the minimum and the standard deviation for each variate. The mean value and standard deviation will have real meaning only for continuously distributed data, such as height, or weight, but they are of use as a method of checking the accuracy of the processing of all the data. The maxima and minima will help to detect impossible values. Another useful screen is that the research worker should specify expected normal limits and examine all those subjects with values outside these limits—to see if errors in recording, transcribing or punching have crept in. The mean value, in conjunction with the range and standard deviation, indicates how the observed values are distributed and the standard deviation shows the amount of scatter in the material; that is, whether the values are closely concentrated around the mean or not. These parameters are a guide to the appropriate statistical tests to be used in further analyses.

The next step is to examine one-way distributions of all items; for discrete or grouped data this is simple. All that is required is a count of the number of observations for each of the possible values for the variate in question (for sex one would want to know the number of males and the number of females in the sample—possibly also the number of intermediate states, queries or 'not known'). For continuous data, the presentation is not quite so simple. If the range is relatively small, it may be practicable to list the values observed and the number of subjects with each observed value. With a wide range and many observations, it will be more appropriate if the data are grouped and the numbers in each group given. With 100 patients it is possible to write out in ascending order the age of each subject, but it is easier to read and digest the number of persons in each of ten-year age-groups. (Note that the groups need not be in equal increments along the scale.) An alternative method of grouping the data is to rank all the observations (that is place them in ascending order) and then divide them into groups of equal size. The choice of number of groups will depend partly on the number of observations, but from three to ten are most usual. Based on the percentage distribution, cutting points for the tenth percentile, lower quartile (twenty-fifth percentile), median (fiftieth percentile), upper quartile (seventy-fifth percentile) and ninetieth percentile are frequently used. The range occupied by successive groups will vary as the inter-group boundaries are arbitrarily chosen in order to obtain an equal number of observations in each of the subgroups.

The above suggestions for the examination of the data have been very superficial, but only when it has been sifted in this way can the worker come to grips with the data, weed out errors in the basic material and attempt a more detailed examination. At this stage, it may be found that 377 subjects have been studied, while the results are only complete for 372—there being some missing values for the other five subjects. If it is impossible to collect the missing data for these five subjects, a decision will have to be taken as to whether or not they should be excluded from further analyses. In certain circumstances, the mean value of the variate in question may be substituted for the missing value.

It is likely that a few errors will be detected in the preliminary analysis, but sometimes a detailed probe of the material will be the first occasion when any logical inconsistencies in the data appear. In some studies there is a greater likelihood that some of the basic items of the patients are amended, perhaps after a review of the basic material, or as the passage of time indicates that some of the original information was erroneous. Therefore, a method is required for correcting or amending the data during processing.

4.5.2 Association between two or more variates

It is best to take the examination of any association in stages, commencing with pairs of variates, and then working round to the more complicated interactions between multiple variates. This stage can be carried out by a joint study between the research worker, the data processor and the statistician. The research worker will be aware of the major divisions in his data and the axes of classification that concern him. The techniques of comparison to be used will depend on the material available, the major factor being whether the variates to be studied are discrete, grouped or continuous.

If, for example, the material collected contains both controls and patients with a disease, it may be of great interest to examine initially whether the two groups are equally balanced for both sex and age. For sex a simple two-way table can be produced thus:

	Males	Females
diseased	52	36
controls	41	47
total	93	83

Inspection of such a table will show whether the sexes are equally represented in the patient and control groups and a simple test may be performed to see if any imbalance between the two groups is greater than would be expected from chance alone. A χ^2-test for difference in proportions may be used; the higher the value of χ^2, the more marked is the difference in proportions for any given number of subclasses of observations. The basic calculation (which is also applicable to tables with more rows and columns than in this simple example) involves the following steps:

(1) Calculate for each cell within the body of the table the expected values (assuming no relationship between sex and disease). This is obtained from multiplying the row and column totals and dividing the product by the grand total.

(2) Obtain the value for $\dfrac{(O-E)^2}{E}$.

(3) Sum the values $\dfrac{(O-E)^2}{E}$ to obtain χ^2.

(4) Compare the results obtained with values in tables of chi-squared, to determine the probability of the results.

	Males	Females	Total
diseased O	52	36	88
E	46.5	41.5	
$O-E$	5.5	-5.5	
$(O-E)^2/E$	0.65	0.73	
controls O	41	47	88
E	46.5	41.5	
$O-E$	-5.5	5.5	
$(O-E)^2/E$	0.65	0.73	
total	93	83	176

$\chi^2 = 2.76$
Degrees of freedom $= 1$
$p < 0.1$

The actual data thus show a relative excess of males, but this does not reach the probability of $p < 0.05$, when the results are considered unlikely to have occurred by chance and are thus referred to as statistically significant.

The influence of age can be examined in a similar way, although the division will not usually be into a two-by-two table, but a two-by-n table (where n is the number of age groups used).

	Age			
	45–54	55–64	65–74	75+
diseased	13	17	21	6
controls	7	15	23	12
total	20	32	44	18

Again, if the age distribution is not exactly the same for the two study groups, a χ^2-test may be used to see whether such a difference might have occurred by chance alone. (The tables now contain more than four cells; the value of the χ^2 for the 5 per cent level of significance increases—depending on the number of cells in the table.)

Instead of giving the absolute number of subjects in each diseased/control age group, the data may be presented as percentages of the row or column totals—this is especially useful when the total numbers of diseased and control subjects are different. Differences in the distribution of age in the two groups will be highlighted by using percentages, although it should be borne in mind that the weight that may be placed on such differences depends on the number of observations.

Another value that might be calculated is the mean age of the diseased and of the control subjects. Assuming the ages are distributed in an approximately normal way, the significance of the difference between the two mean ages may then be tested using Student's t-test (the standard error of the difference will have to be calculated from the raw data). If instead of two subgroups (diseased/healthy) there are several subgroups (healthy/mildly affected/moderately affected/severely affected) the mean age may be given for each of these four subgroups. The appropriate test of significance depends on the distribution of the variates and the nature of the association. (One-way analysis of variance or a test for trend may be suitable.)

With two continuously distributed variates a visual presentation is the best approach, preferably by a scatter diagram, in which one variate is plotted against another. This may be done manually, if computer facilities are not available. A compromise may be reached by grouping the data into a number of groups for instance, and producing a two-way table of the results. The comparison being undertaken here is between two measurements (such as height and weight) that have been recorded for all subjects. If both variates are normally distributed, a correlation coefficient may be calculated (it should be remembered that this varies between $+1$ and -1). The nearer the correlation approaches one, the closer the association, but the scatter diagram should also be examined, since a close association, with just one or two rogue points, may have a low correlation. Again, the significance of the correlation coefficient obtained depends on the number of observations that have been made. The smaller the number of observations the less the weight that can be placed on the result. Where many variates have been recorded, the number of possible pairs of variates rises rapidly; with a computer it is quite easy to produce a complete correlation matrix of all possible combinations, but this should be interpreted with caution.

When the above procedures have all been carried out and the results digested, there may be a number of other approaches that can be made to obtain full value out of the data. It is, however, unlikely that a statistician can be given the data and produce world-shattering results that the investigator has not already suspected or even observed. A general point that requires emphasis here is the need in planning to relate the aim of the study to the method chosen for tackling the problem. Even in the planning stage, consideration should be given to the method of analysis and it is wiser to seek expert statistical advice at this time.

4.5.3 Quantification of validity of data

The way in which data may be analysed in order to comment on the accuracy of the instrument used will now be considered. It is useful to consider the sources of variation in any series of measurements: the subject can show a diurnal, seasonal or secular variation; an individual observer can vary, while there can be an even greater variation between observers; the observer and subject can 'interact' to influence the measure; different 'instruments' for measuring the same item can vary in their accuracy; and there can be other unexplained and random variations. Armitage and Rose (1966) discussed how the use of multiple readings or of multiple occasions on which a reading is taken can reduce the variation in recorded blood pressure.

The concepts of sensitivity and specificity have been developed particularly in relation to screening investigations, where the aim is to categorise the subjects into those with and those without an abnormality that requires intervention. Various statistical techniques have been developed to assist in the interpretation of these aspects of survey instruments.

In a study of the accuracy of responses about circumcision status (Lilienfeld and Graham, 1958), a group of men was questioned and then examined. Table 4.4 shows the results and the way in which the data can be manipulated to show sensitivity, specificity, the index of crude agreement, the index of adjusted agreement and Youden's index. All three indices attempt to combine sensitivity and specificity into one; they may be criticised because they assume that both aspects are of equal value. There is the usual problem that by converting a two-by-two table into a single index, information is lost. Overall the relatively simple calculation of (1) sensitivity and (2) specificity seems justified. This will allow judgements to be made in the light of assessment of the relative importance of false-positive and false-negative errors in specific situations (see Youden, 1950; Newell, 1962; Rogot and Goldberg, 1966; Cochrane and Holland, 1971). The specific data quoted in table 4.4 have been used to illustrate the appropriate statistical handling of such material. A number of studies has followed up the issue of validity of responses about circumcision status from men or their wives. A study of men and women attending a cancer detection centre in Los Angeles recorded appropriate data (responses and independent examination findings). The information given by the men and women was highly accurate, with a Youden's index of 0.87 for both sets of data (Stern and Lachenbruch, 1968). Boyd and Doll (1964), in a study of the aetiology of cervical cancer, had found that data on circumcision status of the women's husbands were of limited value, as about one-third of women failed to provide a definite answer.

Table 4.5 shows actual data from a population survey in which the tension of the eyes was measured by two techniques (Hollows and Graham, 1966). Using an arbitrary cutting point to indentify raised intra-ocular pressure, the

Table 4.4 Comparison of circumcision status reported by subject, and found at examination

Patients' statements	Examination finding	
	Circumcised	Not circumcised
circumcised	37 (a)	19 (b)
not circumcised	47 (c)	89 (d)

Source: Lilienfeld and Graham (1958)

sensitivity
$$= \frac{a}{a+c}$$

$$= \frac{37}{37+47} \times 100 = 44 \text{ per cent}$$

specificity
$$= \frac{d}{b+d}$$

$$= \frac{89}{19+89} \times 100 = 82 \text{ per cent}$$

crude agreement
$$= \frac{a+d}{a+b+c+d} \times 100$$

$$= \frac{37+89}{37+19+47+89} \times 100 = 66 \text{ per cent}$$

adjusted agreement
$$= \frac{1}{4} \times \left(\frac{a}{a+b} + \frac{a}{a+c} + \frac{d}{c+d} + \frac{d}{b+d} \right) \times 100$$

$$= \frac{1}{4} \times \left(\frac{37}{37+19} + \frac{37}{37+47} + \frac{89}{47+89} + \frac{89}{19+89} \right) \times 100$$

$$= 64 \text{ per cent}$$

Youden's index
$$= \frac{a}{a+c} + \frac{d}{b+d} - 1$$

$$= \frac{37}{37+47} + \frac{89}{19+89} - 1 = 0.26$$

subjects were then examined by an ophthalmologist to see if there was any clinical evidence of glaucoma. Although the patients could readily be separated into those with and those without raised pressure, it was found that a number of patients identified as positive had no clinical evidence of glaucoma. By choosing a very high level of pressure, this proportion could be reduced to a minimum. However, this resulted in an increasing proportion of patients, who had defects in the eye, being classified as having 'normal' pressure. It was shown by careful investigation that it was impossible to

Table 4.5   Classification of subjects following to-
nometry and clinical examination of the
eyes

Clinical examination	Pressure on tonometry	
	< 21 mmHg	> 21 mmHg
no glaucoma	3795	397
glaucoma	7	13

Source: Hollows and Graham (1966)

Notes:
(1) This table excludes nineteen subjects with
glaucoma due to angle closure or congenital
anomalies or secondary to other conditions.
(2) Six of the thirteen patients with pressure
> 21 mmHg were already known to have glaucoma,
so the survey detected an equal number of new cases
above and below the cutting point, although the
clinically determined prevalence was much higher in
those with an ocular pressure of 21 mmHg or more.

select a level of pressure at which an appreciable proportion of true cases
were identified as positive, without at the same time identifying a disturbingly high proportion of false positives.

4.5.4   How large a study is required?

At some stage in the planning phase attention must be given to a determination of the size of the study. If raised in such a general way, no progress can
be made. As has already been emphasised (see section 4.2), the aim of the
study must be clear and this should include a specification of the precision of
the answers that are required.

For example, if a survey is to measure the haemoglobin levels of a
subgroup of the population, such as pregnant women, it may be assumed
that the standard deviation is similar to that found in surveys of other
subjects (about 1.25 g/100 ml). The research worker may then specify the
precision of the survey in terms of the required standard error of the
measured haemoglobin (say 0.25 g/100 ml). Then

$$\text{number required in survey} > \left(\frac{1.25}{0.25}\right)^2 = 25 \tag{4.1}$$

If the purpose of the study is to compare the haemoglobin levels of two
subgroups, the argument is similar, requiring specification of the standard
error of the contrast desired from the study (the precision of the comparison). Using the same parameters as in the previous example,

$$\text{number in each sample} > 2\left(\frac{1.25}{0.25}\right)^2 = 50 \tag{4.2}$$

Where the measured item provides a proportion, rather than a continuous variate, a similar approach is used. However, the standard error of a proportion can be directly calculated rather than obtained by estimation. This has the advantage that prepared tables may be consulted, from which the sample size can be directly read (Mainland *et al.*, 1956).

A more sophisticated approach to surveys involving comparisons between two groups of subjects requires specification of (1) the statistical significance that is desired for excluding a chance difference, and (2) the probability required of actually detecting a real difference, should one exist. It is usual to suggest that differences when tested should be significant at the 0.05 level, while the power of the test may be set at 0.95. These figures introduce the constants 1.96 and 1.64 into equation 4.2:

$$\text{number in each sample} > 2\left[\frac{(1.96 + 1.64)\,1.25}{0.25}\right]^2 = 648 \qquad (4.3)$$

It will be seen that these further considerations add appreciably to the suggested numbers for the study. Armitage (1971) discussed these issues, indicating the theoretical approach and some of the practical problems in calculating the number required in any study.

Apart from the lack of background information required for some of these calculations, there may be many constraints on the research design; shortage of time, suitable subjects, facilities or other financial considerations may all be important. Despite pressure from such factors, the research worker must consider whether a small study is likely to result in imprecise or nonsignificant findings. The discipline involved in the type of calculations indicated above may help to guard against an inadequately conceived study.

References

Recommended reading

Abramson, J. H. (1974). *Survey Methods in Community Medicine.* Churchill Livingstone, Edinburgh

Moser, C. A., and Kalton, G. (1971). *Survey Methods in Social Investigation.* Heinemann, London

Moss, L., and Goldstein, H. (1979). *The Recall Method in Social Surveys.* Institute of Education, University of London, London

Stewart, A. (1968). *Basic Ideas for Scientific Sampling.* Griffin, London

Other references

Armitage, P. (1971). *Statistical Methods in Medical Research.* Blackwell, Oxford

Armitage, P., and Rose, G. (1966). *Clin. Sci.*, **30**, 325–35

Armitage, P., Fox, W., Rose, G. A., and Tinker, C. M. (1966). *Clin. Sci.*, **30**, 337–44

Armstrong, A. (1980). PhD thesis accepted by London University

Bernadt, M. W., Mumford, J., Taylor, C., Smith, B., and Murray, R. M. (1982). *Lancet*, **2**, 325–8

Bewley, B. R., Halil, T., and Snaith, A. H. (1973). *Br. J. prev. soc. Med.*, **27**, 150–3

Blackburn, H., Keys, A., Simonson, E., and Rautaharju, P. (1960). *Circulation*, **21**, 1160–75

Bøe, J., Hummerfelt, S., and Wedervang, F. (1957). *Acta. med. Scand.*, **157**, *suppl.* 321

Boyd, N. F. (1978). Observer variation in the interpretation of Xeromammograms. In *Screening in Cancer* (A. B. Miller, ed.), Union International Contra la Cancer, Geneva

Boyd, J. T., and Doll, R. (1964). *Br. J. Cancer*, **18**, 419–34

Cartwright, A. (1978). *Br. med. J.*, **2**, 1419–21

Cartwright, A., and Ward, A. W. M. (1968). *Br. J. prev. soc. Med.*, **22**, 199–205

Chamberlain, J., Ginks, S., and Rogers, P. *et al.* (1975). *Lancet*, **2**, 1026–30

Clausen, J. A., and Ford, R. N. (1947). *J. Amer. statist. Ass.*, **42**, 497–511

Cochrane, A. L. (1954). *Br. med. Bull.*, **10**, 91–5

Cochrane, A. L., Chapman, P. J., and Oldham, P. D. (1951). *Lancet*, **1**, 1007–9

Cochrane, A. L., and Holland, W. W. (1971). *Br. med. Bull.*, **27**, 3–8

College of General Practitioners (1961). *Br. med. J.*, **2**, 973–9

Colombotis, J., Elinson, J., and Lowenstein, R. (1968). *Publ. Hlth Rep.*, **83**, 685–90

Cooper, J. E., Kendell, R. E., Gurland, B. J., Sharpe, L., Copeland, J. R. M., and Simon, R. (1972). *Psychiatric Diagnosis in New York and London—a Comparitive Study of Mental Hospital Admissions*. Oxford University Press, London

Doll, R., and Hill, A. B. (1950). *Br. med. J.*, **2**, 739–48

Doll, R., and Hill, A. B. (1964). *Br. med. J.*, **1**, 1399–1410

Doll, R., and Peto, R. (1976). *Br. med. J.*, **1**, 1525–36

Douglas, J. W. B., and Rowntree, G. (1948). *Maternity in Great Britain*. Oxford University Press, London

Edwards, D. A. W., Hammond, W. H., Healy, M. J. R., Tanner, J. M., and Whitehouse, R. H. (1955). *Br. J. Nutr.*, **9**, 133–43

Edwards, G., Hensman, C., and Peto, J. (1973). *Q. J. Stud. Alc.*, **34**, 1244–54

Enstrom, J. E., and Godley, F. H. (1981). *J. Natn. Cancer Inst.*, **65**, 1175–83

Fairbairn, A. S., Wood, C. A., and Fletcher, C. M. (1959). *Br. J. prev. soc. Med.*, **19**, 175–93

Farr, W. (1841). *Second Annual Report of the Registrar General for Births Marriages and Deaths in England*. H.M.S.O., London

Feinstein, A. R. (1964). *Ann. Int. Med.*, **61**, 1162–93

Fink, R., Shapiro, S., and Lewison, J. (1968). *Publ. Hlth Rep.*, **83**, 479–90

Fink, R., Shapiro, S., and Roester, R. (1972). *Am. J. Publ. Hlth*, **62**, 328–36

Fletcher, C. M., and Tinker, C. M. (1961). *Br. Med. J.*, **1**, 1491–9

Gardner, M. J., and Heady, J. A. (1973). *J. chron. Dis.*, **26**, 781–95

General Register Office (1968). *Census 1961—Great Britain, General Report*. H.M.S.O., London

Godfrey, S., Edwards, R. A. A., Campbell, E. J. M., Armitage, P., and Oppenheimer, E. A. (1969). *Thorax*, **24**, 4–9

Goldstein, H. (1976). A study of the response rates of sixteen-year-olds in the National Child Development Study. In *Britain's Sixteen-year-olds* (K. Fogelman, ed.), National Children's Bureau, London

Gordon, T., and Kannel, W. B. (1968). *The Framingham Study; an Epidemiological Investigation of Cardiovascular Disease*. Sections 1 and 2. National Heart Institute, Bethesda

Graham, N. G., de Dombal, F. T., and Gologher, J. G. (1971). *Br. med. J.*, **2**, 746–8

Gray, P. G. (1957). *Appl. Statist.*, **6**, 139–53

Gullen, W. H., and Garrison, G. E. (1973). *Hlth Serv. Rep.*, **88**, 510–4

Hankin, J. H., Rhoads, G. G., and Glober, G. A. (1975). *Am. J. clin. Nutr.*, **28**, 1055–60

Harris, A. I., Cox, E., and Smith, C. R. W. (1971). *Handicapped and Impaired in Great Britain.* H.M.S.O., London

Heady, J. A. (1973). *Bull. Wld Hlth Org.*, **48**, 243–56

Higgins, I. T. T., and Cochrane, A. L. (1963). *Brit. J. prev. soc. Med.*, **17**, 153–65

Hill, A. B. (1925). *Medical Research Council Special Report Series, No. 95.* H.M.S.O., London

Hill, A. B. (1951a). *J. R. Statist. Soc. A*, **114**, 1–34

Hill, A. B. (1951b). Scientific methods in field surveys. In *Application of Scientific Method to Industrial and Service Medicine*, H.M.S.O., London

Holland, W. W., and Elliott, A. (1968). *Lancet*, **1**, 41–3

Hollows, F. C., and Graham, P. A. (1966). *Br. J. Ophthal.*, **50**, 570–86

Horowitz, O., and Wilbeck, E. (1971). *Am. Rev. resp. Dis.*, **104**, 643–55

Hunt, S. M., McKenna, S. P., and Williams, J. (1981). *J. Epidem. Comm. Hlth*, **35**, 297–300

Husain, O. A. N., Butler, E. B., Evans, D. M. D., MacGregor, E., and Yule, R. (1974). *J. clin. Path.*, **27**, 935–44

International Agency for Research in Cancer. (1977). *Lancet*, **2**, 207–11

Israel, A. C., Raskin, P. A., and Pravder, M. D. (1979). *Addict. Behav.*, **4**, 199–203

Jain, M., Howe, G. R., Johnson, K. C., and Miller, A. B. (1980). *Am. J. Epidem.*, **111**, 212–19

Kannell, C. F., Marquis, A. H., and Laurent, A. (1969). *An Experimental Study on the Effect of Reinforcement, Question Length, and Re-interviews in Reporting Selected Chronic Conditions in Household Interviews.* Survey Research Centre, University of Michigan, Ann Arbor

Kaplan, S., and Cole, P. (1970). *Br. J. prev. soc. Med.*, **24**, 245–7

Kelsey, J. I., and Acheson, R. M. (1971). *Br. J. prev. soc. Med.*, **25**, 177–8

Kemsley, W. F. F. (1975). *Statist. News*, **31**, 16–21

Kemsley, W. F. F. (1976). *Statist. News*, **35**, 18–22

Kemsley, W. F. F., and Nicholson, J. L. (1960). *J. R. Statist. Soc. A*, **123**, 307–28

Kneale, G. W., and Stewart, A. M. (1980). *Br. J. Cancer*, **41**, 222–6

Kozlowski, I. T., Herman, C. P., and Frecker, R. C. (1980). *Lancet*, **2**, 699–700

Kunin, C. M., and Ames, R. E. (1981). *Am. J. Epidem.*, **113**, 55–61

Lambert, P. M. (1972). *Personal communication*

Learmonth, A. (1979). *J. Epidem. Comm. Hlth*, **33**, 270–3

Lilienfeld, A. M., and Graham, S. (1958). *J. Natn. Cancer Inst.*, **21**, 713–20

MacGregor, J. E., Fraser, M. E., and Mann, E. M. F. (1966). *Lancet*, **1**, 252–6

McKennell, A. C. (1980). *Int. J. Epidem.*, **9**, 167–77

Mainland, B., Herrara, L., and Sutcliffe, M. I. (1956). *Statistical Tables for Use with Binomial Samples, Contingency Tests, Confidence Limits, and Sample Size Estimates.* University College of Medicine, New York

Markush, R. E. (1966). *Publ. Hlth Rep.*, **81**, 191–5

Marr, J. W. (1965). *Nutrition*, **19**, 18–24

Meade, T. W., Gardner, M. J., Cannon, D., and Richardson, P. B. (1968). *Br. Hrt J.*, **40**, 661–5

Milne, J. S., and Williamson, J. (1971). *Br. J. prev. soc. Med.*, **25**, 105–8

Mork, T. (1970). *J. chron. Dis.*, **23**, 399–404

Morris, J. N. (1975). *Uses of Epidemiology.* Churchill Livingstone, Edinburgh, p. 46

Morrison, P., and Morrison, E. (1961). *Charles Babbage and his Calculating Engines.* Dover, New York

Mullner, R. M., Levy, P. S., Byre, C. S., and Matthews, D. (1982). *Publ. Hlth Rep.*, **97**, 465–9

Murray, R. M. (1973). *Lancet*, **1**, 554

National Centre for Health Statistics (1965). *Reporting of Hospitalization in the Health Interview Survey*. U.S. Department of Health, Education and Welfare, Washington

Newell, D. T. (1962). *Am. J. publ. Hlth*, **52**, 1925–8

Newland, C. A., Waters, W. E., Standford, A. P., and Batchelor, B. G. (1977). *Int. J. Epidem.*, **6**, 65–7

Nomura, A., Hankin, J., and Rhoads, G. (1976). *Am. J. clin. Nutr.*, **29**, 1432–6

Oakes, T. W., Friedman, G. D., and Seltzer, C. C. (1973). *Am. J. Epidem.*, **98**, 50–5

Office of Population Censuses and Surveys (1973). *The General Household Survey—Introductory Report*. H.M.S.O., London

Osborn, G. R., and Leyshon, V. N. (1966). *Lancet*, **1**, 256–7

Palmer, J. W., Kasap, H. S., Bennet, A. E., and Holland, W. W. (1969). *Br. J. prev. soc. Med.*, **23**, 91–100

Paganini-Hill, A., and Ross, R. K. (1982). *Am. J. Epidem.*, **116**, 114–22

Palta, M., Prineas, R. J., Berman, R., and Hannan, P. (1982). *Am. J. Epidem.*, **115**, 223–30

Pedersen, E. (1966). *Proc. R. Soc. Med.*, **59**, 1189–1214

Philipp, R., Hughes, A. O., Cooper, P., and Rowland, A. J. (1982). *Comm. Med.*, **4**, 196–200

Raftery, E. B., and Holland, W. W. (1967). *Am. J. Epidem.*, **85**, 438–33

Reader, L. G. (1960). *J. Hlth hum. Behav.*, **1**, 123–9

Rogot, E., and Goldberg, I. D. (1966). *J. chron. Dis.*, **19**, 991–1006

Rose, G. A. (1962). *Bull. Wld Hlth Org.*, **27**, 645–58

Rose, G. A., and Blackburn, H. (1968). *Cardiovascular Survey Methods*. W.H.O., Geneva

Rose, G. A., Holland, W. W., and Crowley, E. A. (1964). *Lancet*, **1**, 296–300

Ruiz, L., Colley, J. R. P., and Hamilton, P. J. S. (1971). *Br. J. prev. soc. Med.*, **25**, 165–7

Sansom, C. D., Wakefield, J., and Yule, R. (1970). *Med. Offr*, **120**, 357–9

Scott, C. (1961). *J. R. Statist. Soc. A*, **124**, 143–95

Sharpe, J. E., Poole, O., Lepper, M. H., *et al.* (1965). *Am. Rev. resp. Dis.*, **91**, 510–20

Sheik, K., and Mattingly, S. (1981). *J. Epidem. Comm. Hlth*, **35**, 293–6

Silman, A. J., and Locke, C. M. (1982). *J. Epidem. Comm. Hlth*, **36**, 248–50

Sobell, L. C., Celluci, J., Nirenberg, T. D., and Sobell, M. B. (1982). *Am. J. publ. Hlth*, **72**, 823–8

Stern, E., and Lachenbruch, P. A. (1968). *J. chron. Dis.*, **21**, 117–24

Stewart, A. L. (1982). *J. chron. Dis.*, **35**, 295–309

Stocks, P. (1944). *Proc. R. Soc. Med.*, **37**, 593–608

Stocks. P. (1949). *Sickness in the Population of England and Wales, 1944–7*. H.M.S.O., London

Stuart, A. (1968). *Basic Ideas of Scientific Sampling*. Griffin, London

Tiblin, G. (1965). *Acta med. Scand.*, **178**, 453–9

Todd, G. F. (1966). *Reliability of Statements About Smoking Habits—Supplementary Report*. Tobacco Research Council, London

Todd, G. F. (1978). *J. Epidem. Comm. Hlth*, **32**, 289–93

Todd, J., and Butcher, B. (1982). *Electoral Registration in 1981*. O.P.C.S., London

Tretli, S., Lund-Larsen, P. G., and Foss, O. P. (1982). *J. Epidem. Comm. Hlth*, **36**, 269–73

Vessey, M. P., Johnston, B., and Donnelly, J. (1974). *Br. J. prev. soc. Med.*, **28**, 104–7

Watkins, C. J., Burton, P., Leeder, S., Sittampelam, Y., Wever, A. M. J., and Wiggins, R. (1982). *Int. J. Epidem.*, **11**, 62–6

West, J. F. (1977). *The Times*, 2 February 1977
Whitehead, T. P. (1965). *Progress in Medical Computing*. Elliott Medical Automation, London
Whitehead, T. P. (1974). *Br. med. Bull.*, **30,** 237–41
Wilhelmsen, L., Ljungberg, S., Wedel, H., and Werko, L. (1976). *J. chron. Dis.*, **29,** 331–9
Wilson, P. (1980) *Drinking in England and Wales*. H.M.S.O., London
World Health Organisation (1973). *Report of the International Pilot Study of Schizophrenia*. W.H.O., Geneva
Wright, B. M., and McKerrow, C. B. (1959). *Br. med. J.*, **1,** 1041–7
Yasin, S., Alderson, M. R., Marr, J. W. *et al.* (1967). *Br. J. prev. soc. Med.*, **21,** 163–9
Yerushalmy, J. (1947). *Publ. Hlth Rep.*, **62,** 1432–49
Yorkshire Breast Cancer Group (1977). *Br. med. J.*, **2,** 1196–9
Youden, W. J. (1950). *Cancer*, **3,** 32–5
Yule, R. (1972). *Acta Cytol.*, **16,** 389–90
Yule, R. (1974). *J. clin. Path.*, **27,** 937–8

5 Case–Control Studies

Consideration of case–control studies introduces the first category of study that is essentially hypothesis-testing in aim. (Hypothesis-testing studies may also be referred to as analytic or *a priori* studies.) A major difference from surveys is the requirement to collect information about the past from respondents in case–control studies. The collection of data on the past introduces an additional dimension to the study design and permits a wide range of issues to be explored. At the same time, it has an important bearing upon the validity of the data that can be collected; this is discussed further in subsection 5.2.5. Because the retrospective nature was felt to be an important part of case-control studies and related to major issues of validity, the expression 'retrospective study' was used to describe this method. Unfortunately other terms are also used for such studies: case–referent, case–compeer, and trohoc; such multiplicity of expression can cause confusion and the general use of the term case–control is therefore advocated. ('Retrospective study' can also refer to other categories of study that do not involve controls.)

The primary aim of a case–control study is to explore the aetiology of a given condition, by searching for differences in the prior exposure of the cases and controls to a range of suspect agents or factors. Because development of disease is often the result of a combination of factors (and not just the acute reaction to a particular exposure), a case–control study may often require exploration of a wide complex of factors and their interrelationships in order to comment upon the aetiology. Study of the aetiology of disease includes consideration of genetic and other endogenous factors, and the complete range of exogenous factors that may be either increased or decreased in those who develop a particular disease.

Though case–control studies are often thought of as hypothesis-testing, in many instances there is not just a specific and restricted aetiological factor that is examined; often the study incorporates a (major) element of hypothesis generation. This involves exploring the possible influence of factors that have not hitherto been suggested as having an aetiological role in the disease, or at least for which there does not exist any hard evidence that they have a genuinely causative action.

Section 5.2 discusses the principles involved, and indicates the categories of data that may be collected. A few selected examples of various aspects of method are given in this chapter, but no attempt is made to consider the mass of studies reported in the literature. As with other chapters, the final three sections deal with extensions of the basic method, advantages and disadvantages of the method, and some appropriate statistical techniques.

5.1 Basic Example of a Case–Control Study

Hewitt (1955) examined the vital statistics relating to leukaemia. He drew attention to an unexpected peak of mortality in the third and fourth years of life, which had become much more pronounced in the period 1940–53. Stewart *et al.* (1956, 1958) followed up this observation with a retrospective study in which they approached mothers of children under the age of ten who had died from leukaemia. The identification particulars were obtained from the death certificates provided by the General Register Office. In order to select a sample of children to serve as controls, health visitors' records were used to identify mothers, who had had a child of the same age and sex, living in the same street as each of the index children. The study was co-ordinated by the research workers based in Oxford, but was conducted throughout the country, by contact through the medical officers of health in each of the local authorities. The mothers were interviewed by survey doctors employed by the local health authorities. Among the wide range of information obtained were details of the mothers' exposure to X-rays prior to and during the index pregnancy. Specific questions were posed and an attempt was made to identify the number of X-rays and the parts of the body involved. This was to test the hypothesis that exposure to radiation might have been the relevant aetiological factor. It is important to emphasise that in this retrospective study many other potential aetiological factors were also considered and an extremely extensive range of information was obtained from the mothers of the index cases and controls. Preliminary results from this study were published in 1956. Further work was carried out, with a gradual increase in the number of mothers who were questioned. Consistent findings occurred as the study extended, and a more detailed paper on the results was published later (Stewart *et al.*, 1958).

The principal findings of the study are shown in table 5.1. A significant excess of mothers of leukaemic children had been exposed to X-ray during pregnancy, in particular X-ray examination of the pelvis or abdomen. Such a finding raised a number of important considerations, one of which was that this result might have been a spurious finding due to the method of study.

One issue discussed by a number of authors (Stewart *et al.*, 1956; Court Brown *et al.*, 1960; MacMahon, 1962) was whether the occurrence of leukaemia in the young child and subsequent death had in some way affected a mother's memory and had produced bias in the response from the mothers of index children compared with the control mothers. There was some suggestion that this might be so. In index cases, there was an excess number of X-rays taken prior to pregnancy as well as during pregnancy, but there had been no suggestion that there was any aetiological link between irradiation before pregnancy and leukaemia in a subsequent child. That there was no appreciable bias was demonstrated (Hewitt *et al.*, 1966) by a detailed examination of the medical records of mothers who had given a history of irradiation and a sample of those who had not. Other authors pointed out that X-rays taken in late pregnancy were often required because of complications during pregnancy. The occurrence of such complications could in themselves be associated with a higher risk of subsequent leukaemia; Russell (1970) reviewed this suggestion. If the social class of the mother was associated with poor diet, poor general health, inability to withstand pregnancy well, risk of infection and other complications during pregnancy warranting X-ray examination, then some of these other factors

Table 5.1 Numbers of mothers of children dying from leukaemia and controls who reported X-ray examination of different sites in three periods

| | X-ray examination | | | | | | | | |
| | Abdominal | | | Other | | | Any* | | |
Period	Case	Control	Ratio	Case	Control	Ratio	Case	Control	Ratio
before marriage	44	26	1.69	335	275	1.22	361	296	1.22
between marriage and relevant conception	109	121	0.90	213	184	1.16	304	285	1.07
during relevant pregnancy	178	93	1.91	117	100	1.17	273	184	1.48
any period*	296	215	1.38	531	456	1.16	692	593	1.17

Source: Stewart *et al.* (1958)

*The row and column figures do not equal the totals, because some mothers had X-rays on more than one site or in more than one period.

could be the aetiological agent responsible for the subsequent development of leukaemia in the child rather than the X-rays. Such an argument is, in itself, difficult to disprove but it is an important one to consider in the general interpretation of data; this point will be returned to in subsection 6.5.4. Further work has now excluded this particular source of bias. Stewart and Kneale (1970) demonstrated that the excess cancer risk was directly proportional to the foetal X-ray dose. Mole (1974) reanalysed published data and confirmed that not more than a fifth of the excess cancer in singletons could be due to selection of the cancer-prone for radiography. This topic has been reviewed by Alderson (1980).

Even if the risk had been precisely defined, there would still be the problem of deciding, when dealing with certain complications of pregnancy, whether an X-ray examination of the pregnant woman was justified. The remote risk to the child of subsequently developing leukaemia must be balanced against the risk of the mother and foetus should the complication not be handled appropriately. Since the earlier findings of Stewart and her colleagues were published, the frequency with which mothers have been X-rayed in pregnancy has decreased. Care has also been taken to reduce the amount of radiation to a minimum, and more recently other techniques have been developed, which enable investigation of certain complications to be carried out.

5.2 Principle of Case–Control Studies

Lilienfeld and Lilienfeld (1979) traced the history of case-control studies from comparison studies of different treatments which had begun in the sixteenth and seventeenth centuries and expanded in the nineteenth century. They noted that in the early part of the twentieth century sociologists began to use the method in order to identify the causes of various behavioural problems, such as delinquency.

In a study of 537 patients with epithelioma of the lip attending the Mayo Clinic, Broders (1920) presented data on tobacco use and contrasted these results with data from other patients without epithelioma of the lip. No information is given about the source of these latter patients; their average age was well below that of the cancer patients, but it was suggested this did not invalidate the comparisons. In 1923 the League of Nations Cancer Commission prepared a scheme of enquiry into breast cancer; specific co-ordinated studies were mounted in Holland, Italy and England. A detailed report by Lane-Claypon (1926) presented the results of a case-control study; it was pointed out that observations on cancer patients alone were of relatively limited value and therefore efforts were made to obtain similar information from women who had never suffered from cancer. This report has been cited as the first study using this method; what is remarkable is that it was part of an international collaborative study. Schrek and Lenowitz (1946) compared information for 139 men with carcinoma of the penis admitted to Hines Veterans Hospital in 1931–44, with various categories of control patient (all tumour patients, and various other categories of patient). No discussion of the reasoning behind the method is provided; one might think that by this time such studies were becoming standard practice. The method was clarified in papers by Doll (1959) and Cornfield and Haenszel (1960).

Assuming that the aim has been specified in adequate detail, the first step in the design of a case–control study is to consider the selection of cases and controls; this is discussed in the first two subsections. The third subsection details aspects of matching the cases and controls. As already indicated, a case–control study will usually have the aim of searching for an aetiological relationship. This may have the preliminary aim of searching for any cause and effect relationship; other more specific objectives may be to quantify the strength of the relationship or determine the factors that are responsible for variation in this (i.e. are there any additive, multiplicative, or other interactive effects with other factors?). In order to explore this detail of the items of information to be collected must then be clarified; the fourth subsection deals with this. The final subsection considers aspects of validity of the data collected in this class of study.

5.2.1 Selection of cases

There are three main issues to consider:

(1) What is the diagnostic group that should be studied?
(2) Should the cases include all those occurring in a defined population over a specified period of time?
(3) Should patients be included in the study only shortly after their disease has been diagnosed, or can it include those who were diagnosed and treated some years ago?

As far as the diagnostic group is concerned, the intention should be to define a group of cases that form a homogeneous set and whose aetiology is likely to be similar. For instance, when studying Hodgkin's disease, if it is thought that persons under the age of twenty with a particular type of histology have the form of disease caused by an agent different from that affecting the remainder of the cases, then it is likely that a tighter research design can be formulated by concentrating upon the subset of patients. This point will particularly apply: to cancer where the site is affected by more than one histological type; where there is an appreciable sex-difference in incidence; where the age distribution is markedly discontinuous; where other subsets of patients have very different characteristics.

It is generally argued that the inclusion of all patients in a defined population (i.e. a study of the total incidence of the disease in the community) has the advantage of providing results that are more readily extrapolated to the universe of patients, than are the results provided by a study based on a restricted subset of patients (e.g. those attending one hospital). This theoretical point needs to be carefully weighed against the ease of access to the two categories of patients, differences in response rate and resulting bias, and consideration of the likely use to which the results might be put. For example, if the study is particularly concerned about the influence of coffee drinking upon the risk of bladder cancer (and the main confounding factors can be identified and built into the study design), it is not clear why the use of a restricted subset of patients will prevent the correct answer from being obtained. However, the selected group of patients may be particularly exposed to another bladder carcinogen. If this interacts with the influence of coffee consumption, the distortion that this will produce in the findings depends upon whether the second factor has been identified in the study design and can be allowed for in the analysis. The difficulty is that unless such interaction is suspected and appropriately designated information made available, no amount of statistical treatment will correct for this. It is also not feasible to collect comprehensive information on every item that might conceivably be relevant.

Some conditions may not be always diagnosed in life (e.g., it is suggested that about one-third of new episodes of ischaemic heart disease present with sudden death). To exclude such subjects may bias the findings—if a particular aetiological factor is associated with the more virulent form of the disease. Cole (1979) suggested that to strive for representativeness of subjects to permit generalisations from results was unwarranted, but if this increased the validity of the results (by achieving a less biased group of respondents) then it was desirable.

Quite different is the need to consider if patients who have had their disease for a year or more will be suitable for inclusion in the study (the point arises because there will be usually be the desire to contact as many patients as possible once the study has begun, and the use of 'prevalent' cases will boost the numbers available for study). However, someone who has had a disease for a while may: (1) have thought more about the cause of their disease for this time, which may have altered their recall of the past; (2) have altered their behaviour because of the effect of the disease (given up smoking, reduced calorie intake, changed their job or retired, etc.); (3) have had their way of life affected directly by the treatment in a number of ways. All the differences developing since the diagnosis may influence the responses of the subjects and thus affect the results. They argue for approaching only patients who have recently developed the disease (though patients successfully treated for their disease may be in a more stable state than those who are suffering from the initial symptoms or are just getting over radical treatment). However, even with cancers with quite good survival, inclusion of patients treated several years previously implies the loss of those who did not survive; this will create bias if there is any relationship between the aetiology and prognosis of the disease.

5.2.1.1 Source of cases

The previous chapter indicated that a survey could be the framework for identifying both cases and controls; the suitability of this approach will depend upon the prevalence of the condition and the ease of detection. It could be used for studying a cancer with a very high incidence in a particular population, or perhaps when a very large proportion of the population has been examined—such as in a screening campaign. Rather different would be the use of a survey to detect people with the presence of a precursor of the disease being studied. A population sample, drawn from a private survey of the Rhonda Fach, had their blood pressure recorded (Miall and Oldham, 1955). Particulars were also recorded for all first-degree relatives, and those living within twenty-five miles of the valley were approached. Thus the population sample provided the propositi (some of whom had raised blood pressure), while the information obtained from the initial sample identified the relatives and enabled genetic analysis to be carried out.

Some studies have been carried out on patients who have died from a particular disease; this approach has usually been used when large numbers of patients were sought and it was relatively easy to screen the death certificates for the population to pick out all those who had died from the chosen disease and appropriate controls. For example, Dean *et al.* (1977) obtained identification particulars of a sample of individuals dying from lung cancer, chronic bronchitis, ischaemic heart disease and stroke in the North East of England; the decedents were classified by scrutiny of information available on the death certificate for all persons in the age-range selected who died during the study period.

This information was used to locate the next of kin, who were interviewed in order to obtain information about the decedents' histories of smoking, occupation, residence and other particulars relevant to the aetiology of these diseases. The use of decedents in this way raises specific problems for the collection of valid details about past history for both cases and controls; this is discussed further in subsection 5.2.5. A particular variant of this is discussed in the chapter on occupational studies (see 10.1.1.7), where a prospective study follows up a large cohort of workers, and much more detailed information is obtained about the occupational environment of the relatively small number of individuals dying from the specific disease of interest and controls.

If it is desired to study the complete set of patients developing cancer in a population, some form of cancer register must exist (see 3.1.2). Delay in the registration of patients may create difficulty in those studies where attempts are made to interview the patients soon after diagnosis. Obviously some *ad hoc* arrangement is required for diseases that are not included in any population register. Lee *et al.* (1972) were interested in studying the aetiological factors of carcinoma of the scrotum. They identified a sample of patients with this condition from (1) the records of the regional cancer register and (2) the detailed diagnostic index held by a large radiotherapy centre. Two overlapping sets of data may be used in this way to ensure that as complete a sample as possible is identified.

The basic input into routine morbidity statistical systems can be used for a wide range of case–control studies. In appropriate circumstances cancer registration, congenital abnormality notification, hospital discharge data both from acute and psychiatric hospitals, and notification of infectious disease can all be used to identify 'index' cases for case–control study. These merely require the availability of an accessible diagnostic index with associated identification particulars of the individuals concerned. The important issue of confidentiality of such data will be discussed shortly. Many studies have been carried out using locally maintained diagnostic indexes. These may be available in hospitals or accumulated by general practitioners using 'E' books (Eimerl and Laidlaw, 1969) or some other comparable method. Census data has also been used as a starting point for a few special projects, where the data collection has been carried out by O.P.C.S., the material then being released to the research worker in consolidated statistical tables without any indication of the individuals who had participated in the study.

There is one important point that has to be taken into account prior to definition of such a study. The basic returns for these statistical systems were originally provided on the understanding that the material was confidential. The data-processing system can often provide a list of patients suffering from a particular condition, but prior to the release of such information it is essential that appropriate consideration of this issue of confidentiality is made and that steps are taken to satisfy certain requirements. The Medical Research Council (1973) provided a general statement on this matter and has indicated the appropriate measures to be taken. It is generally accepted that the clinician under whose care the patient has been, the family doctor and the patient should all give their permission in writing for release of this information prior to the research worker contracting the patient. No pressure must be exerted on a patient to participate in such a study. It is preferable if the proposal for the study can come before a committee including representatives of the public and professions in order that the ethical aspects of the study may be judged.

The majority of case–control studies are carried out upon patients identified from hospital sources; a variety of techniques may be invoked to locate such patients, depending upon the organisation of the hospital records systems and the agreement of the clinicians. Scanning may occur at regular intervals of diagnostic indexes of patients recently discharged, operation lists or books, pathological reports or similar records. Interviewers may check at weekly intervals if there are any eligible patients in the particular wards from the participating hospitals. Sometimes clinicians may agree to operate an informal notification system, while for certain conditions (such as blindness, cancer, or tuberculosis) there may be a formal register which can be accessed.

Less frequently used are general practitioners' records. For major life-threatening disease, the incidence is usually such that only a handful of cases will present in a practice each year (and for relatively rare diseases such as childhood leukaemia, only one general practitioner in sixty will see a newly affected child per year in England and Wales). At the other extreme, for common ailments such as acute respiratory disease, or for some of the problems of the elderly, a group practice could form an ideal source of enough patients for a study.

Very occasionally volunteers have been used; they may be contacted for certain types of enquiry through professional or other societies, or by advertising in the press. For example, a series of twins were contacted after a public request for volunteers was broadcast on television (the possible biases are discussed in the subsection 9.2.6.5). Patients with very rare conditions may similarly be contacted through requests for informal notification in the medical press.

Cases of a given disease identified during a prospective study may be used as the focus of a case–control analysis, or as the start point for accumulation of additional historical information, beyond that collected for all subjects in the prospective study. This is an approach particularly suited to certain types of occupational study and the appropriate method is covered in subsection 10.4.1.

5.2.2 Selection of controls

The principles to be considered are: (1) How can subjects be identified who will provide an adequate response-rate (section 4.2.3 has already dealt with the implications of poor response-rate on the validity and interpretation of studies); (2) the bias from information recalled about past behaviour and happenings, and ways of reducing this to an absolute minimum; (3) the need to screen the controls to check that none of them suffer from the disease being studied; (4) the feasibility of the chosen study design versus that of other options (at this stage, this will usually be a consideration of the various types of controls rather than a radical consideration of the suitability of a case–control study versus some other form of study design).

Some of the general principles that lie behind the achievement of an adequate response-rate have already been dealt with; in the present context, it chiefly revolves round the use of controls drawn from a source similar to that for the cases. For instance, if the cases are drawn from current inpatients, it is likely that the same degree of response will be obtained from other patients in the same hospital.

Recall bias is also likely to be kept to a minimum by using patients from the same source as the cases and subjecting them to an identical form of questioning. To interview healthy controls in the general population will probably result in a lower response rate and obtain information from subjects who are less motivated to help with the enquiry and whose memory for past events has been considerably less stimulated than that of the patients who are cases.

Rather more complex to consider is the need for the controls to have attended hospital and undergone the same diagnostic screen as the cases. This has been advocated for three reasons, as follows.

(1) Those patients who attend the medical services may be a biased group of the population—not from the point of prevalence of illness, but from the aspect of utilisers of the service (Are they more affluent, etc.?) and as the cases are attending hospital, it is argued that so must the controls.

(2) If patients have two or more diseases present, there may be a quite different likelihood of their being admitted to hospital; this bias was clearly described in a theoretical example by Berkson (1946), and more recently an actual empirical set of data has confirmed the bias. Because of the attention this issue has received, further details of the points raised are given at the end of section 5.3.

(3) Unless the controls have actually undergone exactly the same diagnostic screen as the cases, there may be a number of latent or undiagnosed patients in the control group. In practical terms, this may cause some dilution in the difference between the cases and controls, but unless the prevalence of the incipient disease in the controls is very high this will have a very minor effect. It has been argued that it is actually preferable to include such incipient cases in the controls, in order to obtain the correct prevalence of the aetiological factor in both cases and controls (Miettinen, 1976), but the logic of this may be disputed. (It will depend on whether the selection procedure has produced an excess of incipient cases.) Using conventional selection of controls, Horwitz and Feinstein (1978) found that the relative risk from oestrogen use was nearly 12 for subsequent endometrial cancer. However, when women who had gynaecological care for uterine bleeding were used as controls the relative risk was only 1.7; they suggested that the conventional approach produces a spuriously high risk due to detection bias. In an attempt to assess the degree of detection bias in endometrial cancer, Horwitz et al. (1981) reviewed autopsies at two United States hospitals. Out of autopsies on 8998 women, 24 revealed unsuspected endometrial cancer; it was argued that this indicated the appreciable detection bias that would occur in case–control studies of endometrial cancer and oestrogen use. This was disputed by Crombie and Tomenson (1981), Hulka et al. (1981) and Merletti and Cole (1981).

The three main classes of controls are: (1) hospital-based, (2) neighbourhood-based and (3) population-based. Some of the points relevant to consideration of the suitability of these different classes have just been discussed, but there are a number of additional points to be borne in mind.

When choosing controls, the known and suspect aetiological factors for the disease being studied have to be listed; other diagnoses should be selected, where there is no suggestion that the same aetiological factors have any bearing on the development of the control diseases. Often it will be easier to negotiate the inclusion of controls from the wards of the same specialists whose patients provide the cases; this matches for certain factors (admission for an operation or referral from the same catchment area around the hospital), but may lead to inclusion of patients with a range of diseases with similar aetiology. There may be planned exclusion (e.g. the avoidance of patients with benign breast-disease lesions when studying the cause of breast cancer), or the deliberate inclusion of patients with a wide range of conditions (so that if the unsuspected or unknown cause of one of them is the same as the disease being studied, this will not grossly distort the overall findings of the study). A wide range of factors have been screened in an attempt to define the aetiology of coronary artery disease. In one study on the role of psychosomatic factors, patients with recent fractures were used as the control group and psychosomatic factors were reported to a greater extent by this than by the index cases. The general conclusion was that this was due to the choice of a particular group of controls and that no conclusions could be drawn about the role of stress in the aetiology of coronary artery disease. In particular, this study serves as a warning against using patients with only one condition as the control group. If hospital patients are used as controls, it is preferable to include those with a range of diagnoses.

The general view has been expressed in the past that the ideal control is alike in all respects to the case, other than in exposure to the causative factor. This has led to the suggestion that neighbourhood controls are suitable; the intention of selecting controls in this way is that they are similar to the cases in terms of broad environment and in such aspects of way of life as are indicated by social class. If the specific aspect that neighbourhood controls introduce can be quantified (for example, particular occupation) then there is no need to utilise this type of control; the factor can be recorded in cases and controls selected from hospital patients and dealt with in the analysis (see subsection 5.5.6). However, if there are other suspect but nonquantifiable factors, the use of the neighbourhood control will 'match' for these without the need to even know that they exist let alone to be able to assess them at interview. If there is a very different response between the cases and controls from the neighbourhood, this may outweigh any theoretical point about increased comparability.

Obviously, population controls will have neither the primed memory of the hospital control, nor the degree of similarity of neighbourhood controls. They have been advocated as they provide a comparison with the distribution of the various suspect aetiological factors in the general population. This will have a particular advantage if the cases are the total incident cases in the defined population. This provides a very simple analysis of the actual difference in the distribution of the aetiological agents in the 'healthy' population and permits calculations of risk factors (see subsection 5.5.5). There are a number of disadvantages to be borne in mind; the response may be poor with such controls. This has a serious effect on the validity of the results, but also will put up the costs (the costs are likely to be higher anyway, because of the increased amount of travelling and the difficulty in contacting the population sample).

There is no simple guide to the choice of optimum control. The following example indicates the repercussions that stem from the (fortuitously) right selection. Case and Hosker (1954) carried out a survey of bladder cancer in chemical workers. As part of an epidemiological survey of this condition in the general population, Birmingham was selected for the study because routine registration data for malignant disease were available and there was no large-scale dyestuff industry present. Examination of this 'control' material resulted in a fortuitous discovery—an unduly large number of patients with bladder tumours had been employed in a large rubber-works. Subsequent investigations (Case, 1966; Davies, 1966) showed that derivatives of the compounds involved in the original study were used as 'hardeners' in the manufacture of rubber. Thus, workers in rubber factories and cable works, where the rubber was used as insulation, were at high risk of developing cancer of the bladder owing to exposure to these compounds.

5.2.2.1 Sources of controls

The three general sources of controls have already been discussed in the preceeding section, but there are a few points of detail that need to be considered. Matching is dealt with in the next section, and the decision on the approach to be taken with matching has a direct impact upon how the controls are selected.

For hospital patients, the same methods as indicated for cases will be used (see subsection 5.2.1.1). Quasi-population controls are sometimes chosen from either hospital staff or visitors to the hospital. Neither of these is recommended, so it is inappropriate to discuss their selection.

The identification of neighbourhood controls will usually need some local visiting, in the absence of complete lists of household members classified by age and sex. The field worker has to contact households in the vicinity of the cases and use some specific plan (such as working up a given street or apartment block, checking the next-highest-numbered residence, or alternate higher and lower ones) until a respondent with the correct match (on age, sex, etc.) is identified, who agrees to participate. It must be borne in mind that visiting during the daytime will permit ready contact with a biased sample (e.g. those not at work for social or health reasons).

Population samples can usually be selected from some formal listing; in the United Kingdom the electoral lists provide a sampling frame of adults eligible to vote (virtually the entire population over the age of eighteen). Such lists are directly available and may be used for this purpose, but have the disadvantage that they are not classified by the age or sex of the subjects. They are also prone to miss individuals who migrate. An earlier section referred to a study by Dean *et al.* (1977) which used death certificates to identify cases; the controls were contacted by visiting households drawn at random from the electoral registers in the study locations. Having identified the household, these were visited and questions asked about all persons over sixteen of either sex. Less suitable are other lists of the public, such as telephone subscribers, unless these are being used in a locality where a very high proportion of the population are subscribers. In some countries bona-fide research workers may have access to the population registers; this may have the advantage of providing classifying information, permitting a specific subsample of the population to be drawn (e.g. males within a narrow age-range, resident in a particular locality).

More restricted lists, which may be suitable in some studies, may be of members of certain professional or other organisations (lists of registered doctors, etc. may be readily available, while union or other nominal roles may be made available in certain circumstances). Obviously, the more restricted the list being considered, the more thought has to be given to the potential bias of the list. (What are the special characteristics of the people that do not possess a telephone? Are union members exposed to unknown confounding factors?)

Whatever the source of the list, some form of random sample will have to be drawn from the names upon it (see subsection 4.2.2 for details).

5.2.3 Matching

In considering the selection of cases and controls, the point was raised that the controls should in some way approximate to the characteristics of the cases, apart from the extent of exposure to the aetiological agent being studied. This is the issue of matching, which is not adequately explained by indicating the need to have some degree of comparability between cases and controls. In order to discuss the rationale for matching of the subjects in a study it is appropriate to consider figure 5.1, which sets out the various aetiological pathways which may be relevant in different chronic diseases; this figure is obviously highly schematic. There is also the disadvantage that it is usually not known, at the time of planning the study, which of the different pathways apply.

If a study was to be mounted of a disease thought to be caused by a single factor, where there was no suggestion of other external factors, that were consistently associated with variation in the degree of exposure, then there would be no need to consider matching of cases and controls. In such circumstances, it would be a simple matter to obtain a direct estimate of the risk of the disease from the exposure of the agent concerned, and also quantify if there was a dose–response relationship.

If the sex of the subjects influences the likelihood of being exposed to the aetiological agent (i.e. if there is a degree of confounding between the factor sex and the exposure to the agent), then there is a need for matching. This was often carried out on a one-to-one basis, leading to the matched-pairs analysis appropriate to this design (see 5.5.4).

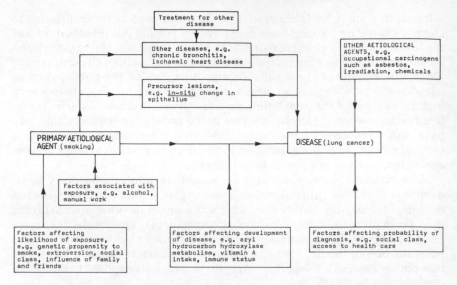

Figure 5.1 Schematic representation of network of aetiological and confounding factors, with examples relating to lung cancer

More complex is the situation where there are two agents responsible, with an action which is not merely additive, but combines in some way (either as multiplication of the risks, or in some more complicated power-relationship). Matching is then not desirable, as it is preferable to explore the influence of the different factors using the more powerful techniques of analysis now available (see 5.5.6).

It has been suggested that both smoking and coffee consumption are independently related to the risk of bladder cancer. However, there is also good evidence that there is an interrelationship between these habits: those who smoke usually also drink more coffee than nonsmokers. This is an example where it is important to disentangle the interrelationship of the two habits from the effect of their independent impacts on the risk of bladder cancer. Close matching of the cases and controls on smoking habits will prevent a full analysis of the effect of the two factors; it is more appropriate to record in some detail the smoking and coffee consumption of these cases and controls and then examine the independent and combined effects of the two agents by the appropriate statistical analysis (see section 5.5.6). In a study of pancreatic cancer, MacMahon *et al.* (1981) excluded smoking-related conditions from those suffered by the controls, arguing that smoking was overrepresented in this group compared with the general population and that also coffee drinking was overrepresented due to the known association between the two facets of behaviour. This point was disputed by others (e.g. British Medical Journal, 1981).

Obviously, the more that is known about the aetiology of a particular cancer, or the distribution of the various suspect agents in the community, the easier it is to plan a satisfactory study. As already indicated, the difficulty comes when there is less information about the background to the topic; there has been a tendency in the past to match for the attributes of age and sex, and also consider marker variables such as social class and neighbourhood (which broadly are related to way of life and thus to aetiological and confounding factors). The danger would come if the sole agent is localised in certain geographical areas; matching on neighbourhood might equalise the chance of exposure of cases and controls and result in very low power of the study to detect the aetiology.

Cole (1980) suggested that matching was desirable where a factor was known to interact with the aetiological agent being studied and thus affected the risk of the index disease. However, he warned of the increased cost if there was difficulty in obtaining matched pairs. Greenland *et al.* (1981) suggested that bias was caused by matching on:

(1) Effects of the exposure
(2) Effects of the disease under study
(3) Intermediate factors in the causal pathway between exposure and disease.

In an exploratory study, if the primary study-factor cannot be identified in advance, then factors which need control will be difficult to identify. Indiscriminate matching may decrease efficiency and increase effort in performing the study.

Where one of the primary goals is to estimate the exposure-specific disease rates in a well-defined target population, Greenland *et al.* (1981) argued, matching is strictly undesirable. This would produce controls which are unrepresentative of noncases in the target population; this may render the estimation of exposure-specific rates impossible. Pike *et al.* (1981) agreed that if matched controls are not freely available then it is not worth attempting to match except on variables that are strongly confounding (such as age and sex for many diseases).

5.2.4 Categories of data

Seven types of information that may be collected are briefly listed below, in what is thought to be a logical order. The list is not exhaustive, but should serve to indicate the major areas that may be explored in an examination of aetiological agents.

Family background. A number of diseases have a clearly defined genetic pattern; study of disease in first-degree relatives may show a higher prevalence than expected. There is considerable difficulty in distinguishing the relative contribution of genetic and home environment, as relatives will share not only genes, but also the micro-environment of the home and its local surroundings; patterns of behaviour will usually resemble those of other members of the family to a greater extent than those of neighbours or population controls.

Further details of the general methods of genetic studies are given in chapter 9, which discusses approaches of several kinds and is not restricted to case–control studies.

Home environment. This will usually require a history of residence, from which some indication of the general environment can be obtained. Of particular concern will be: atmospheric pollution, background radiation, climate, humidity, method of central heating, passive smoking, rainfall and water sources (and thus chemical constitutents of the water). More specific questioning may indicate the degree of overcrowding.

Behaviour. Variations in consumption of alcohol, drugs and tobacco and in diet have all been shown to influence the development of many different cancers. Behaviour in a wider sense, such as sexual habits, hobbies, sports and pastimes can all influence exposure to various harmful agents. An indirect marker of the variation in 'exposure' to these influences may be provided by marital status or terminal level of education. Social class is determined by the occupation held, but is usually employed as a general marker of broad variation in way of life rather than any specific indicator of occupational hazard. Though there are a number of problems with the application of social class based on occupation (see Black, 1980), there are often clearly discernible trends in exposure to hazards (such as smoking), use of services (such as immunisation) and risk of disease (such as chronic bronchitis), so that this measure has continued to be used.

Social and psychological factors. It may be useful to obtain a general picture of an individual's views on life, hobbies, interests and relationships with family and friends. This can be associated with the development of disease, or with the patient's response to disease and the degree of support required.

Race and religion. Culture and thus indirectly many aspects of individuals' way of life are determined by their race or religion. This may be linked to specific proscription of certain foods, smoking or alcohol. Beyond this there may be subtle influences on many aspects of way of life. It should be noted that variates such as race and religion are used in preliminary studies which search for simple markers of variation in risk of cancer; these studies will need to be followed by others which aim to identify the precise mechanism or at least the specific carcinogen involved. For example, when a general association is found between cancer and membership of a particular religion, a more searching study must then be mounted to identify the specific factors of behaviour that are responsible for the initial findings.

Previous illness and treatment. Careful questioning about illness and treatment may identify associations between two conditions, or the risk of subsequent disease following certain treatments.

Occupation. Many studies have been done of the influence of occupation on risk of various diseases. A case–control approach is only one way to study this problem, and further details are given in chapter 10.

5.2.5 Validity of data in case–control studies

The three main study problems are whether there are any (or any appreciable) selection bias, response bias and recall bias in a particular study. Also, the more general aspects of random error in the data must be considered. The latter issue has already been explored, as far as surveys are concerned (see subsection 4.2.6); the points raised there are equally applicable to case–control studies. Feinstein (1979) provided a detailed note on bias in case–control studies—though Sartwell (1979) responded that many of the biases also applied to prospective studies.

(1) Selection bias. The topic of selection bias has already been raised in considering sources of cases and controls, and matching. A simple example of the pitfalls in interpreting data was the initial suggestion that Buerger's disease was more likely to occur in Russian Jews. Reconsideration showed that the cases were reported from Mount Sinai Hospital in New York and this racial–religious category was the pattern of patients referred there (see Morris, 1975). Shapiro (1979) suggested that a doctor might have two women with deep-vein thrombosis (D.V.T.), but send the one who is 'on the pill' to hospital, where the diagnosis could be verified. He pointed out that this biases the proportion of hospital D.V.T. patients who are on the pill, and is one facet of selection bias.

When discussing the increasing reluctance in the United States of hospitals or physicians to permit patients to be included in case–control studies, Herrmann *et al.* (1981) stressed that lack of participation may result in a biased pool of potential cases.

(2) Response bias. Involvement in a personal tragedy may stimulate the willingness of subjects to respond to enquiries, particularly if there is any hope that research may be of benefit to others (perhaps by the introduction of preventive measures). This emotional involvement may have an effect on the recall of specific events, as well as a more general impact on response rate. There is unlikely to be such an influence operating in the controls, especially when this group is a random selection of the general population. Thus bias may be introduced (1) from differences in response rates in the study and control groups and (2) from the variation in recall of past events. This must be considered in the planning phase of the study and then a search should be made for bias during analysis of the collected data. Bartlett (1932) showed that there was a tendency to exaggerate the significance of events as a means of trying to come to terms with illness.

(3) Recall bias. In subsection 4.2.6 the factors influencing the validity of data obtained from respondents by interview or questionnaire were discussed in some detail. The quality of the retrospective information obtained depends on the question, the respondent and the interviewer (or questionnaire). Careful study design and training should reduce random error and avoid bias. One technique for reducing bias is to keep the interviewer 'blind', which is achieved by disguising whether the respondent is in the case or the

control group. As an alternative the interviewer may be trained, but not told of the specific hypothesis being tested. Particularly where the study necessitates development of a new questionnaire or interview schedule, a careful check is required of the reliability and validity of the data collected.

The search for an association between events in the past and current illness may provide a biased examination of the problem. The cause-and-effect relationship extends over a considerable time for many problems. The longer the time lag between the initiating event and the development of the disease, the greater is the chance of errors and biases occurring in the retrospective collection of data. There is always the need to consider whether the retrospective study is being used merely as a screening device to identify particular issues, that then warrant a more protracted, but definitive, prospective study (see chapter 6). The likelihood of bias depends partly on the particular items being collected. As a general rule, these may be considered as a continuum, ranging from very hard, factual information that can be cross-checked—Were you involved in a car accident last week?—to soft, highly subjective information that is to a great extent an assessment by the interviewer of the respondent's attitudes and feelings—Did you have a lot of arguments with your husband last year?

The first example given in this chapter was the search for a fairly factual item (exposure of pregnant women to X-radiation), but even in this situation there was evidence that the mothers' recall was considerably heightened by the death of a child from leukaemia. This example serves as a warning of how the memory may be distorted by such influences. There are ways of checking recall. This is most easily done when the subject does not know the nature of the hypothesis being tested, or is put off the scent by a line of enquiry that is a judicious mixture of relevant and masking questions. As a general rule, careful probing and the selection of supporting detail will increase the validity of the data. For instance, when Lee and his colleagues (1972) were studying the occupational histories of patients with scrotal cancer, a history was collected of all occupations since leaving school by obtaining detailed information on occupations, the name of the employers, the particular tasks on which the individual worked, and dates of such employment; data was then related to other milestones in the history. In this way a more complete picture was obtained.

It has been pointed out that though there are reasons for matching dead cases with dead controls, there was no hard evidence of the bias in obtaining information from the decedents' relatives (Gordis, 1982). Investigation of 297 patients with myocardial infarction, and of matched controls, suggested that unemployment of the fathers for more than a year during the patients' childhood was a risk factor (Barr and Sweetnam, 1980). This indicates the time span over which aetiological factors might be studied.

5.3 Advantages and Disadvantages of Case–Control Studies

Three practical advantages of case–control studies are that they: (1) are relatively quick, (2) be used to study diseases that are relatively rare, and (3) require only the optimum numbers of subjects without the disease to be studied. The duration of the study is closely linked to the speed of recruitment of patients; this is a function of the incidence of the disease and the geographical region that has to be covered in order to accrue enough patients. (The number of patients required to allow significant results is discussed in 4.5.4.) The suitability of this approach for investigating rare disease may perhaps be expressed more forcibly, but indicating that for very rare cancers there is no other type of study that will be practical for investigating the aetiology.

It has already been suggested that many diseases are not the result of exposure to a single overriding aetiological agent; often several agents may act together to cause the disease.

A case–control study is particularly suitable for the investigation of several hypotheses in one study (perhaps with the overlapping interests of testing several old hypotheses, but also seeking preliminary support for other new hypotheses).

The aetiological agent being studied may be a rare one, to which only a small proportion of the general population is exposed; the ability of a case–control study to detect this will depend on the increment in risk that such exposure generates, rather than the fact that a few people have been exposed. (If only one in a hundred thousand of the population are exposed to a given carcinogen but they all develop the cancer and this is the cause of fifty per cent of all such cancers, this should be detected by a case–control study, but it would be very difficult to detect by a prospective study.)

The disadvantages are particularly related to the problems of obtaining valid data from cases and controls; this is due to the issues of selection and recall bias, discussed in subsection 5.2.5. The ways of overcoming this have been indicated in earlier subsections of this chapter, but in many instances it will not be possible to obtain a completely satisfactory study design. A choice will have to be made between the advantages of this approach versus the additional costs or delays that may be necessitated by some alternative approach.

If the agent is widely distributed but only responsible for a small proportion of the disease being studied, a case–control study will not be the most suitable way of defining the effect of such an agent. Crombie (1981) suggested that a case–control study was of limited value for investigating uncommon types of exposures, and was unable to detect small relative risks (e.g. < 1.5) even with widespread exposure to the aetiological factor.

Where the aim is to quantify the contribution of a particular agent, the analysis will often be limited to estimation of the relative disease frequencies in the exposed and the unexposed populations. This is linked to the source of population data on the incidence of the disease and frequency of exposure to the agent in the general population. This is discussed further in subsection 5.5.5 on methods of analysis.

There is a major difference in the range of problems that can be explored by case–control studies, as compared with surveys. By extending the questioning from the present to the past, a very wide range of issues can be examined. These include the natural history of disease, the influence of initiating and promoting factors, the interplay of other confounding factors on the development of disease, and the patient, family or cultural factors that can affect the seeking of medical care. Although the range of problems that can be explored is wide compared with the scope of cross-sectional studies, thought must be given to the quality of retrospective data and the bias in that collected from the study and control groups. A prospective study may be an alternative approach. This requires large numbers of subjects to be screened and followed over a period of time—a slow and expensive study. White and Bailar (1956) suggested that the method of sampling should be considered, rather than the time sequence of enquiry. They are critical of others' use of terminology, but emphasised some aspects of sampling without clearly distinguishing between cross-sectional surveys and questioning of cases and controls about prior exposure. Stewart (1973) suggested that the potential biases in a case–control study should not always lead to a prospective study being considered the most accurate, or the most appropriate way of studying many aetiological problems.

Pearl (1929) examined the records for the first 7500 autopsies performed at the Johns Hopkins Hospital and chose 816 individuals with cancer and 816 controls who were matched for age, sex, race and date of autopsy. Active tuberculosis lesions were found in 6.6 per cent of the cancer patients, compared with 16.3 per cent of the controls. This difference varied in the same way and to the same extent when the material was examined separately according to sex and race. On the assumption that there was an 'antagonism' between tuberculosis and development of cancer, Pearl persuaded others that this negative association was causal and subsequently patients with terminal cancer were treated with tuberculin. Pearl *et al.* (1929) briefly described seven patients with advanced cancer, who had been treated with tuberculin because of the above findings. They suggested that the lives of some, if not all, the patients had been prolonged; further hospitals agreed to try out the treatment.

At the time and more recently it has been queried whether such a negative association can be accepted as evidence that a group with active tuberculosis lesions at some point in time will subsequently be at lower risk of developing cancer than a group without lesions. If the control autopsy group supplied a biased estimate of the prevalence of active tuberculosis among all noncancerous individuals, the answer must be no. A recent review of the original data showed that the control autopsy group included a considerable number of individuals dying from tuberculosis and this would account for the higher prevalence of active tuberculosis lesions than that found in the general population. The use of autopsy material was not the cause of the false conclusions, but the failure to realise that those patients without cancer, who died in hospital, provided a biased estimate of the prevalence of tuberculosis that led to incorrect conclusions (see Lilienfeld, Pederson and Dowd, 1967). In circumstances, a positive association between two conditions can be found: for example, when multiple pathology increases the risk of hospital admission or prolongs the duration of stay (this could account for the recorded association between chronic bronchitis and peptic ulcer).

In a general exposition on this issue, Berkson (1946) demonstrated the limitations of use of hospital data to study either the association between two diseases, or the association between occupations and a disease. He provided mathematical examples of the impact of differences in the probability of admission for the subgroups upon the observed results. Though he was mainly concerned with the association of diseases, he emphasised that it was hazardous to study the occupations of patients with a particular disease, if it was known that the occupations were not represented in the hospital in the proportion they occur in the community. He commented that there did not appear to be any ready way of correcting the spurious correlations. White and Bailar (1956) suggested that Berkson had been the cause of unwarranted concern about the possible bias of case–control studies, though Mainland (1980) felt that curiously little attention was paid to this risk. White and Bailar (1956) also emphasised that there was potential for bias in prospective studies of individuals selected for known exposure or nonexposure to the factor under study. They suggested that use of several different categories of control patients and search for consistency of results was a safeguard against bias; no hard evidence was provided in support for this view.

It was another thirty years before the theoretical issues raised by Berkson were quantified in a study which compared frequencies of diseases in persons in hospital with frequencies in the catchment area populations (Roberts *et al.*, 1978). Boyd (1979) showed that the odds ratio of associations of diseases in inpatients will depend on the hospitalisation rates for the disease and the prevalence of the control-group disease. He derived rules to show under what conditions the results might be due to a 'Berkson-type' bias or a real association between two diseases.

Walter (1980) pointed out that risk factors are not usually independently distributed in the population, as had been an assumption of both Berkson and Roberts *et al.* However, if information was available on the distribution of attributes in the population and the mechanism of hospitalisation, the research worker would have a direct solution to the question a hospital-based study would be designed to answer. Walter (1980) emphasised that in practice the epidemiologist would have to remain wary of the influence of selection bias and use ancillary information to correct for this.

In a review of the role of case–control studies (*British Medical Journal*, 1979) it was suggested that they were less likely to obtain the randomness and independent selection of subjects than in a prospective study. This was disputed by Mann and Vessey (1979) who pointed out that a number of studies had included all cases in a defined population, thus avoiding this criticism.

In a spirited defence of the contribution from case–control studies, Sartwell (1974) pointed out how they could search for attributes associated with disease (which might be permanent, such as blood group, historical such as prior occupation, or current such as medication). Such associations may be aetiological, indicative of host susceptibility, or merely indicate the disirability of further study. He indicated various ways in which bias in selection of cases and controls could be reduced and also methods of overcoming errors in data collection.

It is often suggested that a principal advantage of a case–control study is the speed with which it can be conducted. The *British Medical Journal* (1979) pointed out that this could even lead to embarrassment; if results were made available when an issue was topical and attracting public attention, decisions might be made without adequate reflection on the interpretation of the data.

5.4 Extension of Case–Control Studies

The general design up until now has been concerned with studies restricted to investigation of a single disease, though they may have involved several conditions as sources of controls. An extension of this basic design is to include two or more diseases with a common aetiology: e.g. Alderson *et al.* (1983) studied patients with cancer of the lung, chronic bronchitis, ischaemic heart-disease and stroke when the main focus of interest was the effect of exposure to filter-tip cigarette smoking. Analagous to such a design is the study of intermediate states of disease, such as cancer of the cervix and carcinoma-*in-situ*, and controls without any cervical abnormality. Where it is thought that there is a natural progression from the normal epithelium, through dysplasia and carcinoma-*in-situ* to frankly invasive cancer, with only a proportion of patients moving from one stage to another, a suitable study-design would be to look at the relative risk of each phase of the disease in relation to the various aetiological agents.

Partly owing to the limitations of the original methods of analysis, a common design involved matched pairs; however, earlier sections have indicated the considerable difficulty in defining optimum controls. Some authors have therefore utilised both hospital and neighbourhood controls; if preliminary analyses show no difference in the results using the different groups of controls then the two sources can be combined. In a variant of this, Pike *et al.* (1981) approached individually matched neighbourhood controls and friends of the index cases; no significant differences were found and in the report only the pooled results were provided. A problem arises when an unexpected difference is found in the two sets of controls for which no obvious explanation can be found.

Sometimes there may be readily available controls, which have a specific disadvantage; again this may be an indication to use more than one source of control in order to overcome specific difficulties. A special technique has been evolved to avoid bias introduced by questioning respondents about their history and yet retain two advantages of case–control studies (i.e. starting with cases and controls and the speed of data aquisition). The variation in the technique involves the use of available or retrievable records in order to obtain appropriate historical details. Although such a study entails a search for historical data, these are not obtained by questioning the subjects involved; a number of authors have felt that this technique is more appropriately categorised under prospective studies. The important point to bear in mind is whether or not the subject knew about the outcome when the data on exposure to the aetiological agent have been recorded (i.e. whether or not there was potential for bias due to priming of recall). This approach is particularly suited to occupational studies and is discussed in further detail in Chapter 10.

A simple variant of the above technique is often used in method studies in order to clarify the definition and characteristics of subjects with a particular disease. Such a method study will be required as a preliminary to many epidemiological surveys and will often help in the interpretation of national variation in mortality and morbidity statistics. Thus, such studies warrant description to illustrate the approach.

Twofold differences in the incidence of mortality for cancer of the colon and rectum have been recorded in Denmark and Finland. A sample of death certificates mentioning either disease was obtained and a questionnaire sent to the certifier. A very high response was obtained (94 per cent in Denmark and 100 per cent in Finland), and diagnostic criteria were obtained either directly or through the hospitals providing treatment. It was considered that access to medical aid was similar in the two countries, and a review of the diagnostic material showed no reason for a difference in the national statistics, which was felt to reflect a genuine variation in incidence rather than an artefact (Jensen *et al.*, 1974).

A comparable problem is the definition of a case of tuberculosis. Case histories and X-rays of a representative sample of newly reported patients in eight different areas in Europe, Asia and America were submitted for central review and analysis. Considerable variation was found in the extent of disease, the frequency of cavitation, the average diameter of cavities and the frequency of positive bacteriological findings. Although there was a relationship between positive bacteriology and frequency of cavitation in the different centres, there was little relationship between bacteriology and the extent of disease. It was felt that classification of patients by both bacteriology and radiology was required in order to identify comparable categories of patients; the data were compatible with other material on difference in virulence of the organism and variation in host–agent interaction (Horwitz and Comstock, 1973).

There are problems with requisite sample size when studying a rare disease and the influence of a rare exposure. White (1982) suggested a two-stage procedure; the first determined disease and exposure status in a very large sample and then selected subsamples for intensive study including collection of covariate data. This utilised a large proportion of the rare exposure/disease categories and a small proportion of the nonexposed healthy subjects.

5.5 The Analysis of Case–Control Studies

The analysis of case–control studies involves the use of a number of special techniques that have been evolved specifically for the purpose. The simpler techniques are described in this section, but the analysis of complex files of data are beyond the scope of the book.

This first step is to examine the basic material, using a series of standard procedures for the probing of the descriptive data; this should include (1) presentation of the basic distributions of the material, with the use of tables, graphs and histograms, and (2) calculation of means and standard deviations.

The main use of case–control studies is to test specific hypotheses; the actual mathematical approach will depend on the form of the data collected in the study. The following subsections begin with the simplest analysis of a two-times-two table, cover various intermediate methods, and provide a brief note on the use of complex modelling of the data employing various forms of multivariate analysis.

Though the types of mathematical treatment of the data will depend upon the form in which the material has been collected, there are other issues which influence the final choice of the approach used. Cole (1979) emphasised the needs were to assess bias, confounding, causation and chance. He suggested that the presentation of exposure frequencies and related p-values provided an inadequate examination of the data. This seemed to be associated with a rather restricted view of the role of the epidemiologist in testing hypotheses—which he suggested should be left to legislators and policy makers. However, the value of estimates of p should not be underestimated, as they can provide an invaluable key to discussion and communication of the results from a particular study. Cole (1980) has also emphasised the importance of obtaining a valid estimate of the strength of any causal relationship, rather than being concerned about the generalisation of the results. Equally important is the confidence limits of the measure of the strength of the association. A major element of the succeeding sections is the demonstration of the various techniques for calculation of relative risk for a particular exposure and the confidence limits of this risk. However, such emphasis upon these probes of the data and derived statistics should not divert attention from the prime concern of deciding whether the results from the study have stemmed from aspects of the study design, methods of data collection, or chance fluctuations from the use of relatively small numbers in the study. These issues will be discussed further in chapter 11, where the more general aspects of defining causality are covered.

5.5.1 Relative risk

One of the most important aspects of retrospective studies is the definition of risk to individuals exposed to certain aetiological factors. At its simplest, this is the desire to quantify the risk for those who are, or are not, exposed. An extension of this is the quantification of the risk in relation to the degree of exposure.

Table 5.2 has been derived from an analysis of the pregnancy records of women who subsequently bore a child which was either malformed or healthy. This was part of a continuing examination of maternity and its outcome in Cardiff; abstraction from a paper by Lowe (1973) provided data on the relationship between malformations and a history of the consumption of anticonvulsants by the mother during her pregnancy. The data are laid out

Table 5.2 Number of children with and without congenital malformation, tabulated against history of consumption of anticonvulsants by
mother during pregnancy

History of anticonvulsant therapy	Malformation	Normal
no	868 (a)	30 875 (b)
yes	9 (c)	125 (d)

Source: Lowe (1973)

in a standard way, with the columns relating to the diseased subjects and the controls, and the rows relating to exposure or nonexposure to the aetiological factor. The relative risk may be calculated from such data using the standard formula:

$$\text{relative risk} = \frac{b \times c}{a \times d}$$

Providing the material is laid out in this way, it is a question of multiplying the entries in the diagonals of the table and then dividing one product by the other, that is

$$\text{relative risk} = \frac{30\,875 \times 9}{868 \times 125}$$

In this case the relative risk is calculated to be 2.56; in other words, if a women takes anticonvulsants during her pregnancy, it is suggested that the subsequently born child has about two-and-a-half times the risk of suffering from a congenital abnormality, compared with a child born to a mother not taking such a drug. Although risk is a useful index in considering this problem further, it is important to point out that the presentation of this material and its analysis in this way does not prove that there is a causal relationship. There may be a number of possible explanations: (1) the disease from which the mother suffers may be responsible, rather than the drug; (2) the disease or its treatment may be markers of other environmental or social factors that more directly link to the malformation of the foetus. Detailed consideration of this issue is beyond the scope of this book.

This calculation of the relative risk uses the method advocated by Cornfield (1951); he showed that it was possible to use the relative frequency data from case–control studies to estimate the relative risk (i.e. to provide an estimate of the ratio of the incidence for the groups being studied). He emphasised that the cases and controls had to be representative of the diseased and nondiseased in the population, and this was only so if the disease being studied was of low prevalence in the population. It was argued that this calculation of the relative risk is thus an oversimplification of the exact formula, and is only appropriate where the rates of occurrence of the disease (which generates a and c) are low. The index should also more correctly be called the odds ratio, as it represents the ratio of the odds of the disease's occurrence in the exposed and nonexposed subgroups of the population. Miettinen (1972) demonstrated how the risk ratio could be partitioned into (1) a measure of the strength of confounding, and (2) an estimate of the residual risk ratio. Examples were given of the application to both case–control and cohort studies.

Having obtained the value for the relative risk, the next step is the testing of the significance of the ratio (is it significantly different from unity?) and the calculation of the confidence interval of the ratio. Miettinen (1976) showed that the concern about the rarity of the disease was unnecessarily restrictive and he demonstrated that it was possible to estimate the exposure-specific incidence rates and risks from conventional case–control studies. He introduced a method, coupled with this, of calculating estimates of the confidence limits for the ratio.

Greenland and Thomas (1982) have discussed the 'rare disease' assumption and its relation to estimates of risk. Fleiss (1979) discussed various methods of estimating the confidence limits for the odds ratio from a fourfold table: intervals based on the sample odds-ratio; intervals based on the logarithms of the odds ratio; Cornfield's method for an approximate confidence-interval. He suggested that Cornfield's method was extremely accurate and the additional calculation, as compared with the simpler but more inaccurate methods, was warranted. Finney (1979) was even more critical of the simpler methods for calculating intervals; Miettinen (1979) pointed out that his test-based procedure became easier to apply when dealing with multiple two-times-two tables.

Using the abbreviations S.N.D. = standard normal deviate, S.E. = standard error, R.R. = relative risk, var = variance and C.I. = confidence interval, the steps in the calculations are:

(1) $S.N.D. = \dfrac{\log_e R.R.}{S.E. (\log_e R.R.)}$

$\log_e R.R. = \log_e 2.56 = 0.940$

$var (\log_e R.R.) = \dfrac{1}{868} + \dfrac{1}{30\,875} + \dfrac{1}{9} + \dfrac{1}{125}$
$= 0.1203$

$S.E. (\log_e R.R.) = \sqrt{0.1203} = 0.3468$

$S.N.D. = \dfrac{0.940}{0.3468} = 2.710, p < 0.01$

(2)   95 per cent C.I. for $\log_e R.R.$

$C.I. = \log_e R.R. \pm 1.96 \times S.E. (\log_e R.R.)$
$= 0.940 \pm 1.96 \times 0.3468$
$= \text{from } 0.260 \text{ to } 1.620$
$= \text{from } 1.297 \text{ to } 5.05 \qquad \text{taking exponentials}$

Finney (1979) cautioned that the odds ratio may not reflect a constant effect in different segments of the population. The statistical convenience of this measure may lead to overreliance upon it, when it may fail to provide useful information.

5.5.2 Two-times-n tables

Smulevitch *et al.* (1979) have discussed these issues and emphasised that the first phase should be a descriptive study of the risk ratio followed by an analytic study of the 'dose-effect' and of the interactions of the data. Obviously there is very limited information in any two-times-two table; where the exposure can be divided into two or more levels a more powerful probe of the data can be carried out. This can occur with ordinal data which rank subgroups of the study population in some sequence of 'degree of exposure'; it is also appropriate where continuous data have been grouped by appropriate cutting points. Table 5.3 provides an example of ordinal data derived from a national survey of perinatal mortality carried out in England and Wales in 1958. This survey provided an extensive range of material and only one small facet of this is shown in the table; the table is an over-simplification of material presented in the full report (Baird and Thomson, 1969).

Table 5.3   Distribution of perinatal deaths and control live births by occupational grouping of father

Occupation	Perinatal death	Control live birth	Relative risk Incremental	Relative risk Relative to professional
professional	630 (a)	2162 (b)	—	1.00
nonmanual	561 (c)	1733 (d)	1.11	1.11
skilled	2580 (e)	6811 (f)	1.17	1.30
semi- or unskilled	1950	4315	1.19	1.55
remainder	530	1264	0.93	1.44

Source: Baird and Thomson (1969)

When examining the relationship between the occupation of the father and perinatal mortality, these authors also took into account the age of the mother and her parity. In table 5.3 the occupation of the father is classified into one of four subgroups together with a remainder (chiefly relating to parents where the paternal occupation was not known and to unmarried mothers). As before, the table has been laid out in a standard way, with the columns relating first to the 'disease' group and then to the controls; the rows are in the conventional order in which occupational category is presented. The material in this table can be used to provide two different indices of risk. The first is the relative risk of one occupational subgroup against the top one—in this example the professional group. The calculation of the risk of perinatal death for the nonmanual subgroup in relation to professional families is exactly the same as in the previous example; that is:

$$\text{relative risk in nonmanual families} = \frac{b \times c}{a \times d}$$

$$= \frac{2162 \times 561}{630 \times 1733}$$

$$= 1.11$$

The preceding occupational category to nonmanual is professional, therefore both the incremental risk and the risk relative to professional occupations are identical.

A modification is then introduced by calculating the risks for skilled occupations. In order to calculate this incremental relative risk against the preceding category of nonmanual workers, the two rows nonmanual and skilled are handled as above; that is

$$\frac{\text{perinatal death in skilled families}}{\text{relative to nonmanual}} = \frac{d \times e}{c \times f}$$

$$= \frac{1733 \times 2580}{561 \times 6811}$$

$$= 1.17$$

For the second type of calculation, the skilled row is directly compared with the professional row; that is

$$\frac{\text{relative risk compared with}}{\text{professional families}} = \frac{b \times e}{a \times f}$$

$$= \frac{2162 \times 2580}{630 \times 6811}$$

$$= 1.30$$

This pattern is continued for the other two subgroups and the results of the calculation are shown in the right-hand columns of the table. It is important to remember that the standard layout is required in order to copy this approach directly.

It can be seen from the table that no result is entered for the incremental risk against professional, and the relative risk of course is 1.00. Examining the subsequent incremental risks, the first three are raised by between 10 and 20 per cent, the fourth has dropped to below 1—the relative risk of the 'remainder' subgroup is less than that of the semi- or unskilled parents. The correct placing of this category can more readily be identified from an examination of the extreme right-hand column, which shows the risk in relation to the professional subgroup. It can be seen that the risk rises for the first three, and then the final subgroup has a value between the skilled and the semi- or unskilled parents.

Analysis can in this way often provide an index that facilitates interpretation of the data. It must be emphasised that a relative risk cannot be directly interpreted, without some thought being given to its significance or reliability. The following indicates the method whereby the significance of the relative risk can be tested, and then a confidence interval provided. The algebra is similar to that used in a two-times-two table; it merely requires selection of the appropriate values from the standard layout.

(1)
$$S.N.D. = \frac{\log_e R.R.}{S.E.\,(\log_e R.R.)}$$

To test the relative risk for skilled workers, the values are inserted in the above formula as follows:

$$\log_e R.R. = \log_e 1.30 = 0.262$$

$$S.E.\,(\log_e R.R.) = \left[\frac{1}{630} + \frac{1}{2162} + \frac{1}{2580} + \frac{1}{6811}\right]^{1/2}$$

$$= 0.0508$$

$$S.N.D. = 5.157, p < 0.0001$$

(2) The 95 per cent confidence interval can be calculated, in a similar way to that required for the basic two-times-two table, via the use of $\log_e R.R.$:

$$C.I. = 0.262 \pm 1.96 \times 0.0508$$
$$= 0.262 \pm 0.0996$$
$$= \text{from } 0.1624 \text{ to } 0.3616$$

Therefore, for the original R.R. of 1.30, the confidence interval is from 1.1763 to 1.4356.

The above is the conventional method for the two-times-n table, where there is a logical rank-order for the different subgroups and it is appropriate to consider one of the subgroups as a base with relative risk equal to unity. An alternative is to use the total data as the base, calculating the relative risk from the ratio of cases to controls in the subgroup divided by that for all subjects in the study. For the material in table 5.3, the results are as follows:

	Source of base	
	Professional	Total data
professional	1.00	0.76
nonmanual	1.11	0.84
skilled	1.30	0.99
semiskilled	1.55	1.18
remainder	1.44	1.09

Though the absolute values are different, the ordering is very similar, and the relative increase in risk comparable (e.g. for semiskilled compared with professional $1.18/0.76 = 1.55$).

Where the two-times-n table represents n levels of exposure to some aetiological factor (such as cigarette smoking), it is possible to test the relative risks for the presence of a trend—which might indicate a dose–response relationship. This is beyond the scope of this section, but has been described by Breslow and Day (1980).

Mantel et al. (1977) emphasised the interest in probing the influence of a factor on risk of disease, to see whether this is arithmetically equal in populations with different baseline incidence levels of the disease, or if there are unequal (heterogeneous) effects. They cautioned about the use of logarithmic scales (also referred to as multiplicative scales), which may provide results that are invalid. Mantel *et al.* stressed that primary concern should be with inspection of the data, to search for homogeneous effects, rather than automatic application of tests for interaction. Other extensions of the basic method have been described by Hakulinen (1981).

5.5.3 Combining several two-times-two tables

There are several techniques for combining the results from two-times-two contingency tables. Before deciding to combine such data, it must be borne in mind that it may be misleading to try to combine a series of results that are very different; one may mask an important trend across the subsets of data, or be pooling results that are not compatible (for instance, owing to subtle differences in study design). In certain circumstances, the simple addition of results from two studies can introduce a spurious result, as shown in the following fictitious example:

	Case	Control	
study I	2	1	
	10	5	R.R. = 10/10 = 1.0
study II	5	10	
	1	2	R.R. = 10/10 = 1.0
pooled data	7	11	
	11	7	R.R. = 49/121 = 0.40

Mantel (1963) provided guidance on analysing multiple two-times-two contingency tables; Mantel and Haenszel (1959) described a method which is now widely used to combine estimates of relative risk from two or more two-times-two tables from case–control studies. There are other techniques available, such as the calculation of an average $\log_e$ R.R. or a weighted

Table 5.4   Numbers of cases with bladder cancer and controls who did and did not report use of artificial sweeteners in four recent papers

Authors	Cases Sweetener use		Controls Sweetener use	
	Yes	No	Yes	No
Hoover and Strasser (1980)	909	1349	1723	2554
Wynder and Stellman (1980)	76	226	80	222
Morrison and Buring (1980)	101	224	113	193
Howe *et al.* (1977)	73	407	47	433

average R.R. However, the Mantel–Haenszel method is described below as it is simple to calculate, is analagous to standardisation, readily provides a test of the significance of the R.R., and is satisfactory if the numbers in some of the cells are small or even zero.

$$\text{R.R.}_{\text{MH}} = \frac{\Sigma \, a_i d_i / n_i}{\Sigma \, b_i c_i / n_i}$$

where i denotes each of the studies being amalgamated from 1 to n. For the data set out in table 5.4, this can readily be transferred to the following matrix for the calculation of the pooled R.R.:

	1	2	3	4	Σ
$a_i d_i / n_i$	355.3	27.9	30.9	32.9	447.0
$b_i c_i / n_i$	355.7	29.9	40.1	19.9	445.6

$$\therefore \quad \text{R.R.}_{\text{MH}} = 447.0/445.6$$
$$= 1.00$$

The significance of this R.R. may be tested by the formula:

$$\chi^2 = \frac{[\Sigma \, a_i - \Sigma \, E(a_i)]^2}{\Sigma \, \text{var} \, (a_i)} \qquad \text{on one degree of freedom}$$

The expected values are obtained by the usual method for a two-times-two table (i.e. row total × column total ÷ grand total), while the variance of a is given by

$$\text{var} \, (a_i) = n_{1i} n_{2i} m_{1i} m_{2i} / [n_i^2 (n_i - 1)]$$

The actual steps in the calculation can be followed by setting out the data for the four studies used in table 5.4 in the following matrix:

Study	a_i	n_{1i}	n_{2i}	m_{1i}	m_{2i}	n_i	$E(a_i)$	var (a_i)
1	909	2258	4277	2632	3903	6535	909.42	355.53
2	76	302	302	156	448	604	78.0	28.98
3	101	325	306	214	417	631	110.2	35.38
4	73	480	480	120	840	960	60.0	26.28
Total	1159						1157.6	446.17

$$\chi^2_{\text{MH}} = \frac{(1159 - 1157.6)^2}{446.17}$$
$$= 0.004$$

Note: The particular example chosen is a topic where there has been appreciable variation in the estimates of the risk from artificial sweeteners, but these four recent papers show no indication of a hazard.

5.5.4 Analysis of a matched case–control study

A separate problem in the statistical handling of case–control studies occurs when the controls have been matched on one or more variates prior to the collection of data. The reason for matching has already been discussed earlier (see 5.2.3). McNemar (1947) and Mantel and Haenszel (1959) suggested appropriate techniques for examining such data.

Table 5.5 Counts of pairs of myocardial infarction patients and matched controls questioned about their previous exposure to stress

Controls	Myocardial infarction patients	
	Stress present	Stress absent
stress present	37 (r)	12 (s)
stress absent	26 (t)	19 (u)

An example is set out in table 5.5. These fictitious data represent an investigation in which a sample of patients with a myocardial infarction and an equal number of matched controls have been questioned about exposure to stress. It is important to emphasise that the table contains counts of the pairs of cases and controls allocated to the four possible categories of response. Either member of a pair can answer yes or no to a question about exposure to an agent; thus there are only four possible results—both yes (r), case yes and control no (t), case no and control yes (s), or both no (u). This is rather different from tables 5.2 and 5.3, which contained counts of individuals and where tests of association could be carried out by the conventional χ^2 test. McNemar's test can be applied in order to check whether there is a significant excess of cases reporting exposure to the aetiological agent compared to the controls. This test is simpler to apply than the conventional χ^2 test and it is important to bear it in mind when dealing with data of this nature. The reason for this simplification is that those pairs in which the case and the control have both either been or not been exposed to the aetiological agent provide no relevant information to test the hypothesis. It is only those pairs whose answers have been different which contribute useful data. The examination depends on the relative balance between the number of pairs with positive responses from cases and those with similar responses for controls. Thus

$$\chi^2 = \frac{(s-t)^2}{s+t}$$

$$= \frac{(-14)^2}{38}$$

$$= 5.16$$

Degrees of freedom = 1 $p < 0.05$

The next issue is the determination of the relative risk. This again can be calculated directly from the answers presented in table 5.5. Again, only two of the four values are required and the relative risk is easily estimated as follows:

$$\text{relative risk} = \frac{t}{s}$$

$$= \frac{26}{12}$$

$$= 2.17$$

The 95 per cent confidence interval is calculated as in the previous example of the Mantel–Haenszel method:

$$95 \text{ per cent C.I. of R.R.} = \text{R.R.}^{1\pm(\text{S.N.D.}/\chi)}$$

$$= 2.17^{1\pm(1.96/\sqrt{5.16})}$$

$$= 2.17^{0.137} \text{ to } 2.17^{1.863}$$

$$= 1.11 \text{ to } 4.23$$

Again it will be seen that the confidence interval is not symmetrical about the calculated R.R. and does not include 1, which is compatible with the test of significance already calculated.

The above example has been presented to illustrate the calculation of the R.R., the test of the null hypothesis, and calculation of the confidence interval of the relative risk. The place of the appropriate test of significance for matched pairs has been stressed by Pike and Morrow (1970). However, the example used above is for a very simple situation; a real study will often be complicated by the use of more than one control, by a variable number of controls, or by separation of exposure into multiple levels (see for example, Pike et al., 1975).

The types of matched data that can be presented in table form and analysed using elementary methods are limited. With studies involving multiple controls, multiple levels of exposure, and several exposure variables, other approaches have to be considered. These are discussed in the next section.

5.5.5 Relative risk and attributable risk

The attributable risk has been used to provide an indication of the impact that control or removal of the aetiological agent will have upon the prevalence of the disease in the community. However, it must be emphasised that extension of the findings in this way assumes that studies used to calculate the attributable-risk percentage are a satisfactory basis from which to generalise, and that there has already been agreement that there is adequate proof of causality.

The following measures may be calculated:

$$\text{attributable risk in the exposed} = \frac{\text{R.R.} - 1}{\text{R.R.}}$$

$$\text{population attributable risk} = \frac{p(\text{R.R.} - 1)}{(p \times \text{R.R.}) + (1 - p)}$$

Where R.R. = relative risk, p = proportion of the population exposed.

The confounding risk ratio measures the degree to which the effect of one factor is confounded by the effect of another factor; it is rather different from the above indices and is beyond the scope of the present contribution. It is discussed fully by Breslow and Day (1980).

$$\text{relative attributable risk} = \frac{\text{A.R.}_2 - \text{A.R.}_1}{1 - \text{A.R.}_1} \div \frac{\text{R.R.} - 1}{\text{R.R.}}$$

where A.R._1 = attributable risk for factor 1,
          A.R._2 = attributable risk for factor 2

A number of points should be noted about the above indices:

(1) Where the attributable risk is calculated from data which do not incorporate a self-evident baseline of non-exposed, but require selection of the lowest category of a continuous variate, the actual choice of the cutting point may have a marked effect on the calculated relative and absolute risks.

(2) The relative attributable risk may be used to avoid the preceeding difficulty, as it is much less sensitive to change in the definition in the base level used.

(3) Where more than one factor is associated with a given disease and their combined effect is at least additive, the sum of the separately calculated attributable risks may then exceed 100 per cent, indicating the individual and combined attributable risks must be interpreted with caution.

It was implicit in the original paper of Cornfield (1951) that the ratio of the disease incidences in the exposed and nonexposed individuals could be estimated directly from a case–control study. When hospital patients are used as the source of cases and controls no information on the magnitude of these incidences will be obtained. However, where information is available on the exposure levels in the population and incidence of the disease being studied is known, it is possible to calculate the population attributable risk of the disease. This may be illustrated using the data from table 5.2:

$$I = I_e p_e + I_0 p_0$$

where I = population incidence of disease
          i_e = incidence in those exposed
          p_e = proportion of the population exposed
          I_0 = incidence in the nonexposed
          p_0 = proportion of population nonexposed.

This is a self-evident statement that the overall incidence in the population is the sum of the respective incidences in the exposed and the unexposed population, weighted for the proportion who are and are not exposed. However, the incidences in the exposed and unexposed differ by the size of the relative risk:

$$I_e = \text{R.R.} \times I_0$$

Substituting in the first equation gives

$$I = (\text{R.R.} \times I_0 p_e) + I_0 p_0$$

$$\therefore I_0 = \frac{I}{(\text{R.R.} \times p_e) + p_0}$$

Usually, information will be required from a population survey to solve this equation; however, table 5.2 gives the following values (as this was based on a population study of cases and controls):

$$I = 27.51 \text{ per } 1000$$

$$p_e = (9 + 125)/31\,877 = 0.004$$

$$p_0 = (868 + 30\,875)/31\,877 = 0.996$$

$$\text{R.R.} = 2.56 \qquad \text{(already calculated in 5.5.1)}$$

$$\therefore \qquad I_0 = \frac{27.51}{(2.56 \times 0.004) + 0.996}$$

$$= 27.34 \text{ per } 1000$$

$$I_e = 27.34 \times 2.56$$

$$= 69.99 \text{ per } 1000$$

$$\text{A.R.} = 69.99 - 27.34$$

$$= 42.65 \text{ per } 1000$$

However, even in the absence of data on the population incidence of the condition, an estimate can be made of the increment in the disease from exposure, using the following approach:

$$I_0 = \frac{I}{(2.56 \times 0.996) + 0.004}$$

$$= 0.3916I$$

$$I_e = 2.56 \times 0.3916I$$

$$= 1.0025I$$

$$\text{A.R. per cent} = \frac{1.0025I - 0.3916J}{1.0025I} \times 100$$

$$= 60.9 \text{ per cent}$$

This may be compared with the simpler calculation for the attributable risk in the exposed:

$$\text{A.R. per cent} = \frac{\text{R.R.} - 1}{\text{R.R.}} \times 100$$

$$= \frac{1.56}{2.56} \times 100$$

$$= 60.9 \text{ per cent}$$

This result is the same, owing to the very small proportion of the population that are exposed and the fact that rounding therefore obscures any minor difference.

There are thus three ways of handling this aspect of aetiological data:

(1) Estimate the relative frequency with which the exposed and nonexposed individuals will develop the condition being studied.
(2) Estimate the magnitude of the problem as far as this affects the general population.
(3) Estimate the magnitude of the problem as far as the exposed population is concerned.

The data requirements for calculating attributable risk have been set out by Walter (1978), who provided a number of worked examples. The nomenclature of risk assessment was reviewed by Waltner-Toews (1982), who provided references to recent papers covering about twenty various statistical methods.

5.5.6 Multivariate analyses

A recent text by Breslow and Day (1980) has set out in a comprehensive fashion the newer techniques that may be used for handling data from more complex studies. They emphasise that, as a preliminary to the more sophisticated analysis, there should be extensive probing of the basic data using tabular and graphical methods.

For unmatched data Breslow and Day describe an unconditional logistic regression which fits a linear logistic regression model to the data. This is based upon a logit transform of the probability of disease in each exposure category, which is presented as a linear function of the regression variables. The authors demonstrate (1) how this model, which was initially used in prospective studies, can be adopted for case–control studies, (2) the combination of several two-times-two results, (3) the adjustment in the regression model for confounding, (4) the advantages of using continuous variables rather than categorised data, (5) how the regression coefficients may be interpreted, and (6) the study of interaction between different risk and 'nuisance' variables.

Where matched case–control studies have been carried out, with fine stratification of some of the variables, analysis by conditional logistic regression may be preferable. Breslow and Day (1980) point out that the various types of study for matched data discussed above can now be analysed using conditional likelihood (e.g. matched pairs with dichotomous or polytomous exposure; varying numbers of controls with single or multiple levels of exposure; combination of a series of two-times-two tables). They emphasise that whenever matching occurs in the study design, it should be accounted for in the analysis. Stratification of the data can occur during the analysis, even if this was not incorporated in the study design—for instance, when population controls have been used.

It is often desirable to standardise the risk ratios for the distribution of some confounding factor. A method for so doing was proposed by Miettinen (1972); this involved use of an explicitly identified standard from within the study data. The results obtained were mutually comparable within any given study and could provide a relative risk adjusted for the influence of the confounding factor. The more powerful techniques indicated above provide an approach to examining the influence of confounding factors; Berry (1980) has described how the modifying effects of two variates can be explored. He pointed out that not all biological models have an exponential dose–response relationship and there could be difficulty in fitting a factor having a protective effect into the model. He concluded that these techniques should be used to examine the influence of matching factors.

Cornfield and Haenszel (1960) expressed a preference for post-stratification in the analysis as apposed to matching in the study design, as the former gave greater flexibility in studying interactions. However, Mietti-nen (1979) pointed out that matching was more likely to satisfy critical colleagues than was reporting a post-stratification analysis. Cole (1980) described the reasons for and against matching and emphasised that now there were efficient ways to control confounding in the analysis, the need for matching in design required reassessment.

Even if matching has been carried out, it is still possible to examine the influence of interaction of the various factors. Rothman (1974) discussed the situation where two agents both act as causes of a disease and modify the effect of each other in causing the disease. He applied probability theory to discover if the risk attributable to a combined exposure exceeds the sum of the risks attributable to each of the exposures separately; this was called positive interaction or synergy. The concept was extended to three causes (such as two known causes being studied, and all others counted as a third category). Rothman (1976) set out the method of estimating this interaction and provided an example of the application of the method.

Using rather a different approach, Walker (1981) set out a method for analysis of the interaction of two aetiological factors, which was based upon the additivity of the attributable risks. He stated that this was justified when the purpose was to provide a basis for making decisions about personal risk or public-health intervention.

Greenland (1981) presented three approaches to the derivation of exposure-specific incidence from case–control data by means of mul-tivariate modelling. These permitted derivation of the joint confidence limits for exposure-specific incidence estimates; however, the importance of bias-free data in interpreting such estimates was stressed.

Wicken (1966) presented data on all persons aged thirty-five and over who had died in Northern Ireland in the period 1960–2 from lung cancer, and a control group matched for age and place of residence who had died from nonrespiratory disease. Material from a sample survey of all house-holds was used to provide information about the population's smoking habits, social class and place of residence in an attempt to identify those individuals at particular risk of dying from lung cancer. Buck and Wicken (1967) performed a discriminant analysis on the data, which identified those variates most closely associated with lung cancer. A further analysis was then carried out to investigate more closely the relationship of the variates. It was presumed that individuals exposed to the influence of a number of factors had a greater risk of dying from lung cancer. A mathematical model was used to examine how the place of residence, smoking habits and history of a morning cough combined to establish the 'risk' of dying from lung cancer. It was postulated that there was an interaction between smoking and morning cough, and that this multiplied by the place of residence indicated the risk of lung cancer.

Buck and Wicken presented data that indicated that the factors did combine in such a fashion. There are a number of ways in which such data can be handled (see Armitage, 1967), but discussion of the mathematics involved is beyond the scope of this book. The important issue is that single-factor analyses of the determinants of a disease, even if standardised or controlled for the influence of a combination of factors, provide a limited examination of real life. Berry *et al.* (1972) in examining the effect of smoking and exposure to asbestos dust suggested that, particularly in women, these two carcinogenic factors have a multiplicative effect in determining the development of lung cancer. Other work (Brown *et al.*, 1957) suggested that the influence of social-class factors on the development of chronic bronchitis was apparent only in smokers. These examples indicate the need to consider the matter when analysing comparable data. Exploration of the way in which a number of relevant items combine may provide a more appropriate description of observed data and lead to improved definition of those at risk of developing a particular disease. However, such an approach does not enable a confident judgement to be made about causality (see discussion in section 11.3).

References

Recommended reading

Truelove, S. C. (1975). *Medical Surveys and Clinical Trials*. Oxford University Press, London

Other references

Alderson, M. R. (1980). *Adv. Cancer Res.*, **31**, 2–76
Alderson, M. R., Lee, P., and Wang, R. (1983). Work in progress
Armitage, P. (1967). *Appl. Statist.*, **16**, 203
Baird, D., and Thompson, A. M. (1969). In *Perinatal Problems—The Second Report of the 1958 British Perinatal Mortality Survey* (N. Butler and E. D. Alberman, eds), Livingstone, Edinburgh, pp. 16–35
Barr, M. L., and Sweetnam, P. M. (1980). *J. Epid. Comm. Hlth*, **34**, 93–5
Bartlett, F. C. (1932). *Remembering: a Study of Experimental and Social Psychology*. University Press, Cambridge
Berkson, J. (1946). *Biomet. Bull.*, **2**, 47–53
Berry, G. (1980). *J. Epidem. Comm. Hlth*, **34**, 217–22
Berry, G., Newhouse, M. L., and Turkok, M. (1972). *Lancet*, **2**, 476–9
Black, D. (1980). *Inequalities in Health*. D.H.S.S., London

Boyd, A. V. (1979). *J. chron. Dis.*, **32**, 667–72
Breslow, N. E., and Day, N. E. (1980). *The Analysis of Case–Control Studies.* International Agency for Research in Cancer, Lyon
British Medical Journal (1979). *Br. med. J.*, **2**, 884–5
British Medical Journal (1981). *Br. med. J.*, **283**, 628
Broders, A. C. (1920). *J. Am. med. Ass.*, **74**, 656–64
Brown, R. G., McKeown, T., and Whitfield, A. G. W. (1957). *Br. med. J.*, **1**, 555–62
Buck, S. F., and Wicken, A. J. (1967). *Appl. Statist.*, **16**, 185–210
Case, R. A. M. (1966). *Ann. R. Coll. Surg. Engl.*, **39**, 223-35
Case, R. A. M., and Hosker, M. E. (1954). *Br. J. prev. soc. Med.*, **8**, 39–50
Cole, P. (1979). *J. chron. Dis.*, **32**, 15–27
Cole, P. (1980). In *The Analysis of Case–Control Studies* (N. E. Breslow, and N. E. Day, eds), International Agency for Research in Cancer, Lyon, pp. 15–41
Cornfield, J. (1951). *J. Natn. Cancer Inst.*, **11**, 1269–75
Cornfield, J., and Haenszel, W. (1960). *J. chron. Dis.*, **11**, 523–34
Court Brown, W. S., Doll, R., and Hill, A. B. (1960). *Br. Med. J.*, **2**, 1539–45
Crombie, I. K. (1981). *J. epidem. comm. Hlth*, **35**, 281–7
Crombie, I. K., and Tomenson, J. (1981). *Lancet*, **2**, 308–9
Davies, J. M. (1966). *Proc. R. Soc. Med.*, **59**, 1247–8
Dean, G., Lee, P., Todd, G. F., and Wicken, A. J. (1977). *Report on a Second Retrospective Study in North East England. Part I*, Tobacco Research Council, London
Doll, R. (1959). In *Medical Surveys and Clinical Trials* (L. J. Witts, ed.), Oxford University Press, London, pp. 64–90
Eimerl, T. S., and Laidlaw, A. J. (1969). *A Handbook for Research in General Practice*, 2nd edn, Livingstone, Edinburgh
Feinstein, A. R. (1979). *J. chron. Dis.*, **32**, 35–41
Finney, D. J. (1979). *J. chron. Dis.*, **32**, 78–9
Fleiss, J. L. (1979). *J. chron. Dis.*, **32**, 69–77
Gordis, L. (1982). *Am. J. Epidem.*, **115**, 1–5
Greenland, S. (1981). *J. chron. Dis.*, **34**, 445–54
Greenland, S., Morgenstern, H., and Thomas, D. C. (1981). *Int. J. Epidem.*, **10**, 389–92
Greenland, S., and Thomas, D. C. (1982). *Am. J. Epidem.*, **116**, 547–53
Hakulinen, T. (1981). *Am. J. Epidem.*, **113**, 192–7
Herrmann, N., Amsel, J., and Lynch, E. (1981). *Am. J. publ. Hlth*, **71**, 1314–9
Hewitt, D. (1955). *Br. J. prev. soc. Med.*, **9**, 81–8
Hewitt, D., Sanders, B., and Stewart, A. (1966). *Mon. Bull. Minist. Health*, **25**, 80–5
Hoover, R. N., and Strasser, P. H. (1980). *Lancet*, **1**, 837–40
Horwitz, O., and Comstock, G. W. (1973). *Int. J. Epidem.*, **2**, 145–52
Horwitz, R. I., and Feinstein, A. R. (1978). *New Engl. J. Med.*, **299**, 1089–94
Horwitz, R. I., Feinstein, A. R., Horwitz, S. M., and Robboy, S. J. (1981). *Lancet*, **2**, 66–8
Howe, G. R., Chambers, L., Gordon, P., Morrison, B., and Miller, A. B. (1977). *Am. J. Epidem.*, **106**, 239
Hulka, B. S., Grimson, R. C., and Greenberg, B. G. (1981). *Lancet*, **2**, 817
Jensen, O. M., Mosbech, J., Salaspuro, M., and Jhamaki, T. (1974). *Int. J. Epidem.*, **3**, 183–6
Lane-Claypon, J. E. (1926). *A Further Report of Cancer of the Breast, with Special Reference to its Associated Antecedent Conditions.* H.M.S.O., London
Lee, W. R., Alderson, M. R., and Downes, J. E. (1972). *Br. J. Indust. Med.*, **29**, 188–95

Lilienfeld, A. M., and Lilienfeld, D. E. (1979). *J. chron. Dis.*, **32,** 5–13
Lilienfeld, A. M., Pedersen, E., and Dowd, J. E. (1967). *Cancer Epidemiology: Methods of Study*. Johns Hopkins Press, Baltimore
Lowe, R. (1973). *Lancet*, **1,** 9–10
MacMahon, B. (1962). *J. Natn. Cancer Inst.*, **28,** 1173–91
MacMahon, B., Yens, S., Trichopoulos, D., Warren, K., and Nardi, G. (1981). *New Engl. J. Med.*, **340,** 1605–6
McNemar, Q. (1947). *Psychometrica*, **12,** 153–7
Mainland, D. (1980). *Br. med. J.*, **280,** 330
Mann, J. I., and Vessey, M. P. (1979). *Br. med. J.*, **2,** 1507
Mantel, N. (1963). *J. Am. statist. Ass.*, **58,** 690–700
Mantel, N., and Haenszel, W. (1959). *J. natn. Cancer Inst.*, **22,** 719–48
Mantel, N., Brown, C., and Byar, D. P. (1977). *Am. J. Epidem.*, **106,** 125–9
Medical Research Council (1973). *Br. med. J.*, **2,** 213
Merletti, F., and Cole, P. (1981). *Lancet*, **2,** 579
Miall, W. E., and Oldham, P. D. (1955). *Clin. Sci.*, **14,** 459–88
Miettinen, O. S. (1972). *Am. J. Epidem.*, **96,** 168–72
Miettinen, O. S. (1976). *Am. J. Epidem.*, **103,** 26–35
Miettinen, O. S. (1979). *J. chron. Dis.*, **32,** 80–2
Mole, R. H. (1974). *Br. J. Cancer*, **30,** 199–208
Morris, J. N. (1975). *Uses of Epidemiology*. Livingstone, Edinburgh
Morrison, A. S., and Buring, J. E. (1980). *New Engl. J. Med.*, **302,** 537–41
Pearl, R. (1929). *Am. J. Hyg.*, **9,** 97–159
Pearl, R., Sutton, A. C., and Howard, W. T. (1929). *Lancet*, **1,** 1078–80
Pike, M. C., Casagrande, J., and Smith, P. G. (1975). *Br. J. Prev. Soc. Med.*, **29,** 196–201
Pike, M. C., Henderson, B. E., Casagrande, J. T., Rosario, I., and Gray, G. E. (1981). *Br. J. Cancer*, **43,** 72–6
Pike, M. C., Hill, A. P., and Smith, P. G. (1981). *Int. J. Epidem.*, **10,** 393–4
Pike, M. C., and Morrow, R. H. (1970). *Br. J. prev. soc. Med.*, **24,** 42–4
Roberts, R. S., Spitzer, W. O., Delmore, T., and Sackett, D. L. (1978). *J. chron. Dis.*, **31,** 119–28
Rothman, K. J. (1974). *Am. J. Epid.*, **99,** 385–8
Rothman, K. J. (1976). *Am. J. Epid.*, **103,** 506–11
Russell, J. G. B. (1970). *Br. J. Hosp. Med.*, **3,** 601–5
Sartwell, P. E. (1974). *Ann. int. Med.*, **81,** 381–6
Sartwell, P. E. (1979). *J. chron. Dis.*, **32,** 42–4
Schrek, R., and Lenowitz, H. (1946). *Cancer Research*, **7,** 180–7
Shapiro, S. (1979). *J. chron. Dis.*, **32,** 32
Smulevitch, V. B., Bulbulian, M. A., and Katsnelson, B. A. (1979). *J. occ. Med.*, **21,** 11–4
Stewart, A. (1973). *An Epidemiologist Takes a Look at Radiation Risk*. Department of Health, Education and Welfare, Maryland
Stewart, A., and Kneale, G. W. (1970). *Lancet*, **1,** 1185–8
Stewart, A., Webb, J., Giles, D., and Hewitt, D. (1956). *Lancet*, **2,** 447
Stewart, A., Webb, J., and Hewitt, D. (1958). *Br. med. J.*, **1,** 1495–508
Walker, A. R. M. (1981). *Int. J. Epidem.*, **10,** 81–5
Walter, S. D. (1978). *Int. J. Epidem.*, **7,** 175–82
Walter, S. D. (1980). *J. chron. Dis.*, **33,** 721–5
Waltner-Toews, D. (1982). *Int. J. Epidem.*, **11,** 411–3
White, J. E. (1982). *Am. J. Epidem.*, **115,** 119–28
White, C., and Bailar, J. C. (1956). *Am. J. publ. Hlth*, **46,** 35–44

Wicken, A. J. (1966). *Environmental and Personal Factors in Lung Cancer and Bronchitis Mortality in Northern Ireland, 1960–2*. Tobacco Research Council, London

Wynder, E. L., and Stellman, S. D. (1980). *Science*, **207**, 1214–6

6 Prospective Studies

Prospective studies require an approach very different from that for case–control studies and serve as a more direct test of a specific hypothesis on aetiology. Also, these studies require considerably more investment of resources than case–control studies and they would mainly be carried out when case–control studies have produced conflicting results, or where the topic is of considerable importance to the health of the general population. There are a number of developments of the technique, some of which require extremely complex organisation, such as longitudinal (cohort) studies. However, routine data, combined with *ad hoc* surveys or linked to other data, can provide the high efficiency associated with prospective studies relatively cheaply and speedily. Such an approach requires extremely careful consideration and will be discussed in section 6.4

A prospective study includes a consideration of time, degree of exposure to the aetiological agent and usually a range of other factors. Additional problems of analysis and interpretation arise because of this. Some of the techniques for handling such material are discussed in section 6.5.

6.1 Basic Example

The use of case–control studies to examine the prevalence of smoking in patients with and without lung cancer was hinted at in the previous chapter, but the extensive literature on this topic was not indicated. The majority of these studies showed that the relative risk of developing lung cancer was appreciably higher in smokers, and particularly in heavy smokers. However, this is an extremely important issue, because a large proportion of the population smokes and the mortality due to lung cancer and other diseases thought to be associated with smoking has been rapidly rising. There was felt to be a need for further studies.

An extensive prospective study was mounted among doctors by Doll and Hill (1954). In 1951 they wrote to all practitioners on the medical register in the United Kingdom and included a very brief self-completion questionnaire about smoking habits. This material was then collated with subsequent information on the mortality of the respondents. One of the advantages of selecting a professional group, such as doctors, was that it became relatively easy to set up a system for obtaining the death certificates of all respondents. The Registrars General in the United Kingdom co-operated by automatically providing all death certificates on which the deceased's profession was identifiable as a doctor. Also the authorities responsible for maintaining the register of doctors collaborated. The latter provided a regular list of details of those doctors whose names had been removed from the medical register because of death. Cross-checking these two sources of material enabled the death certificate to be traced and the doctor certifying the cause of death was then approached directly if the certificate mentioned lung cancer.

168

The main interest of the study was the examination of the relationship between smoking habits on entering the study and subsequent mortality. Initial results of a twenty-nine-month follow up are presented in table 6.1. The data are presented for nonsmokers and three categories of smokers, the latter being classified by the amount of tobacco smoked per day (one ounce of tobacco per week was taken as equivalent to 4 g per day). It can be immediately seen that there was a deficiency of deaths from lung cancer in nonsmokers, and an excess among the heavy smokers. In addition, data was available for ex-smokers and for those smoking pipe tobacco. The mortality rates for these groups of smokers were between those of nonsmokers and cigarette smokers.

Table 6.1 Observed and expected numbers of deaths from lung cancer by smoking category among 24 389 male doctors followed over 29 months

| | | Smokers Daily consumption (g) | | | |
	Nonsmokers	1–14	15–24	25 +	Total
observed deaths	0	12	11	13	36
expected deaths	3.77	14.20	10.73	7.33	36.03

Source: Doll and Hill (1954)

χ^2 for trend = 7.7
Degrees of freedom = 1
$p < 0.01$

The doctors were then followed for a much longer period and further analyses of the mortality data were published after continuing the study for ten years (Doll and Hill, 1964). The variation in death-rates from lung cancer, standardised for age, are shown in figure 6.1 compared with numbers of cigarettes smoked daily at the start of the study (men smoking pipes and cigars, and ex-smokers have been excluded). A linear dose–response is shown. An even more crucial point in the argument was the examination of the mortality among the ex-smokers; this is shown in figure 6.2. There was a high mortality due to lung cancer in those who had just given up smoking, with a lower mortality in those who had not smoked for many years (the mortality approximates to that of the nonsmoker in those who had not smoked for twenty years).

Some general points can be made using the above example. Data on the risk factor were collected in as simple a way as possible; the self-completion questionnaire had very few questions on it and merely provided a guide to current smoking habits. The population chosen might be motivated to respond and was a group that facilitated follow up. Mortality was obtained by use of two routine sources of data, one a by-product of the officially held records for a particular professional group. These factors assisted the prospective study; although having said this, it should be pointed out that the study required a very large number of subjects (60 000) and some encouragement was needed to boost the response rate. (It is interesting to note that

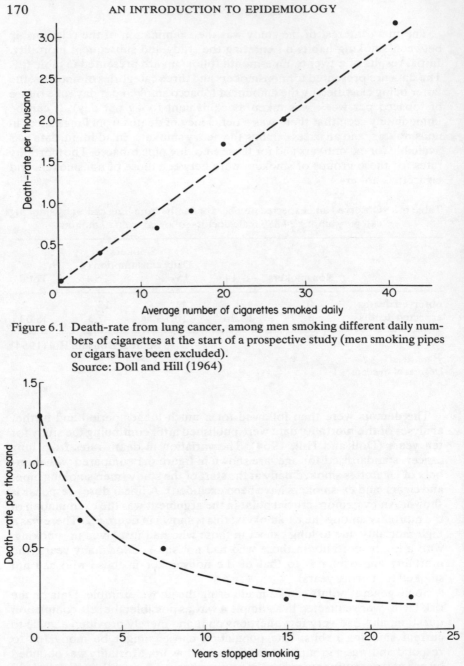

Figure 6.1 Death-rate from lung cancer, among men smoking different daily numbers of cigarettes at the start of a prospective study (men smoking pipes
or cigars have been excluded).
Source: Doll and Hill (1964)

Figure 6.2 Death-rate from lung cancer, men continuing to smoke cigarettes and
men who have given up smoking for different periods (men who had
regularly smoked pipes or cigars as well as cigarettes have been excluded).
Source: Doll and Hill (1964)

the response rate was only 68 per cent of those approached.) In order to collect sufficient numbers of events (that is, deaths from lung cancer) the 40 000 subjects enrolled in this study had to be followed up for two years before sufficient material had been collected to warrant a preliminary analysis. Only after such a period was it possible to calculate mortality rates according to the category of smoking; the main analysis used a twenty-years follow-up period for men and twenty-two years for women (Doll and Peto, 1976; Doll *et al.*, 1980).

Such a study classified material on smoking, which enabled the respondents to be classified by this variate and then followed over a period of time to see who died from lung cancer. The smoking histories were therefore collected predominantly from healthy subjects, who were divorced from any direct bias of the relationship between smoking and presence of lung cancer. Care was required in the interpretation of the material. There was a possibility that those reporting themselves as nonsmokers were in this category because of the recent development of acute disease, for which they had been advised to give up smoking. There was also no proof that the smoking histories were valid. There may have been a tendency to exaggerate or underestimate present levels of smoking—but no obvious reason why such variation in the recording of smoking history should have been associated with subsequent disease in a way that could bias the interpretation of data. If random, such error would merely reduce the strength of any true association.

The above example demonstrates the use of prospective studies to test hypotheses (in this case, that there is a causal relationship between smoking and lung cancer). Another application is as a descriptive study to demonstrate the natural history of disease. In 1956, during the repeat of a mass X-ray survey in one part of Bergen, the opportunity was taken to screen the population for diabetes. 2796 male and 4645 women were X-rayed; 2273 and 3637, respectively, participated in the diabetes study. Out of this group 510 subjects were identified as suspicious on the basis of preliminary urinalysis and blood-sugar levels—but forty of these subjects were known diabetics already receiving treatment. The remaining 470 underwent a glucose-tolerance test, together with a sample of those who gave negative results on screening. Depending on the results of the glucose-tolerance test, the 470 'suspected' subjects were classified as latent diabetics (70), borderline diabetics (82), glycosuric (54), and nondiabetic (218), and forty-six were not further tested.

In 1966–8 follow up of these people was carried out. Death certificates were obtained for those who had died and re-examination of the remainder was attempted. Standardised biochemical tests were used and the subjects were classified according to strict World Health Organisation criteria (W.H.O., 1965). Asperik and his colleagues (1974) found that the mortality had been high in the latent-diabetes group (60 per cent had died) and the borderline group (34 per cent of the males and 37 per cent of the females had died). There remained 176 'suspected' subjects in the four categories identified above. These subjects and a sample of persons found to be normal in 1956 were invited to attend for examination; only 78 per cent responded.

Table 6.2   Results of re-examination ten years after a population survey for diabetes

Classification in 1956	Number re-examined	Found to have diabetes number	Found to have diabetes per cent
latent diabetes	23	21	91
borderline	41	8	20
glycosuric	41	5	12
nondiabetic	36	2	6
normal	68	7	10

Source: Asperick *et al.* (1974)

Table 6.2 shows the basic results from the re-examination. It can be seen that nearly all those classified in 1956 as latent diabetics were now suffering from overt diabetes, sixteen of whom were controlled by diet alone and only two required insulin. Somewhat more surprising is the fact that seven out of sixty-eight subjects found to be normal in 1956 were classified as diabetics ten years later. The authors discussed whether some bias had occurred in those responding in the two examinations—there was no clear indication of how this could account for such an incidence of diabetes in the ten-year follow-up period.

This study has been described as an example of the use of population samples to mount prospective studies, and the way such studies can contribute to an appreciation of the natural history of disease. Diabetes is a condition where screening can identify an appreciable proportion of subjects in a borderline category—much further knowledge is required before the suitability of intervention can be defined. The use of controlled trials will be briefly mentioned in subsection 7.4.1.

6.2 Principles of Prospective Studies

The aim of prospective studies is, in most cases, to examine the influence of a specific aetiological factor on the incidence of, or mortality from, a particular disease. In planning such a study the first point is to define the population that will be surveyed and followed up. As has already been mentioned (see subsection 4.2.3), there is a need to identify a group of the population in which an adequate response-rate can be anticipated or ensured by various techniques, and for which the nonrespondents can be identified. Several research workers in the United Kingdom have used various occupational groups for a wide range of studies. The main point in this approach is that by going to a particular organisation one can obtain a list of employees to use as a sampling frame. This approach is desirable in the absence of a population register for use as a sampling frame. The use of occupational groups in this way is quite different from the study of occupationally induced disease that is discussed in chapter 10. Various approaches have been made to postmen

(Reid and Fairbairn, 1958), telephone men (Holland and Stone, 1965), London Transport Board and civil servants (Morris *et al.*, 1966), light engineering and clerical workers (Fletcher *et al.*, 1970) and twenty-four factories of light, medium and heavy industry (Rose *et al.*, 1980).

Another sampling frame can be the executive council (family practitioner committee) lists. These are not automatically available because of considerations of confidentiality. Also, the physical arrangements for holding the records do not enable lists of subgroups of the population according to age, sex and marital status to be provided.

Nearly seventy thousand volunteer workers of the American Cancer Society were used in 1959–60 to enroll over a million men and women in a prospective study with particular emphasis on smoking and health (Hammond, 1966). The study covered twenty-five states in the U.S.A. and care was taken to include all segments of the population except: (1) migrant workers or others that could not be traced and (2) persons in long-term medical institutions. Enrolment was by household; any household was eligible if there was at least one person over the age of forty-five. All members over thirty were asked to complete a questionnaire. The subjects were traced annually; every two years they were asked to complete a brief questionnaire. Whenever a death was reported, a copy of the death certificate was obtained from the appropriate health department.

When considering any specific subgroup of the community for a prospective study thought must be given to the use of the results. For example, there may be certain factors affecting the chosen group, which prevent extrapolation of the findings to the general population. There may be an interrelationship between smoking and a specific occupational group, either through the influence of the occupation on the amount of smoking, or because of an occupational hazard that has a synergistic effect on, for example, the risk of lung cancer. The selection of such a population for a study would be unwise.

Having identified a population suitable for the study, there is then the need to consider the most appropriate way of collecting the basic information. As discussed earlier (subsection 4.2.5), data may be collected by questionnaire, interview, examination or investigation. These baseline data must be collected in such a way that they provide a valid and unbiased classification of the 'exposure' of the individuals to the aetiological agent. A consideration of the collection of valid data has already been covered, and the points that have been raised (see 4.2.6.1–4) are as relevant to prospective studies as to other forms of investigation. The main advantage of the prospective study is that 'healthy' subjects are approached and asked to participate in the study, and material, including the quantification of exposure to potential aetiological factors, is collected from them. Often the approach to the subjects is in fairly general terms, particularly if the hypothesis is very tentative. For example, in a study on leisure activity it would be inadvisable to publicise that the intention of the study was to examine the relationship between the amount of physical labour undertaken and the incidence of or fatality from coronary heart disease.

It is much less likely that bias will enter into the classification of exposure to the factors under study when the material is collected from individuals who are not necessarily aware of the cause-and-effect relationship of the study. It is of course self-evident that the study of a 'healthy' population means that the mortality and morbidity of the respondents will be somewhat lower in the first few years of the follow up, because the study will have automatically excluded those individuals who were ill at the time of survey. Doll (1959) suggested that extension of the period of follow up allowed this bias due to the initial exclusion of the sick to wear off. In support of this he quoted the work of Jordan (1952), and pointed out that it was a common actuarial experience that the effect of screening out sick persons by medical examination was relatively slight after the third year, and that for all practical purposes it disappeared altogether after five years.

Having collected valid data from the chosen population, there is then the need to organise some system for follow up of the population, in particular to collate data on the chosen end-point or outcome. There are two main approaches to collecting follow-up material. The first involves the painstaking recontact of all the individuals at regular intervals. This technique is particularly necessary when the index of outcome being sought is not necessarily the development of overt disease, but the more subtle identification of various changes in individuals or their way of life. Where the index of outcome is more clear cut, such as registration of malignant disease, admission to hospital because of a particular condition, performance of an operation or death from a certain condition, other approaches to the collection of follow-up material may be considered. This can be done by linking the basic data collected on the sample with an outcome identified from routine morbidity or mortality data. Examples of the various ways of collecting follow-up data will be discussed in section 6.4.

Prospective studies rely on the natural variation that occurs on exposure to a given aetiological agent. Although certain studies have been termed natural experiments, they are essentially observational and quite different from the intervention studies discussed in the next chapter. The analysis of a prospective study can test the hypothesis that smokers are at higher risk of dying from lung cancer, but this does not constitute proof that smoking is a cause of lung cancer. In a well-designed study, the degree of association between the aetiological factor and the outcome may be quantified. The smoking study discussed in section 6.1 showed the measured mortality-rate in relation to the amount of smoking on entering the study. Further surveys have replicated these findings and explored the confounding factors; the complex of aetiological factors has thus been steadily unravelled. The various techniques for the analysis and statistical testing of such data will be discussed in section 6.5. Consideration will then be given to the derivation of interferences. These can lead to the identification of specific hazards, and the posposal of preventive measures. The consideration of these important issues is far beyond the realm of epidemiology. Once a decision has been made to change the exposure to a particular hazard (such as by altering the environment or changing people's way of life), there is a need to establish planned intervention studies, which will be discussed in the next chapter.

6.3 Advantages and Disadvantages of Prospective Studies

When discussing the enquiry about antenatal X-ray examinations of women whose children had subsequently died from leukaemia, it was pointed out that the traumatic experience of the child's death had probably affected the mother's recall. A prospective study provides an opportunity to collect data on an aetiological factor in an unbiased way. However, this advantage has to be balanced against some extremely important drawbacks. Where the condition being studied is relatively rare, it will be necessary to study a large number of subjects and follow them up over a considerable number of years before sufficient events have occurred in the cohort to enable an adequate analysis. For example, if only one in 15 000 individuals develops leukaemia each year and it is felt that approximately 100 leukaemia patients are required to provide sufficient material for comparison, 1 500 000 years of experience will need to be accumulated in the prospective study. Such person years of experience can be accumulated either by having a large number of subjects or extending the follow up over a long time. In general, prospective studies require a large number of subjects to be investigated and followed over a relatively long period of time; this approach is expensive and results are not quickly available. It is also evident from the preceding remarks that the vast majority of the subjects who enter the study can contribute relatively little to the testing of the hypothesis; this depends on how small a proportion of the subjects develop the disease.

Because of the volume of data that is collected in prospective studies there are variants in design to avoid the full costs of processing this material. In some studies the cases identified on follow up are matched with a sample of the healthy subjects and only data for this restricted number of individuals are processed. Because of the major task of coding records, in a study of leisure activity and subsequent health those subjects developing ischaemic heart disease, matched controls, and a twenty per cent sample of the total study population had their initial material coded (Morris *et al.*, 1980). In a study of the relationship of Epstein Barr virus infection to risk of Burkitt's lymphoma, blood samples were obtained and stored from about forty-five thousand children in Uganda; the rather complex virus studies were only carried out on the handful of children developing the lymphoma and selected controls (de Thé, 1978).

Although it has been suggested that the prospective study should enable data on possible aetiological factors to be collected in an unbiased way, it is possible that the initial investigation and subsequent follow up automatically modify the behaviour of participants. For example, a question that has been explored over the past twenty years is whether the dietary patterns of individuals influence their likelihood of developing heart disease. Case–control studies are suspect because the collection of such dietary histories is of questionable validity and the actual occurrence of heart disease may have affected appetite and attitudes to diet. Therefore, the collection of dietary data from 'healthy' subjects and their follow up have been considered. However, investigating an individual's diet can immediately affect the actual food that they eat, particularly when the study involves weighing the portions of food that are put out on the plate at each meal. Such a direct examination of an individual's behaviour can make him reconsider his need for a second helping, whether this is plum pudding or whisky! It is quite possible that such influence on dietary behaviour may not affect all the potential respondents in the study to the same extent, thus introducing bias. This is a particular aspect of observer error.

White and Bailar (1956) placed emphasis on the potential for bias where subjects were selected because they were known to have been or not to have been exposed to a specific factor. They suggest that the fact of exposure may have been linked to other characteristics that determine likelihood of disease. However, they do not stress that this is a rather atypical form of prospective study (though one that can occur in the occupational field—see subsection 10.4.2).

A further problem occurs in prospective studies in which contact with the individuals is made on several occasions over a period of time. The greater the number of contacts with each individual that are required or the longer the period of follow up, the more difficult it becomes to achieve a complete or nearly complete collection of data. The subjects who 'fall by the wayside' are extremely likely to be biased. This requires a careful balance to be maintained between the desire to extend the data collection and the possibility of over-contact, resulting in withdrawal of some of the subjects. The problem of bias from nonresponse has been discussed in subsection 4.2.3.4; in a prospective study, the drop-out rate is likely to be more crucial than the initial response rate. In the Honolulu heart program, 8006 Japanese men completed a questionnaire and were examined, 1871 only completed a questionnaire, while 1259 failed to respond at all. After ten years it was possible to compare the mortality of responders and nonresponders. The examined men had a significantly lower risk of death for all causes, cancer and stomach cancer; they had a nonsignificant increase in prostate cancer. Review of the cumulative incidence of discontinued follow-up among 5454 patients known to a thyroid disease register over an eight-year period varied between 5.4 and 8.4 per cent in different Scottish locations. This was due to patient movement, patient noncompliance or general-practitioner or clinician withdrawal of patients from the system. There was evidence of weakness in the usual method of communication (Jones *et al.*, 1981).

It has been suggested that a prospective study overcomes one of the disadvantages of a case–control study—the influence of past events and present health on memory. Attention has also been drawn to the effect of follow up on behaviour and drop out. In addition to these issues, the general points on the accuracy of epidemiological data raised in subsections 4.2.6.1–4 must be borne in mind in the planning, execution and interpretation of the results of a prosective study.

During the 1950s and 1960s a number of large prospective studies were initiated to study heart disease, chronic respiratory disease and cancer. Some of these studies have been mentioned in this chapter, while the major ones in the United Kingdom were reviewed by Alderson and Dowie (1979).

Findings are now appearing on twenty-year follow up, such as in the work in South Wales (e.g. Cochrane *et al.*, 1980), and ten-year mortality of civil servants (Jarrett *et al.*, 1982). In the past ten years there has been a tendency to pursue hypothesis-testing via case–control studies, or to extend prospective studies on chronic disease topics to major 'population intervention studies'. Projects involving change in diet, smoking, exercise, and detection and treatment of hypertension have been mounted in England and Wales (Rose *et al.*, 1980), Finland (Tuomilehto *et al.*, 1980), Norway (Hjermann *et al.*, 1981), and the United States (Hypertension Detection and Follow-up Program Cooperative Study Group, 1979); the English study was extended under the auspices of W.H.O. to Belgium, Italy, Poland and Spain (W.H.O. European Collaborative Group, 1974). This extension to intervention raises aspects of method that are further discussed in the next chapter.

6.4 Extension of the Method of Prospective Studies

The example discussed in section 6.1 was a study in which the survey had been carried out using a very simple questionnaire to classify subjects according to risk (in that case smoking habits). Two routine systems of notifying death and cause of death were combined in order to provide a semi-automatic collection of data on outcome. This section describes six different ways in which the entry and end-points in a prospective study may be obtained. Obviously where the study utilises retrievable data, rather than carrying out *ad hoc* field work to follow subjects, the scope for such work will vary from country to country and depend on (1) the information systems available, (2) the storage of retrievable data other than in conventional information systems and (3) attitudes to confidentiality.

6.4.1 Initial survey plus automatic end-point

In a number of follow-up studies, it is possible to link the basic data collected about individuals with routinely collected incidence data. For example, Rimington (1968) carried out a mass X-ray survey on a large number of subjects, and questioned them about their smoking habits and the prevalence of symptoms of chronic bronchitis. Following examination of the cross-sectional data, he studied the relationship between symptoms of chronic bronchitis and the subsequent incidence of lung cancer (Rimington, 1971). A list of subjects from the survey with chronic bronchitis was matched against an alphabetical list of patients with lung cancer registered in the region, which automatically provided incidence data for the study population. This use of routine morbidity or mortality data for the identification of the end-point in a prospective study is an extremely useful approach, since it avoids the necessity for extensive *ad hoc* follow up of the subjects.

Mention has been made in chapters 2 and 3 about the use of mortality and morbidity data for providing an automatic end-point in prospective studies.

An example has been given above of the use of cancer registration particulars to provide data on development of the malignant disease in the years following a mass X-ray survey. A more general end-point may be the recording of a death (with or without the cause of death). The N.H.S. Central Register can play a vital part in such work. This register exists for the purpose of assisting Family Practitioner Committees (F.P.C.s) to carry out the registration work of the N.H.S., by acting as a clearing house for the transmission of documents and information between F.P.C.s. The register has an alphabetical section (in order of surname and forenames), and a numerical section (in order of N.H.S. number) for the population of England and Wales. Provided that the N.H.S. number or full identification particulars (surname, forenames, maiden name, date of birth and address) are known, the register can be used to trace individuals. It is highly desirable if such tracing is to be carried out that the appropriate steps are taken in the planning phase of the study. With the permission of the subjects and the Registrar General, each individual can be traced on the register, and details of death provided automatically. Newhouse and Williams (1967) described the use of the N.H.S. Central Register, the records branch of the Social Security division of the D.H.S.S., the electoral roll, the national death register and the records of F.P.C.s in epidemiological studies. A specific example of this will be given in section 6.4.5.

The facilities available for the automatic tracing of samples of people or individual patients varies in different countries. A national follow-up study was carried out on all patients who had been detained in hospital for acute myocardial infarction in Denmark during two months in 1963. 646 patients were discharged after varying lengths of stay, all but four of whom were subsequently traced. The number of deaths recorded in the central files up until 1969 was 343. The remaining patients were traced using the population files, and a further fourteen deaths were identified up to 1969 and forty-two in the following years. Copies of the death certificates were obtained (since 1966, in Denmark, these have included a note of the autopsy findings), together with supporting data when there was insufficient on the death certificate. This material enabled the natural history of the survivors from infarction in 1963 to be quantified. The overall mortality was three times that expected—based on national rates according to age and sex. The influences of sex and age in 1963 and the total number of infarctions on subsequent mortality were also analysed (Geismar et al., 1973).

6.4.2 Ad hoc follow up

For many studies it is not possible for the outcome data to be derived automatically from routine mortality or morbidity systems. In these circumstances, it is necessary to arrange for a specific follow up. Truelove (1959) suggested that anyone who can make an unplanned follow up by assembling and analysing routine case-histories of patients with a particular disease can much more easily conduct a planned follow up. It is possible to identify a proportion of patients in whom follow-up data may be derived from available records. There is then a problem of tracing the remainder. Writing letters to the subjects will not provide many answers—there is no reply to some and others are returned marked 'gone away'. As soon as a response of 75 per cent has been obtained, the real work of follow up begins.

A second letter should be sent to those who had not replied, and the defaulters should then be traced using a variety of means. Those who might be dead could possibly be traced through local registrar's files or the Registrar General's quarterly alphabetical lists of deaths. For this one needs to know the approximate date of death because records for each quarter's deaths are bound separately. Visits should be made to the last known address of the untraced subjects and a door-to-door enquiry made. Use can be made of neighbours, the local post office and shops to yield some clue. When eventually the numbers of untraced subjects is reduced to a handful, considerable ingenuity and patience is needed to trace any further patients.

The sources of such information will obviously vary from one country to another. Modan (1966), in a study in the United States, found that patients initially treated by seven medical centres could be traced via hospitals (44 per cent), local physicians (16 per cent), letters to the subjects (13 per cent), relatives (8 per cent), health departments (7 per cent), neighbours (4 per cent), local authority (2 per cent), postmaster (1 per cent) and various other ways (including employers, military and federal archives, churches and funeral directors). As discussed with surveys (see subsection 4.2.3.4), an important aspect is whether the first 70 per cent who are traced are a biased group. This is likely to depend on the nature of each specific study.

Many studies of patients using this approach have provided interesting information about the long-term natural history of the disease and indicated some of the factors associated with successful outcome. For example, Easson and Russell (1968) reported on the curability of various cancers; Honey and Truelove (1957) identified the prognostic factors in myocardial infarction; Prior et al. (1970) followed patients with Crohn's disease for up to thirty-eight years to determine their mortality rate. Sims (1973) recently discussed the approaches used in a long-term follow up of a sample of neurotic patients.

Brunner et al. (1974) reported the incidence of coronary heart disease in a population followed up over fifteen years in fifty-eight collective settlements in Israel. Members of the kibbutzim were engaged in different types of work and it was possible to classify over 5000 men aged forty to sixty-four and an equal number of women by physical activity at work. In each kibbutz food is prepared centrally and eaten in a communal dining room; the job performed does not in any way affect the income or standard of living of the members. A sample of sedentary and nonsedentary workers was investigated. There were no differences in leisure activities, obesity or blood lipids concentrations of the subjects. Follow-up data were obtained from the physician attending each kibbutz; details were available of symptoms, signs and investigations, including autopsy following sudden death. This enabled angina, myocardial infarction and death from ischaemic heart disease to be identified. There was a two to fourfold excess of five categories of coronary disease in all age groups of sedentary males; similar findings occurred in the females. These results were obtained from a review of the clinical records of the patients. The study was only possible because of the special living conditions, stable population and availability of high-standard medical care in the kibbutzim.

6.4.3 Resurvey

In some studies the aetiological factors have been checked against the incipient development of the disease. In such cases, it is necessary to collect baseline information from the respondent and then, after an appropriate interval, to resurvey the subjects in order to detect symptoms, signs or positive investigations indicating development of the disease.

Morris and his colleagues (1966) examined a large number of busmen working for the London Transport Board. Material was collected on a number of postulated aetiological agents. For example, the subjects were questioned about symptoms of coronary artery disease using standard questionnaires and they were examined. Investigations recorded included an E.C.G. and blood-lipids levels. After an interval of about six years, a further survey of the subjects took place, which led to the identification of 'new' cases of coronary heart disease, some being symptomless but with evidence of a silent infarct on E.C.G. A detailed analysis of this material was then carried out in order to identify the contributory factors for coronary heart disease and their relative importance. Thus, such a study may involve a preliminary investigation of the respondents followed, after an interval, by a re-examination.

Some studies have extended this principle and the subjects have been re-examined a number of times. Two population surveys carried out in America at Framingham and at Tecumseh endeavoured to include in the survey all members within a defined age-range in a specific population. At regular intervals, the subjects were re-examined, in a longitudinal survey that continued over many years. Repeat contact with the subjects provided a more specific indication of any change occurring in a population over a period of time and a more precise quantification of the natural history of disease. Truett *et al.* (1967) analysed data on seven risk factors in relation to the development of coronary heart disease over a twelve-year period. This showed a striking gradient in risk when the combined effect of all seven factors was determined. Epstein *et al.* (1970) reviewed the design, progress and perspectives of the Tecumseh study, whose detailed results have been published in a range of papers.

6.4.4 Longitudinal study

Resurveying in its simplest form may be used in studies aimed at clarifying one particular problem. A comparable but more extensive approach is a longitudinal cohort survey in which a selected group of subjects is followed up over many years and contacted at regular intervals—but during this time the field of interest may change, and a number of different problems may be investigated in a series of overlapping studies.

The classic example in the United Kingdom was the study made by Douglas and his colleagues, who began by following up all babies born in a single week in 1946. Initially the material was used for examination of the problems of childbirth, including the risks of perinatal mortality in relation to the characteristics of the mother and her family (Douglas and Rowntree, 1948). The liveborn children, who were scattered throughout the country even at the start of the study, were followed up until they approached middle age. In its early stages, a large number of tests were used to collect information about the physical, mental and emotional development of these young children (Douglas and Blomfield, 1958). This was a considerable undertaking, which was facilitated by the provision of a large amount of routine and specially collected data from schools, including information on educational progress. Information was also derived from health examinations (Douglas, 1964). The children, who were followed through adolescence and after leaving school, have now entered adult life; many have married and begun to raise their own families. With such an extensive and long-running survey, there is the need for very careful planning in the initial stages and enthusiastic leadership of the research team in order to maintain motivation for the project over such a wide span of time.

There have been two other major longitudinal studies started in this country since the work of Douglas began. These are the National Birthday Trust projects which have been following up large numbers of children born in 1958, and again in 1970 (see Butler and Bonham, 1963; Kellmer Pringle et al., 1966; Butler and Alberman, 1969; Davie et al., 1972; Chamberlain, 1973). The work of the National Birthday Trust has been briefly referred to in section 5.5, where comment was made about the calculation of relative risk of perinatal mortality according to the father's occupation. A study of a similar nature was mounted in Newcastle upon Tyne, where 1000 families to whom children were born in two months in 1947 were followed up (Spence et al., 1954; Miller et al., 1960; Miller et al., 1974).

Goldstein (1979) has described cohort studies of the growth and development of children. Some aspects which he covered are of general interest, such as sampling, some of the practical considerations (e.g. tracing and gaining cooperation) and data processing.

6.4.5 Automatic entry and end-point

The fundamental principle of a prospective study is that individuals are classified according to the degree of exposure to aetiological factors before the long-term outcome of this exposure is assessed. Provided that the classification of the individual takes place before the onset of the disease being studied, it is generally maintained that the study has been documented in an unbiased way. Reference has already been made under case–control studies to the ability to conduct a prospective study economically (see section 5.4). This is an extremely valuable technique, and one that warrants careful consideration. Some people disagree that the approach can genuinely be classified as prospective, while others have used the rather inelegant term 'retrospective/prospective study'. Leaving aside this semantic issue, the basic approach is to retrieve routine material, that has been recorded at the time of exposure of individuals to potential risk, and then to match these data against the results of follow up.

Alderson and Jackson (1971) used this approach to examine the mortality rate from leukaemia in women who had been treated by irradiation for menorrhagia. Routine records from the Christie hospital were used to identify patients who had had this treatment, and these patients were traced through the N.H.S. Central Register. (This procedure of tracing individuals has already been described in subsection 6.4.1.) The particulars available from the initial hospital records enabled a very high proportion of the patients (96.2 per cent) to be identified on the national register. Moreover, the register indicated those patients who had died, and it was possible to obtain a copy of the death entry from the O.P.C.S. Using the standard technique for the calculation of the years at risk, and taking into account age and calendar period, it was possible to calculate the expected number of deaths by cause and to relate this number to the observed number of deaths (the statistical technique has been dealt with in subsection 3.5.2). In this way a combination of two routine sources of data—the hospital's records of those who had been given this specific treatment and the N.H.S. Central Register entry identifying the death registration particulars and hence the cause of death—provided an 'automatic' prospective study. The average period of follow up was 14.6 years, but the technique used enabled the total study to be completed in a relatively short period.

The case of tracing individuals through official registers obviously depends on how these records are organised. Westlund and Schulz (1972) traced patients who had been admitted to the infectious diseases hospital in Oslo for scarlet fever in 1918–25 and for diphtheria in 1920–3. To obtain a precise denominator each patient was traced in the Oslo population register until migration, death or residence on 1 January 1969. The cause of death was obtained from the national alphabetical lists of deaths, available from 1951 onwards. This clerical exercise enabled the mortality rates for hypertension-associated causes to be examined for the two diagnostic groups of patients and to be compared with expected figures based on national age and sex-specific mortality. There was no evidence of abnormal mortality in either the scarlet fever or the diphtheria patients.

One rich source of information for such studies is from members of unions or employees in organisations that maintain detailed records of recruitment of individuals, specific job locations, sickness absence, retirement and mortality. With the permission of the union and employer, access to such records can greatly facilitate prospective studies.

6.4.6 Automatic entry and survey

There are, of course, a number of variants of this general approach. Hill and his colleagues (1958) used sickness-absence routine records to identify women who were absent from work due to an infectious disease. These records were matched with a list of women who drew maternity benefit over the ensuing months. In this way, the routine data were used to identify pregnant women who had had an infectious disease during early pregnancy and who were possibly at risk of delivering a child with a congenital abnormality. This material was used to trace the mothers and contact them through their family doctor. Provided that the mother agreed she was visited and her child examined. Thus, by a detailed survey the research workers were able to identify the number of children suffering from congenital abnormalities with an adequate degree of certainty. This study combined two sets of routine data to identify those at risk, and then provided the follow up material by a specific survey to identify the outcome.

Another point of interest in this study was the special technique used to preserve confidentiality. The central authority wrote directly to the family doctor concerned and advised him that an approach might be made by a research team in regard to one of his patients. The patient was named in this correspondence, but, of course, this was only information of which he was already aware. The research workers did not know the patient's name but only that of the family doctor. They then wrote to the doctor saying that they would like to study a particular child recently born to a mother, who had had an infection in early pregnancy. Only if both the family doctor and the mother consented to the study were the identification particulars released to the research team.

6.4.7 Case–control within a cohort study

Section 6.3 has already touched on restriction of data handling to cases and matched controls identified within a prospective study. The point there was to economise on data handling costs of information stored on the complete cohort. Rather different is the concept that the prospective study should be limited to baseline information about all subjects who are then followed; in those developing the outcome of interest, and matched controls, detailed information may then be collected from (1) the individuals themselves, (2) their next-of-kin, (3) occupational or medical records and/or (4) other sources of retrievable data on potential aetiological factors. In this way the collection of detailed data is kept to a minimum within the overall framework of the prospective study.

6.5 Statistical Techniques

This section begins with a note on the quantification of attributable risk in prospective studies, using a simpler approach than is required for case–control studies. Life-table technique may be used in the analysis of data from prospective studies. Actuarial data may also be applied to measure the survival compared with a national or local standard and then to judge whether a 'cure' has occurred. Many prospective studies have been used to examine the factors determining onset of or fatality from disease. Brief mention will be made of the use of predictive techniques in this field.

6.5.1 Attributable risk

This measure can be derived by subtracting the rate of disease among unexposed persons from the corresponding rate among exposed individuals. This is much simpler than calculating this index for case - control studies. An important assumption is that other causes of the disease operate equally upon those exposed and unexposed to the primary factor being studied.

Table 6.3 Age-adjusted death-rates per 100 000 men per year from four diseases in nonsmokers and heavy smokers, with rate ratio, attributable rate and attributable rate per cent

	Death rates				
	Non-smokers	Heavy smokers	Rate ratio	Attributable rate	Attributable rate %
lung cancer	10	251	25.1	241	96
chronic bronchitis and emphysema	3	114	38.0	111	97
ischaemic heart disease	413	792	1.9	379	48
cerebral thrombosis	86	137	1.6	51	37
all causes	1317	2843	2.2	1526	54

Derived from Doll and Peto (1976)

Table 6.3 presents data from the prospective study of British doctors (Doll and Peto, 1976); age-adjusted death-rates are given for four major causes of death for (1) nonsmokers and (2) heavy smokers (i.e. consuming more than twenty-four cigarettes daily). These data are converted into (a) a ratio of the mortality-rates, (b) an attributable rate (the increment in the death-rate associated with heavy smoking) and (c) an attributable-rate percentage (the increment as a percentage of the death-rate in the heavy smokers). The rate ratio can be thought of as the risk to the individual of heavy smoking, and the attributable rate as that increment in the burden of disease on the population from heavy smoking. Comparison of the relative magnitude of these two indices presents the health problem in quite different perspectives: as far as the individual is concerned, the risk of dying from chronic bronchitis is increased to the greatest extent, while for the population, heavy smoking adds the greatest burden from heart disease and lung cancer.

Other aspects of the use of attributable risk have been discussed by Walter (1978). Morgenstern et al. (1980) pointed out that the measures of disease incidence used in epidemiological research were not quite so readily calculated or interpreted as is usually thought. They distinguish between the two concepts of risk and rate, indicate procedures for calculating these measures, and indicate considerations to be borne in mind before choosing the appropriate indicator of incidence. Tarone (1981) provides two summary estimates of relative risk that can be used for prospective studies with stratified data.

6.5.2 Life tables

Brief reference has already been made to life tables when discussing 'future years of life lost' (see 2.5.5), while further comment is made on statistical testing of differences in survival in the next chapter (see 7.5.3).

One of the common problems in a prospective study is to examine the distribution of mortality from one or more diseases in a cohort of subjects over a period of time. A simple approach is to present the fixed-interval incidence or mortality for the study population. For example, where a number of men have been screened on entry to a survey and checked a year later for the development of coronary artery disease, the material can be presented as the percentage developing the disease within one year. A prospective study will usually be comparative; the percentage of subjects developing the disease is compared in those who have and those who have not been exposed to the aetiological agent. Then, a relatively simple test of significance can be applied to check whether the proportion developing the disease in the exposed group is significantly greater than the proportion in the control subjects. (The appropriate test has already been mentioned in section 2.5.3.)

For many prospective studies, however, such a limited analysis would not be applicable; the date of entry to the study is constant and the survey is continued over a variable and often lengthy period. The follow-up period may not be a constant because some subjects leave the study for a specific reason, such as emigration. A method is therefore required that will enable this variation in follow-up time to be handled. The appropriate technique is the life-table method. This calculates for each specific increment in the follow-up period the number entering the period, the number leaving during the period and the number developing the disease. It is assumed that an individual not completing the follow-up period is exposed for half of this period, thus enabling the data for those 'leaving' and those 'staying' to be combined into the appropriate denominator. This is then used to calculate the percentage developing the disease, and the relatively simple calculation is repeated for each succeeding interval of follow up. Table 6.4 demonstrates the method of calculation; the technique has been described by Merrell and Shulman (1955). The important point is that this approach enables the material to be handled even if some subjects have been involved in the survey for only a short period and others for an extended period.

There are various reasons for incomplete follow up; these require consideration. The first is that some patients may be entered into the study a long time after others, and consequently are only studied for a short time. The technique allows their data to be included for this limited period, thus making available larger numbers of results for the first few times intervals. The advantages of this technique were stressed by Cutler and Ederer (1958), who pointed out that this approach improved the precision of the results. Incomplete follow-up in other patients may be because of development of the disease being studied, or due to death from this or any other disease. A third category is the subjects who are lost to follow up because of known migration or other reasons preventing continued contact. It is assumed that it is satisfactory to include such subjects in the study up until

Table 6.4 Life-table calculations for males with asthma

Follow-up interval in years (x)	Living at start of interval (O_x)	Withdrawn in interval (W_x)	Died in interval (D_x)	Probability of death during interval (q_x)	Probability of survival during interval (p_x)	Percentage surviving to beginning of interval (l_x)
0 –	762	4	106	0.139	0.861	100
5 –	652	7	41	0.063	0.937	86.1
10 –	604	3	56	0.093	0.907	80.7
15 –	545	186	46	0.102	0.898	73.2
20 –	313	238	21	0.108	0.892	65.7
25 –	54	46	3	0.097	0.903	58.6
30 +						52.9

Method

x = intervals chosen to best represent the attrition of the study population; unequal intervals permissible

O_x = initial figure is the number entering the study; subsequent figures are previous interval living less withdrawals and deaths

W_x = withdrawals in the interval (see text for definition of withdrawal)

D_x = deaths in the interval

$$q_x = \frac{D_x}{O_x - \frac{1}{2}W_x}$$

$$p_x = 1 - q_x$$

$l_x = 100 \times$ each p_x down to interval x

$$\text{S.E. } l_x = l_x \left(\sum_{x=1}^{n-1} \frac{D_x}{(O'_x)(O'_x - D_x)} \right)^{1/2}$$

the date that they were last known to be alive. This assumption is only acceptable if the proportion of such subjects is less than 10 per cent of the total number in the study group. If their incidence of disease or fatality is high shortly after they leave the survey, this will bias the results.

The percentage incidence or mortality is derived for each interval to follow up and plotted on a graph, the results providing a simple picture of the distribution of events in the study group over a period of time. Figure 6.3 shows how the results, in this case the survival of men with asthma, may be plotted. It is conventional to plot the results as the percentage remaining free from the disease or the percentage surviving, and it is usual to locate 100 per cent at the top of the ordinate.

The figure also indicates the confidence limits of the survival curve, that is, the limits within which there is a 95 per sent chance that the survival curve in an infinite sample would lie. The method of calculating this is discussed by Merrell and Shulman (1955). Though the method of calculation is indicated at the foot of table 6.4, it is not essential to master the algebra—as computer production of such statistics is now likely (rather than 'hand calculation'). The important point to appreciate is that the standard error at any point is based partly on the data available for earlier points; thus the confidence limits are narrower than if the curve had been based upon only the known deaths and survivors (and had ignored those 'withdrawn').

6.5.3 Assessment of cure

An extremely important issue, particularly for those involved in the treatment of malignant disease, has been the development of statistical techniques for identifying cure. Some malignant diseases are fatal for the majority

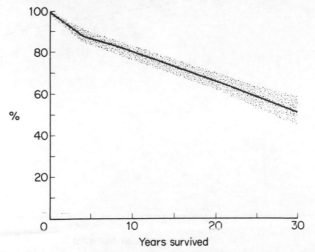

Figure 6.3 Survival curve and 95 per cent confidence band for 764 men with asthma
followed over a varying period.
Source: Alderson (1977)

of patients in a relatively short time, despite modern treatment. In contrast, patients treated for breast cancer have had a comparatively good survival rate throughout the present century. However, even after twenty years a patient may develop a recurrence of the disease and die. This chronicity of such a malignant disease makes assessment of cure extremely difficult. Two techniques have been used for examining this issue in large-scale studies.

One is based on the observed survival of a group of patients, calculated as indicated in the preceding subsection. Such data are plotted on semi-log graph paper. Immediate comparison is possible if a second curve of the expected survival of a group with the same age and sex distribution as the treated group is superimposed on the initial graph. The method used was explained by Lane (1968). The use of semi-log paper enables one to search for parallelism in the two curves, which would indicate that the subsequent death-rate in the two groups was identical. It has been suggested by Russell (1958) that this parallelism indicates cure—the treated group have achieved the same death-rate from all causes as the normal population.

A comparable approach is to convert the observed survival into an age-corrected survival, which is achieved by dividing the actual survival in each interval of follow up by the expected survival for members of the general population of the same age and sex composition. This 'age- and sex-corrected' survival may then be plotted on arithmetic graph paper, the point at which the curve becomes horizontal being referred to as the point of definitive cure (Berkson, 1942).

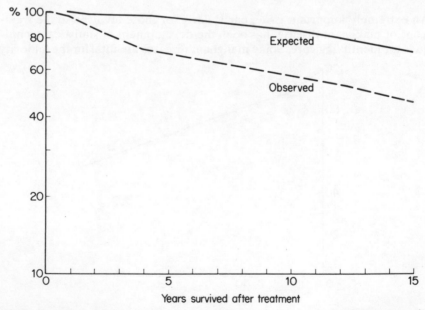

Figure 6.4 Comparison of observed and expected survival rates for 262 women with stage 1 cancer of the cervix followed for a fifteen-year period.
Source: Easson and Russell (1968)

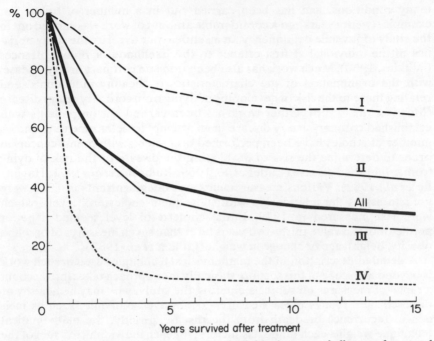

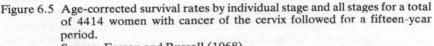

Years survived after treatment

Figure 6.5 Age-corrected survival rates by individual stage and all stages for a total of 4414 women with cancer of the cervix followed for a fifteen-year period.
Source: Easson and Russell (1968)

A number of examples of these two approaches to the identification of cure have been provided by Easson and Russell (1968) in a comprehensive review of statistics for patients treated at the largest radiotherapeutic centre in the United Kingdom. The two approaches to presentation of such data are shown in figures 6.4 and 6.5.

6.5.4 Prediction

Prospective studies can be used to examine the feasibility of prediction in various situations. The aim of prediction is to relate the characteristics of an individual to future events. In many of the present-day problems, whether these are the study of chronic disease, emotional disorders or even infection, there is a need to disentangle the relative influence of multiple aetiological factors and to quantify the influence of those on the natural history of the disease.

The usual technique for the development of a predictive instrument requires the identification of risk factors, and placing them in order of their impact on outcome. The independent effect of each of these risk factors and the degree to which they are present must then be related to outcome. Such work is a necessary preliminary to the planning of intervention studies for many conditions, and has been carried out in a number of fields. For example, twenty years ago a considerable amount of work was carried out in the study of juvenile delinquency, in an endeavour to relate the characteristics of the individual at first offence to the likelihood of repeat offences (Wilkins, 1960). Much work has also been done on coronary artery disease, with the examination of the characteristics of 'healthy individuals' and relating these to the risk of developing or dying from coronary artery disease (Morris *et al.*, 1966). Other work has been carried out on patients with established coronary artery disease in an attempt to determine outcome. A number of studies have been performed on patients with breast cancer, in order to determine the risk of developing the disease or the risk of dying from established disease (Cutler *et al.*, 1969; Bulbrook *et al.*, 1971; Haybittle *et al.*, 1982). Various measurements on college entrants in 1947 were used to assess the relationship with subsequent cholesterol levels, which were last measured in 1979. Initial cholesterol level seemed a better predictor of the value thirty-two years later than seven measures of baseline obesity, height, age or change in weight (Gillum *et al.*, 1982).

A detailed description of the mathematical techniques used in such work is beyond the scope of this section. Basically the approach takes into account a range of measures on subjects entering the study, who may be healthy or diseased, and relates these measures to observed outcome, such as incidence, recurrence or death from the disease. Briefly, the mathematical technique weights each of the risk factors; for each individual, the sum of the products of the observed value for each factor times the weight is determined. The distribution of totals is closely related to the distribution of outcome for the individuals. However, subsequent studies usually show that the relationship between 'prediction' and outcome is not as close as in the preliminary study. Armitage *et al.* (1969) stressed, in a discussion on breast cancer, that the prediction is likely to be less effective on subsequent data than it appears for the data from which it was derived. The techniques are only likely to be satisfactory when the available data 'account' for an appreciable proportion of the variation in outcome. If all the independent factors together still leave a major component of outcome unexplained, it is extremely unlikely that any satisfactory predictive instrument can be derived. The inability to explain the outcome in such an analysis may be due to a combination of factors. These include bias in the data collection, random errors in the measurement of various items, failure to collect data for a factor that is known to be relevant to outcome, failure of studies to have identified other major factors determining outcome and random variation in outcome. Also, the mathematical technique for disentangling the material may be forcing the data into a mathematical model that does not accurately demonstrate the biological relationship of the various factors and outcome. This problem can only be overcome by an appreciation of the issues involved and application of the technique only to appropriately selected variables with interrelationships that are understood.

Woodbury *et al.* (1981) have discussed the implications of the commonly used logistic multiple regression, indicating some of the properties that make it unsuitable for analysis of prospective data on onset of chronic disease (e.g. where the probability of incidence of the disease is very low).

They indicated how the appropriateness of the approach can be assessed and compared with other statistical techniques.

6.5.5 Determining the size of prospective studies

Some longitudinal studies are descriptive in nature; the issue to resolve is therefore the precision required of the various descriptive statistics. This involves an approach similar to that discussed in subsection 4.5.4; Schlesselman (1973) has set out the approach for such prospective studies, dealing with sample size, frequency of measurement and duration of study.

The ultimate comparison in a prospective study for hypothesis testing will usually involve comparison of the rates of incidence (or mortality) in the exposed and unexposed subjects. For simplicity the following comments refer only to incidence; it is assumed that there is one specific disease being studied, and the subjects are divided solely into exposed and unexposed categories (ignoring the additional information provided by variation in 'dose' of exposure). In the unexposed population the number of persons developing the disease will depend on their age distribution, the age-specific incidence, and the number of years of follow up. In the exposed population the relative risk of developing the disease directly influences the number of events. The other aspect affecting the power of a study to detect a significant increase in the exposed subjects is the proportion of the initial cohort who have been exposed to the aetiological factor.

The calculation to determine sample size is beyond the scope of this book, but is analogous to those required for intervention studies (see subsection 7.5.1). Lilienfeld (1976) presented a table showing numbers required; as a warning of the size that may be involved, where the relative risk is 2, and the annual incidence 1 in 1000, then 100 000 exposed and an equal number of unexposed individuals would be required for a 10-year follow-up period to detect a difference significant at 5 per cent. At the other extreme, with a relative risk of 10, and annual incidence of 1 in 100, then 100 subjects in each group would only need to be followed for one year.

References

Recommended reading

Goldstein, H. (1979). *The Design and Analysis of Longitudinal Studies: Their Role in the Measurement of Change*. Academic Press, London

Other references

Alderson, M. R., and Dowie, R. (1979). *Health Surveys and Related Studies*, Pergamon, Oxford

Alderson, M. R., Jackson, S. M. (1971). *Br. J. Radiol.*, **44**, 295–8

Armitage, P., MacPherson, C. K., and Copas, J. C. (1969). *J. chron. Dis.*, **22**, 343–60

Asperick, E., Jorde, R., and Raeder, S. (1974). *Acta med. scand.*, **196**, 161–9

Berkson, J. (1942). In *Carcinoma of the Stomach* (W. Walters, H. K. Gray, and J. T. Priestley, eds.), Saunders, New York, ch. 22

Brunner, D., Manelis, G., and Modan, M. (1974). *J. chron. Dis.*, **29**, 217–33

Bulbrook, R. D., Hayward, J. L., and Spicer, C. C. (1971). *Lancet*, **2**, 395–8

Butler, N. R., and Alberman, E. D. (1969). *Perinatal Problems—The Second Report of the 1958 British Perinatal Mortality Survey.* Livingstone, Edinburgh

Butler, N. R., and Bonham, D. G. (1963). *Perinatal Mortality—The First Report of the British Perinatal Mortality Survey.* Livingstone, Edinburgh

Chamberlain, R. (1973). *Lancet*, **2**, 1037–8

Cochrane, A. L., Moore, F., Baker, I. A., and Haley, T. J. L. (1980). *Br. med. J.*, **1**, 1131–3

Cutler, S. J., Black M. M., Mark, T., Harvei, S., and Freeman, S. (1969). *Cancer*, **24**, 653–67

Cutler, S. J., and Ederer, S. (1958). *J. chron. Dis.*, **4**, 699–712

Davie, R., Butler, N., and Goldstein, H. (1972). *From Birth to Seven: Second Report of the National Child Development Study.* Longman, London

de Thé, G., Geser, A., Day, N. E., *et al.* (1978). *Nature*, **274**, 756–61

Doll, R. (1959). Retrospective and Prospective Studies. In *Medical Surveys and Clinical Trials* (L. J. Witts, ed.), Oxford University Press, London

Doll, R. Gray, R., Hafner, B., and Peto, R. (1980). *Br. med. J.*, **280**, 967–71

Doll, R., and Hill, A. B. (1954). *Br. med. J.*, **1**, 1451–5

Doll, R., and Hill, A. B. (1964). *Br. med. J.*, **1**, 1399–1410

Doll, R., and Peto, R. (1976). *Br. med. J.*, **1**, 1525–36

Douglas, J. W. B. (1964). *The Home and the School.* McGibbon and Kee, London

Douglas, J. W. B., and Blomfield, J. N. (1958). *Children Under Five.* Allen and Unwin, London

Douglas, J. W. B., and Rowntree, G. (1948). *Maternity in Great Britain.* Allen and Unwin, London

Easson, E. C., and Russell, M. H. (1968). *The Curability of Cancer in Various Sites.* Pitman, London

Epstein, F. H., Napier, J. A., Lock, W. D. *et al.* (1970). *Arch. Environ. Hlth.*, **21**, 402–7

Geismar, P., Iverson, E., Mosbech, J., and Dreyer, K. (1973). *Int. J. Epidem.*, **2**, 257–63

Gillum, R. F., Taylor, H. L., Brozek, J., Anderson, J., and Blackburn, H. (1982). *J. chron. Dis.*, **35**, 635–41

Goldstein, H. (1979). *The Design and Analysis of Longitudinal Studies: Their Role in the Measurement of Change.* Academic Press, London

Hammond, E. C. (1966). In *National Cancer Institute Monograph No. 19*, U.S. Dept of Health, Education and Welfare, Bethesda, pp. 127–204

Haybittle, J. L., Blamey, R. W., Elston, C. W., *et al.* (1982). *Br. J. Cancer*, **45**, 361–6

Heilbrun, L. K., Nomura, A., and Stemmermann, G. N. (1982). *Am. J. Epidem.*, **116**, 353–63

Hill, A. B., Doll, R., Galloway, T. McL., and Hughes, A. P. W. (1958). *Br. J. prev. soc. Med.*, **12**, 1–7

Hjermann, I., Velve Byre, K., Holme, I., and Leren, P. (1981). *Lancet*, **2**, 1303–10

Holland, W. W., and Stone, R. W. (1965). *Am. J. Epidem.*, **82**, 92–101

Honey, G. E., and Truelove, S. C. (1957). *Lancet*, **1**, 1155–61 and 1209–12

Hypertension Detection and Follow-up Program Cooperative Study Group (1979). *J. Am. med. Ass.*, **242**, 2562–76

Jarrett, R. J., Shipley, M. J., and Rose G. (1982). *Br. med. J.*, **285**, 535–7

Jones, S. J., Hedley, A. J., Young, R. E., Dinwoodie, D. L., and Bewsher, P. D. (1981). *Comm. Med.*, **3,** 25–30

Jordan, C. W. (1952). *Life Contingencies.* Society of Actuaries, Chicago

Kellmer Pringle, M. L., Butler, N. R., and Davie, R. (1966). *11,000 7-year olds. First Report of the National Child Development Study (1958 cohort).* Longmans, London

Lane, H. R., (1968). In *The Curability of Cancer in Various Sites* (E. C. Easson and M. H. Russell, eds.), Pitman, London, pp. 129–39

Lilienfeld, A. M. (1976). *Foundations of Epidemiology.* Oxford University Press, New York

Merrell, M., and Shulman, L. E. (1955). *J. chron. Dis.*, **1,** 12–32

Miller, F. J. W., Court, S. D. M., Knox, E. G., and Brandon, S. (1974). *The School years in Newcastle-upon-Tyne 1952–62.* Oxford University Press, London

Miller, F. J. W., Court, S. D. M., Walton, W. S., and Knox, E. G. (1960). *Growing Up in Newcastle-upon-Tyne.* Oxford University Press, London

Modan, B. (1966). *Am. J. Epidem.*, **82,** 297–304

Morgenstern, H., Kleinbaum, D. G., and Kupper, L. L. (1980). *Int. J. Epidem.*, **9,** 97–104

Morris, J. N., Everitt, M. G., Pollard, R., and Chave, S. P. W. (1980). *Lancet*, **1,** 1207–10

Morris, J. N., Kagan, A., Pattison, D. S., Gardner, M. J., and Raffle, P. A. R. (1966). *Lancet*, **2,** 553–9

Newhouse, M., and Williams, J. M. (1967). *Br. J. prev. soc. Med.*, **21,** 35–9

Prior, P., Fielding, J. F., Waterhouse, J. A., and Cooke, W. T. (1970). *Lancet*, **1,** 1135–7

Reid, D. D., and Fairbairn, A. S. (1958). *Lancet*, **1,** 1147–52

Rimington, J. (1968). *Br. med. J.*, **1,** 732–4

Rimington, J. (1971). *Br. med. J.*, **2,** 373–5

Rose, G., Heller, R. F., Tunstall Pedoc, H., and Christie, D. G. S. (1980). *Br. med. J.*, 747–51

Russell, M. H. (1958). Symposium on presentation of results of cancer treatment. Seventh International Cancer Congress, London. Quoted by Lane (1968)

Schlesselman, J. J. (1973). *J. chron. Dis.*, **26,** 553–70

Sims, A. C. B. (1973). *Lancet*, **2,** 433–5

Spence, J., Walton, W. S., Miller, F. J. W., and Court, S. D. M. (1954). *A Thousand Families in Newcastle-upon-Tyne.* Oxford University Press, London

Tarone, R. E. (1981). *J. chron. Dis.*, **34,** 463–8

Truelove S. (1959). Therapeutic trials. In *Medical Surveys and Clinical Trials* (L. J. Witts, ed.), Oxford University Press, London, pp. 134–47

Truett, J., Cornfield, J., and Kannel, W. (1967). *J. chron. Dis.*, **20,** 511–24

Tuomilehto, J., Nissinen, A., Salonen, J. T., Kottke, T. E., and Puska, P. (1980). *Lancet*, **2,** 900–4

Walter, S. D. (1978). *Int. J. Epidem.*, **7,** 175–82

West, J. F. (1977). *The Times,* 2 February 1977

Westlund, K., and Schulz, C. (1972). *J. chron. Dis.*, **25,** 469–72

White, C., and Bailar, J. C. (1956). *Am. J. publ. Hlth.*, **46,** 35–44

World Health Organisation. (1965). *Technical Report Series No. 310.* W.H.O., Geneva

W.H.O. European Collaborative Group. (1974). *Int. J. Epidem.*, **3,** 219–24

Wilkins, L. T. (1960). *Delinquent Generations.* Home Office Research Unit report, H.M.S.O., London

Woodbury, M. A., Manton, K. G., and Stallard, E. (1981). *Int. J. Epidem.*, **10,** 187–97

7 Intervention Studies

A classic intervention study carried out over 200 years ago will be discussed. Although this is an example of a therapeutic trial, the principles involved in preventive, therapeutic and medical-care studies are comparable. It may seem rather surprising to find discussion of clinical trials in a text on epidemiology; however, there are several issues that require consideration in just the same way as in a prospective study. The actual introduction of a preventive or therapeutic measure adds little to the complexity of a study. The important points are the collection of baseline data, the separation of the subjects into two, or more, similar groups and then the collection of unbiased accurate data on outcome. Separation into groups involves similar issues to the selection of samples in case–control or retrospective studies.

Epidemiologists have been closely connected with the development of techniques used in clinical trials. Initially this was through involvement with preventive trials and now with intervention studies in the medical-care field. This chapter is provided to cover the basic principles and a number of the points relevant to planning, execution, analysis, and interpretation of intervention studies. This is particularly so that these principles can be applied to medical care studies; because epidemiologists should be familiar with the techniques involved, they may also contribute to the design and interpretation of clinical trials.

7.1 Basic Example

More than 200 years ago Lind (1753) carried out a trial of alternative forms of treatment for scurvy:

> On 20th May, 1747, I took 12 patients in the scurvy, on board the Salisbury at sea. The cases were as similar as I could have them. They all in general had putrid gums, the spots and lassitude with weakness of their knees. They laid together in one place being the proper treatment for the sick in the forehold; and had one diet common to all, the water gruel, sweetened with sugar in the morning; fresh mutton broth often for dinner, at other times light pudding, boiled biscuits with sugar and for supper barley and raisins, rice and currants, sago and wine, or the like. Two of these were ordered each a quart of cider a day. Two others took 25 drops of elixir vitriol three times a day upon an empty stomach; using a gargle strongly acidulated with it for their mouths. Two others took two teaspoonfuls of vinegar three times a day upon an empty stomach, having the gruel and other food well acidulated aith it, and also the gargle for their mouths. Two of the worse patients were put on a course of sea water. Of this they drank half a pint a day and sometimes more or less as it operated by way of gentle physic. Two others had each two oranges and one lemon given them every day. These they ate with greediness at different times,

194

upon an empty stomach. They continued for six days under this course, having consumed the quantity that could be spared. The two remaining patients took the bigness of a nutmeg three times a day of an electuary recommended by a hospital surgeon, made of garlic, mustard seed, *Rad. Rapham.*, balsam of Peru and gum of Myrrh, using for drink barley water well acidulated with tamarinds; by a concoction of which with the addition of cream of tartar they were gently purged three or four times during the course.

The consequence was that the most sudden and good effects were perceived from the use of oranges and lemons, one of those who had taken them being at the end of six days fit for duty. The spots were not indeed by that time quite off his body, nor his gums sound; but without any other medicine, than a gargarism of elixir virtriol, he became quite healthy before we came into Plymouth, which was on the 16th June. The other was best recovered of any in his condition, and being now deemed pretty well, was appointed nurse to the rest of the sick.

7.2 Principles of Intervention Studies

Despite the lead set by Lind, the introduction of formal trials was slow. Bull (1959) in a comprehensive review of the historical development of clinical therapeutic trials, has suggested six reasons for this delay: (1) reverence for authority, (2) the doctor–patient relationship, (3) the paucity of records, (4) the lack of facilities for investigation, (5) polypharmacy and (6) lack of active remedies. Some of these still apply today. In the early part of this century the experimental techniques were clarified in a quite different sphere—that of agriculture. An important contribution was made by Fisher (1966) to the method of experimental design. The Medical Research Council (M.R.C.) set up a Therapeutic Trials Committee in 1931; the role played by the M.R.C. extended after the Second World War, with the advent of many new treatments ardently extolled by their developers. A major contribution to the development of an acceptable method for trials of preventive or therapeutic agents was the work of Hill (1962). Any discussion of this pioneer work acknowledges the contribution made to the general acceptance of randomised controlled trials. Hogben was also responsible for clarifying the design of prophylactic and therapeutic trials (see Hogben and Wrighton, 1952).

The conduct of intervention studies requires consideration of the characteristics of the study population. Some mechanism of allocation to the alternative forms of intervention is needed; aspects of these issues will be dealt with in subsection 7.2.2, although there is further consideration of random allocation (see subsection 7.5.2). Assuming that an agreed protocol for the intervention can be drawn up and implemented, there then remains the task of collecting valid data on the outcome. These issues will be covered at the end of this section.

The points dealt with are all relevant to planning a study; apart from consideration and discussion with colleagues, computer simulation has been used to aid the design of clinical trials (see Madsen *et al.*, 1978).

7.2.1 Definition of the study population

The aim is to obtain two groups of subjects similar in all respects other than the introduction of the preventive or therapeutic measure to one group. Whether or not some subsidiary form of treatment is provided for the second group depends on the circumstances of the study. All the subjects are then followed up and, after an appropriate interval, data are collected to assess the outcome.

The first main point is to achieve two groups that are equal in all respects. In the past, the usual approach was to study the effect of prophylactic treatment on volunteers and to contrast the health of these volunteers after treatment to that in other subjects. This creates major problems, as was shown in the introduction of typhoid vaccine for use by the British Army. The success of this was supported by Professor Sir Almoth Wright, but at the beginning of this century an eminent statistician, Pearson, was asked to comment on the data. Records of the incidence of and fatality from typhoid among volunteers who had been inoculated were contrasted to similar statistics for other groups of the army in South Africa. Pearson (1904) stated that the greatest care ought to be taken to get homogeneous material, that is men of like proportion subjected to the same environment. He suggested that a request should be made for volunteers for immunisation, and a register of the subsequent health of these volunteers should be kept. Furthermore he advised that only every second volunteer should be inoculated. A sharp and fascinating correspondence ensued in *The Lancet*, with all the letters written by Wright (1904) challenging the views of Pearson and each of these letters drew a reply from the statistician. In three of his letters Pearson returned to the point that there had been no proper controlled experiment to determine whether a spurious association of immunity and inoculation had existed. It seems remarkable that it was a further fifty years before a controlled field trial of typhoid inoculation was reported (Cvjetanović, 1957).

For any intervention study it is usually essential to draw up criteria of eligibility for the trial. The aims of these criteria are usually to identify a group of people or patients in which the influence of various extraneous factors can be avoided. Thus, subjects in a restricted age group may be examined, leaving aside young children or the elderly. If the intervention study involves providing treatment for a disease, it is essential to have some method of classifying the extent of the disease, so that cases of similar severity are involved. Also, if there are known factors that can influence a subject's response to treatment, other than the severity of the disease, it is important to consider these and take them into account in defining the eligibility for a study. It is essential that all the relevant baseline information is collected for each patient. The necessity for this is partly to confirm that the two groups in the trial are in fact similar. It is then a relatively simple matter as a preliminary to the analysis of the trial data to check whether this is so. In addition to having this assurance about comparability, the collection of data on other factors enables a more detailed examination to be made of the results of the trial in a search for confounding factors and their interaction with the treatment under test.

7.2.2 Methods of allocation

Having identified the subjects that are suitable for inclusion in the trial, it is necessary to introduce a technique for the random allocation of the subjects into the treatment and control groups. Random allocation is a process comparable to the selection of a random sample discussed in cross-sectional studies (see subsection 4.2.2). Within a series of numbers, individual numbers can be allocated to either of the groups at random and the information stored. As each new patient volunteers and is found to be suitable, he can be given the next number in the series and automatically allocated to one of the groups in the study. In certain circumstances, it is appropriate to allocate the patient to a group without either the doctor or the patient knowing whether they are receiving the new treatment, an older, possibly less effective treatment, or a placebo.

In many trials, there may be a number of subsidiary factors that are known to influence the outcome or response to a specific treatment. If a heterogeneous set of patients are accepted into a trial, it may be an advantage to match the patients allocated to treatment and control groups. This can be achieved by a modified method of randomisation, by stratifying the trial into the suborders and then allocating the patients at random to treatment or control groups within the strata. For example, in trials concerning breast cancer where stage-one and stage-two patients may be included in the same trial, it is possible to stage the patients prior to their entry into the study and then allocate them to treatment groups within each stage. Extension of matching to several factors adds to the complexity of the trial and may create difficulty owing to small numbers in some categories. Peto *et al.* (1976) indicate that allowance can be made for prognostic factors in the analysis phase and there is hardly any need to stratify at entry in large trials.

In some therapeutic trials a 'crossover' design is used in which patients receive drug (A) and then drug (B), or vice versa. Hill and Armitage (1978) have discussed the design criteria and methods of analysis of such trials.

7.2.3 Standardisation of intervention

In the planning phase the study protocol must be drawn up and should include a section on standardisation of the regimes in the treatment groups. The aim of this is to reduce the uncontrolled variation in the treatment given to individuals in the study. Particularly in cases where the intervention involves treatment by a number of different members of staff (surgeons, physicians, psychiatrists, or ancillary staff) working in one or more centres, the standardisation becomes an important issue. Apart from variation in dosage in relation to the characteristics of the subjects (such as an agreed dose per unit of body weight), random differences in treatment should be reduced to a minimum, and where appropriate, mechanisms for the calibration and checking of conformity should be instituted.

7.2.4 Collection of outcome data

Assessment of each subject must involve a bias-free accurate measure of outcome. The approach to this may, of course, differ considerably according to the study. The outcome measure may range from a factual piece of information that can be recorded, such as the death and the date of death, to much more subjective measurements, such as variations in the level of depression for patients receiving antidepressants in psychiatric trials. The points that have been raised in subsections 4.2.6 and 5.2.5 on the collection of valid data are equally relevant to intervention studies. Wright and Haybittle (1979) have identified how the design of forms used in a trial can affect the validity of the recorded data.

Withholding information from the patients about the specific treatment groups to which they have been allocated may reduce the bias that may occur if the patients believe they are, or are not, on the more effective therapy. The observers, who ultimately record the response to therapy, can also be influenced if they are aware of the exact nature of the treatment that the patients are receiving. It is usual to refer to trials in which both the patients and the observers are unaware of the allocation as 'double-blind'. Some trials are termed as 'single-blind', with only one of the parties being aware of whether or not the new treatment is being carried out on a particular subject. Of course, if the treatments being compared are a major operation and radiotherapy, there is no possibility of withholding information from the patient or the observer. However, if the trial involves comparing two forms of mastectomy (such as radical versus modified radical or extended simple mastectomy) the patient may be unaware of the difference between these operations, and it may also be arranged that the observer collecting the follow-up information is unaware of which treatment the patient has received.

When considering the need to keep patients and observers 'blind' in the assessment of clinical trials, it is useful to examine a study reported by Batterman and Grossman (1955) who examined the influence of treatment in musculo-skeletal conditions. They studied the effect of aspirin and a placebo on the relief of discomfort and on causing adverse side effects. Initially, using a double-blind controlled trial, they found that a similar proportion of the patients taking the placebo reported relief and a slightly lower proportion reported adverse effects compared with those receiving aspirin or salicylamide. The initial results are shown in table 7.1. The authors' interpretation of these results was that a double-blind controlled trial was inappropriate in such a situation, because it had artificially boosted the effects of the placebo. They then carried out a trial in which initially only the patients were 'blind', and subsequently another in which the patients were 'psychologically prepared'. The patients receiving aspirin therapy were

Table 7.1 Variation in the effect of a placebo in patients with musculo-skeletal conditions on relief and adverse effects, depending on study design

Study design	Drug	Patients reporting		Number of patients
		Effective relief	Adverse effects	
double-blind	placebo	60%	17%	57
patient-blind	placebo	46%	12%	41
open	placebo	35%	21%	43
double-blind	aspirin	56%	25%	55

Source: Batterman and Grossman (1955)

informed that this was a new, very powerful drug and was the best treatment that could be obtained. Table 7.1 shows these further results. The authors concluded that it was necessary to have an open trial, in order to obtain a valid assessment of the effect of treatments. This was a most remarkable suggestion, since normally a double-blind trial is aimed at identifying the 'placebo effect', thus enabling one to check if there is any additional benefit from the new treatment. A more reasonable interpretation of the data is that there is little basic difference between the placebo and the therapy tested, until the patients' responses were biased by both the observers and the patients becoming aware of the design of the trial. This report suggested that if the doctor was not 'blind' in the assessment of both the relief of discomfort and the generation of adverse effects, he was likely to adjust his scoring of the measurements.

A very interesting example of this phenomenon was recorded by Heaton Ward (1962) who reported on a trial of a nialamide (a monoamine oxidase inhibitor) used in the care of mongols. The patients were divided into two groups and were assessed frequently by psychologists and nurses. Any changes in behaviour and mental age were noted. A placebo and the therapeutic agent were each given a code number and administered to groups of patients. Halfway through the trial the treatments were apparently switched—the declared intention being that each group should spend half the trial time on each treatment. However, unknown to all the other observers, Heaton Ward switched the code numbers on the containers halfway through so that the group of patients that had been receiving nialamide in the first half of the trial continued to take it in the second half, and similarly the initial control group still received the placebo. The observers thought that the treatment had been switched and this appears to have affected the results. Statistical analysis showed that the monoamine oxidase inhibitor was significantly superior to the placebo in the first half of the trial, and that the placebo was equally superior to the therapeutic agent in the second half. Presumably the drug had been correctly spotted early in the trial because of its side effects and the observers' bias in its favour had been carried through into the second half of the trial. This study provides a salutary warning of the bias that can creep into the observers' assessments.

At a simpler level, some of the outcome responses can be influenced even by the variation in the size, colour or taste of different preparations given in a trial. Hill *et al.* (1976) has indicated the difficulty that there is in obtaining preparations that are indistinguishable. This serves as a warning about assessing outcome from regimens that are obviously very different (when this is obvious to subjects and observers alike).

7.2.5 When is a formal study required?

In testing pharmaceutical agents there is a recognised path from laboratory work on the chemistry of the compounds, animal testing and human pharmacology, through clinical studies to general use of the agent. It is now conventional to refer to four phases of human study, in which phase I and II are exploration of the pharmacology, first on healthy subjects and then on patients (checking on the potential therapeutic effect and the side effects); phase III is the formal randomised controlled trial, while phase IV involves the more general use of the drug in familiarisation trials (by extended use of the agents in conventional practice, without randomised controls, but continuing to monitor outcome and side effects).

It has been pointed out that in the field of surgery there is need for a preliminary testing and learning phase with any new technique (see Dollery, 1978; van der Linden, 1980). The definitive technique may evolve over a number of years and premature exposure in a formal clinical trial may result in inappropriate rejection of the new method. This is really arguing for a parallel to the four phases of trials for pharmaceutical agents. This can be extended to all fields of intervention studies—preventive, therapeutic and medical care. There is a need to advance cautiously from the initial indication that the new regimen is potentially useful, through clarification of detail of the new approach, and assessment of its efficacy, safety and costs in comparison with conventional care. Only at the optimum time should the randomised controlled trial be carried out, i.e. after the learning period has been completed but before there is reluctance to expose patients to a control regime.

7.3 Advantages and Disadvantages of Intervention Studies

It is sometimes suggested that the problems of organising a trial, in particular the delay in mounting it, carrying it through and then analysing the results, are such that this approach is not warranted. Delay can occur at any stage, from the preparation of the protocol to the interpretation of the results. However, the history of medicine is scattered with examples of treatments that have been extensively used and have exposed patients to a range of side effects, but have been of no therapeutic value. The claims for benefit from such treatments have often stemmed from their use in conditions where the natural history is so varied that the patient may spontaneously improve, or where the placebo effect and the bias of the observers have resulted in spurious findings. Some argue that, in such a variable situation as the treatment of human beings, statistics cannot quantify the genuine response to treatment. However, it is in this very situation—where judgement of cause and effect is so difficult—that the carefully defined trial and the appropriate statistical analysis are required to rule out chance findings and the influence of some of the confounding factors. There is the problem of quantifying the multiple responses to treatment, particularly where the patients' response may involve a number of aspects, such as a general feeling of well-being, the relief of symptoms, an absence of side effects, and possibly, a decrease in mortality. In such a situation, only by carefully discussing the most appropriate measures of outcome and defining the precise way in which these can be assessed, recorded and quantified is it possible to judge the outcome of the trial and convey this to other practitioners in the field.

One reaction to proposals for a trial is that no comparison is possible because it would be unethical to expose patients to a less effective treatment than the standard one. Obviously the use of placebos raises serious ethical considerations, both for the treating physician and for the patients. *The Lancet* (1979) discussed this issue and emphasised that in many circumstances a trial will compare a new regime against the best alternative available. Lindley (1975) indicated how analysis can best be carried out when ethical considerations override aspects of statistical design. Hart (1946) discussed the exaggerated claims that had been made for gold treatment in the treatment of tuberculosis from 1925 to 1935 without any proof of the drug's effect having been obtained from formal trials. Reference will be made in subsection 7.4.3 to a trial of home versus hospital treatment (initially in an intensive-care unit) for myocardial infarction (Mather *et al.*, 1971; Cochrane, 1972). In the first report, after a few months of the trial, it was shown that there was a slightly greater death-rate for those treated in hospital compared with those treated at home. Someone reversed the figures and showed them to an advocate of treatment in an intensive-care unit, who immediately declared that the trial was unethical and must be stopped at once. However, when the table was shown to him the correct way round, he could not be persuaded to declare that intensive-care units were unethical! The argument that it is unethical to test certain treatments can in fact be phrased the other way round; the proponents of clinical trials would advocate that it is really unethical to introduce or to continue to apply treatments that have not been exposed to clinical study.

When a clinical trial has shown that a new treatment is not significantly better in its effects, it is sometimes suggested that there is a subgroup of patients for whom the new drug is particularly effective. An extension of this argument is that variation in dosage or drug combinations can influence the outcome. This aspect can only be studied by increasing the size of the trial and by extending the trial to different categories of patients and treatment regimes, so that the interaction of treatment and confounding factors can be quantified. In certain circumstances, where there is strong opposition to comparing a new treatment with a placebo, it may still be considered ethical by the clinicians concerned in the trial to use a homeopathic dose, or some other form of treatment that does not directly affect the issue being studied.

The following subsection will mention one of the original Medical Research Council trials on whooping-cough vaccination. In this study it was thought ethical to give the control subjects an injection of an antiviral vaccine. This had no effect whatsoever on whooping cough, but enabled the parents, children and observers to remain blind and was thought to be an ethical approach to providing an injection in the control group.

One particular problem occurs when studying rare conditions. It has already been pointed out that in designing a study thought must be given to the number of subjects required and that this number depends on the magnitude of difference between the outcome measurements in the two comparison groups (see subsection 4.5.4). Where a rare condition is being studied, particularly if the new treatment is unlikely to have any dramatic impact on the outcome, there is a need to continue the study for many years until sufficient patients have been entered into the trial. A long trial poses a number of problems. There is often difficulty in maintaining the enthusiasm of the staff involved, particularly when they hear no results about the actual outcome of their study. At the same time, if the trial continues for many years, other published research is likely to supersede the views prevalent at the time of planning the trial and this can make the issue being studied irrelevant in the light of advancing knowledge.

The number of patients available for a trial can be increased by using several centres, but this adds to the complexity of organisation and control of the trial. It is usually accepted that different centres may introduce some local bias, even if careful attempts are made to standardise the procedures for the assessment of subjects entering the trial, the treatment regime and the measurement of outcome. The important issue to consider is whether the variation between the centres is greater or less than the variation between the different treatment regimes; as long as the former is small compared with the anticipated treatment effect it is unlikely to prevent an adequate answer being obtained from the study.

Even for relatively common conditions, for which adequate numbers can be entered into a trial, there may still be a considerable delay before the results are available if a long interval is required before the outcome of treatment can be appropriately assessed. For example, such a situation exists in the treatment of breast cancer. Although it is possible to examine the five-year survival rate of this condition, owing to the relative chronicity of the disease and the tendency for relapse to occur after a long latent period, follow up for up to fifteen years may be required to identify any minor differences in outcome as the result of different treatments. It is, of course, extremely difficult to maintain enthusiasm for a clinical trial lasting for as long as this.

In some of the studies of medical care, the 'treatment' regimes may be very different and this can create difficulties in drawing up a protocol that clearly specifies the variation in all details. In the dietary study mentioned in subsection 7.4.1, there was considerable difficulty in organising the study so that (1) the subjects could be advised about their change in diet, (2) this could be tested at monthly intervals, and (3) an independent check could be maintained of the results obtained. Throughout the period of follow up, which extended over a number of years, it was necessary to supervise the subjects and their wives in the control of the diet and exhort them to continue the recommended regime.

It is inevitable in such studies that a degree of drop out occurs. Provided that the drop out has been anticipated in the design of the study, this should still leave adequate numbers of participants remaining in the treatment and control groups to provide an appropriate comparison. The analysis of the results becomes more complex where, in addition to drop out, there is a tendency for certain subjects to switch from one regime to another, for example, those subjects in the control (normal) diet group might hear about the advantages of low-saturated-fats diet and gradually change their diet themselves to conform to the treatment regime. This adds to the complexity of planning and analysing a study, but it is important to remember that these changes in behaviour are in fact representative of real life and attention must be paid to the number of subjects who either drop out or change their behaviour over a period of time. Such information is of great value when assessing the suitability of the treatment for general use.

A particular example of this problem has been the failure of patients to take drugs. The difficulty occurs when the patients maintain that they are taking the drugs, when in fact they are forgetting to do so or are even throwing them down the lavatory (see Schwartz *et al.*, 1962; Reynolds *et al.*, 1966; Gatley, 1968; Bonnar *et al.*, 1969). In many clinical trials independent checks have been applied to test whether the patient is in fact taking the drug. This issue has been raised by Porter (1969) who reviewed the literature and carried out studies on drug defaulting among patients under his care. He has strongly urged the necessity of checking medication in trials on ambulant patients.

The Coronary Drug Project Research Group (1980) discussed the difficulty in analysing results when there is considerable variation in adherence to the planned regimen. Even if patients take their prescribed drugs there can be subject variation in bio-availability of some drugs (see for example Shepherd, 1970). This may require modification of the basic design of a therapeutic trial.

Some workers advocate the use of other approaches to a formal controlled trial. They argue that comparison can be obtained in one of the following ways.

(1) With the use of historical data.
(2) With the use of volunteers receiving the new treatment who are compared with other subjects not coming forward for special treatment.
(3) By comparison of the results of the new treatment with national routine morbidity and mortality rates.
(4) By comparison between hospitals or between doctors—suggesting that, for instance, material may be collected from hospital A or from the patients of doctor X and compared with the results from hospital B or the patients of doctor Y.

Alderson (1974) discussed problems with these four sources of comparative data. It is usually argued that historical data, material from other patients under the care of the same doctor or from other hospitals, or national morbidity-rates are immediately available and that analyses can be carried out without the delay caused by mounting a prospective clinical trial.

Cranberg (1979) strongly advocated the heterodox view of the use of retrospective controls. Much as one sympathises with the wish to obtain a quick answer about the effect of new treatments, review of all such approaches suggests that they may be used to provide background information, but a definitive answer can only be obtained by a carefully designed and executed trial.

It must be emphasised that a trial may not reflect the real-life problems and standards of care. The trial situation may result in very careful selection of patients, greater numbers of staff and facilities for providing and monitoring the treatment and raised morale of patients and staff. The results of the study can show that in such special circumstances treatment A is better than treatment B; this only gives an indication of the long-term effects of introducing treatment A into routine practice for a wider range of subjects. Although this suggests that the trial situation may be artificial, it does not indicate that merely drawing up a protocol will result in a smooth-running trial—the pitfalls are numerous and it has been proposed that everything that could conceivably go wrong will, plus a few other things! A successful outcome necessitates close supervision of all aspects of the trial.

Schwartz and Lellouch (1967) discussed the general background to the planning of therapeutic trials and emphasised the need to consider two different approaches. One is the explanatory approach that endeavours to discover whether a difference exists between two treatments which is specified by strict and usually simple definitions. The second type of study involves a pragmatic approach, aimed at a decision. It seeks to answer the question, which of the two treatments should we prefer? The definition of the treatments is flexible and usually complex; it takes into account auxiliary treatments and the possibility of withdrawals. The criteria on which the effects are assessed should take into account the interests of the patient and costs in the widest sense.

7.4 Extension of the Method of Intervention Trials

The initial example in section 7.1 deliberately dealt with a trial that occurred many years ago; however, the application of this technique has only blossomed in the past thirty years.

The techniques used may involve preventive, clinical or medical-care trials. Attention is drawn to the extension of the principles involved in each category of study, in particular where this amplifies points made in the preceding section on the advantages and disadvantages of invention studies. It must be emphasised that the following examples are provided to illustrate and do not necessarily reflect the latest thinking on any specific topic (such as the control of heart disease by dietary and other measures, which is beyond the remit of a chapter on study method).

7.4.1 Preventive trials

Prevention is a term that may be used in a number of different ways. It has become customary to refer to primary prevention—the prevention of onset of disease in healthy subjects; secondary prevention—the treatment and cure of established disease; and tertiary prevention—the alleviaiton of discomfort and disability in established chronic disease that cannot be cured. This section deals with primary prevention. The first two examples are concerned with immunisation of healthy volunteers and automatic exposure of a defined population to prophylaxis. The third example is different in that it refers to protection of those 'at risk' or with precursors of disease.

From the 1930s the prevention of whooping cough has been attempted by vaccination; there have, however, been conflicting results from the many studies. In 1946, a Medical Research Council committee planned an extensive trial to test vaccine from three manufacturers in ten separate field trials (Medical Research Council, 1951). Parents were advised that such a study was needed and that some children would be inoculated with a substance that was not whooping-cough vaccine; parents and observers did not know until the conclusion of the trial which group the individual children were in. Those children between six and eighteen months who were entered into the trial were randomly allocated into two groups of approximately equal size. The vaccine was given in three monthly injections and the children were then followed up at monthly intervals by a health visitor to detect the occurrence of whooping cough. One-fifth of the children were visited within two or three days of inoculation to determine the severity of the reaction to the inoculation. 3801 children were vaccinated, and 149 developed whooping cough. The control group consisted of 3757 unvaccinated children, and 687 of these developed the infection. This gave an attack rate of 1.45 per 1000 child months in the vaccinated group of 6.72 per 1000 child months in the control group—a difference that was clearly significant. With few exceptions, there were no severe local or general reactions after inoculation, and in about two-thirds of the clinical cases microbiological confirmation was obtained. One particular manufacturer's batches gave a considerably greater degree of protection than the others. This trial was followed up by further tests of vaccines prepared in the United Kingdom, and also studies to examine the relationship between laboratory tests of immunising potential and their prophylactic value in the field.

In 1952 the British government sent a mission to the United States and Canada to study fluoridation and to advise whether fluoride should be added to water supplies in the United Kingdom. Acting on the mission's recommendation, the government decided to investigate methods of fluoridation suitable for use in Britain, to organise research to confirm the absence of hazards to health and to conduct a series of demonstration studies of fluoridation in selected communities. The major difference between these studies and the preventive ones discussed above was that communities were involved and not individuals. Fluoride was administered to a complete segment of the population by introducing it into the water supply for certain localities, and the study did not rely on volunteers individually agreeing to participate.

Three study areas were selected. Anglesey was divided into two zones, one of which was supplied with fluoridated water and the other with soft unfluoridated water. Watford, a mainly residential town just north of London, was supplied with naturally hard water softened before distribution and with fluoride added. This was contrasted with Sutton, another residential area, where no fluoride was added. Two Scottish towns, Kilmarnock and Ayr, were slected; both had soft waters of similar composition, but fluoride was added to the former. Baseline dental examinations were carried out to establish the prevalence of dental decay in children in study and control areas before fluoridation was started.

The preliminary report of the study (Ministry of Health, 1962) noted a very substantial improvement in the state of the teeth of three- and four-year-old children in the study areas; this was not apparent in the control areas, where only a slight change was observed. It was found that the three-year-olds had a reduction by two-thirds and the four-year-olds a reduction by half in the dental decay. Substantial improvements were also found in the dental health of five-year-old children—that is, children born before fluoridation commenced, and who would not be expected to show the same degree of benefit as the younger children. A second report (Department of Health and Social Security *et al.*, 1969) confirmed improvement in the temporary teeth of six- and seven-year-olds and in the permanent teeth of children of eight, nine and ten who had lived in fluoridated areas since their birth. There was also some information on the reduction in dental caries among older children who had not been exposed to fluoridation since birth. A particularly interesting aspect of the report is the material for Kilmarnock. After six years of fluoridation the burgh council reversed its decision and fluoridation ceased. Up until that time there had been a decline in the amount of dental decay, but subsequently there was a rise in the prevalence of decay. Both reports contained data on the possibility of side effects occurring in the population from the addition of fluoride to the water supplies; no evidence was found that there was any harmful effect from this action.

Jackson and his colleagues (1975) showed a twofold difference compared with controls in the permanent teeth (decayed, missing and filled) of fifteen-year-olds from Anglesey, with less marked differences among those aged five in 1974. This finding was due to the improvement in the dentition of the control children aged five from 1961 to 1974.

Wynne Griffith (1956) indicated some of the problems in obtaining support from the local authority in Anglesey for this study in the face of organised opposition from an anti-fl024oride pressure group. The influence of worry and rumour was also evident from the flow of complaints received after a council decision, when some members of the public mistakenly thought that fluoridation had already commenced. There has been a sad lack of progress in the implementation of the findings from this work. Wofinden (1974) showed how the actual demonstration of the alarming state of children's teeth could influence the appropriate local authority committee of the need for action.

Over the past thirty years there has been increasing interest in the primary prevention of coronary heart disease. Much work has been done to identify the various aetiological factors. The current philosophy is to identify those subjects at risk due to the prevalence of high values for one or more aetiological agents, or precursors of overt disease. Preventive measures are then concentrated on such subjects. This usually involves treatment of the precursors of disease, such as obesity, hypertension or raised serum lipid levels. However, smoking is associated with an increased risk of coronary artery disease and this is an aetiological agent that can be attacked directly. The complexity of the issues involved and the difficulty in providing clear-cut results, have hampered progress in this field.

A number of extensive trials have been mounted and a very clear description of the general method of one of these was provided by Heady (1973). This report deals with a multicentre trial in Edinburgh, Prague and Budapest aimed at the prevention of ischaemic heart disease by lowering the blood cholesterol levels by means of a daily dose of clofibrate. Samples of the male population aged from thirty to fifty-nine were screened with detailed history, examination and investigation; certain categories of patient were not included (such as those with previous heart disease or diabetes). This detailed examination collected in a standardised way information on some of the confounding factors associated with development of coronary artery disease. The rationale behind the trial was explained to the subjects, and men in the top third of the distribution of blood cholesterol levels plus half those in the bottom third were invited to participate in the trial. The aim was to enter about 5000 subjects in three centres. Half of the men in the top third of the cholesterol distribution were entered into the treated group, while the other two groups served as controls. The reason for including some subjects with low serum cholesterol was twofold. The men could be reassured that they had not all been entered into the trial because they were at high risk and also to provide a comparison group that should have a near-normal incidence and fatality from coronary artery disease.

After initiation of treatment the patients were followed up at six-monthly intervals for two years and then annually until five years had elapsed. At each contact they were questioned, examined and investigated; the purpose of the follow up was to identify any new events (such as the onset of angina, myocardial infarction or other disease). The opportunity was taken to analyse blood samples to check that the subjects in the treatment group were taking the appropriate drug. Some patients were removed from the trial for medical reasons (such as the development of coronary artery disease or diabetes). As anticipated a proportion of the patients dropped out of the trial for some reason; there was no evidence that the side effects of the therapeutic drug played a major part in this, but in one centre about a quarter of the subjects had withdrawn from the trial by the end of five years. (The subsequent results showed a higher mortality in the treated group, which could not be readily explained; discussion of this is beyond the scope of the present chapter—see Committee of Principal Investigators, 1980.)

Rose (1970) described a proposed trial for the prevention of heart disease. Reid and his colleagues (1974) reported progress in screening of over 12 000 civil servants, with associated randomised controlled trials among (1) those at risk of cardiorespiratory disease given vigorous anti-smoking counselling, and (2) those with border-line diabetes treated by diet and oral hypoglycaemic drugs. Other studies of this nature have been discussed at the end of section 6.3.

An important point to bear in mind is that the subjects involved in the above studies have some evidence of abnormality, but not of overt disease. This is an aspect of the search for precursors of disease, in the hope that intervention will arrest development of disease. The main epidemiological approach in defining the natural history of disease has already been discussed in chapter 6; the detailed considerations that are required before accepting a screening programme as national policy will be referred to in section 8.7.

It is now accepted that a rigorous investigation should precede introduction of screening for any condition; whenever possible this should involve a formal intervention trial (see Chamberlain, 1982).

7.4.2 Clinical trials

An example has already been given of a clinical trial carried out 200 years ago; since then the general application of intervention studies has been widely explored throughout the range of medical, surgical and psychiatric treatment. The aim of such studies is to clarify the influence of intervention on recovery from the disease in question or the ability to influence the recurrence of and mortality rate from the condition (secondary prevention). Rather than choose a restricted example dealing with the testing of a new therapy or surgical procedure, the problem of preventing a recurrence in coronary artery disease by a controlled trial of subsequent diet will be discussed.

Morris *et al.* (1968) reported a controlled dietary study carried out on male patients under sixty who had recovered from their first myocardial infarction. The aim was to determine whether a diet in which saturated fats were replaced by polyunsaturated fats would reduce the incidence of re-infarction. Specific criteria for inclusion in the study were drawn up. Only men under sixty with a first infarction confirmed by appropriate clinical detail were accepted. There were various criteria for exclusion covering a range of other conditions and the inability to co-operate in the dietary plan. Subjects entering the trial were allocated, at random, within the four participating hospitals to a diet regime or a control group. Those placed on the diet regime were instructed by dieticians to remove saturated fats from their diet, take 3 oz of soy-bean oil daily and control the intake of other fat to 35 g daily. The control group ate the diet that they would normally have. Data was collected at follow up of the subjects and this material was assessed by a review committee for any evidence of a relapse. The patients in both test

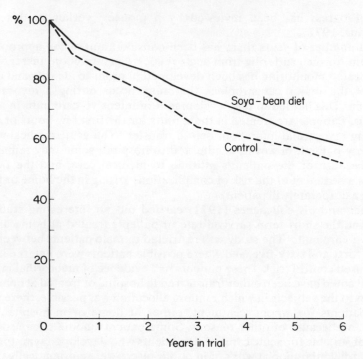

Figure 7.1 Percentage of men remaining free from relapse of myocardial infarction among those on a soya-bean diet and a control diet.
Source: Morris *et al.* (1968)

and control groups were supervised by the dietician and a regular weighed dietary survey was carried out.

Of the 199 patients on the test diet, five lapsed partially and twenty-five lapsed completely (this represented 11 per cent of the total possible time in the trial for the test-group subjects). There was an immediate, highly significant fall (22 per cent) in the serum cholesterol levels in the test group, with a steady rise from this low point to the end of the fifth year of the trial. From an almost identical starting point, the level in the control group fell by 6 per cent in the first six months and also showed a rise later. Figure 7.1 shows the percentage of men remaining free from relapse in the treatment and control groups. Sixty-two men on the soya-bean diet suffered at least one relapse compared with seventy-four in the control group. Of the first relapses in the test group forty were major compared with thirty-nine in the control group. None of the differences was significant.

7.4.3 Medical-care intervention studies

Over the past few years there has been increasing interest in the extension of randomised control trials from clinical studies to more general medical-care issues. Progress has been reviewed by a pioneer worker in this field (Cochrane, 1972).

For a number of years there has been consideration of the appropriate treatment for men suffering from acute myocardial infarction. Increasingly sophisticated monitoring has been developed in order to identify and avert some of the major catastrophies that may occur during a myocardial infarction. This has led to the development of intensive-care units in many hospitals. Patients are treated in these units for the first few hours or days following myocardial infarction, before transfer to an acute medical ward. Not every patient, however, is admitted to hospital; some may remain at home because of the patient's attitude to medical care, and the family doctor's assessment of the risk of complications arising in the home or from moving a desperately ill patient.

Mather and his colleagues (1971) carried out an interesting study to determine the short-term survival rate of patients treated at home and in intensive-care units. The study was restricted to male patients between the ages of forty and sixty-five, and where possible patients were entered into a randomised control trial. These patients had evidence of myocardial infarction and could have been either transferred to hospital or treated at home. In addition to the subjects in which random allocation was possible, there were some patients for whom treatment, either at home or in hospital, was decided on because of other reasons. Some patients' home circumstances were not suitable for acute care, while patients who developed symptoms of a myocardial infarction at work or in public places were automatically taken straight to hospital. Admission to hospital was not arranged for others, because the patients expressed a strong preference for treatment at home.

Basic particulars were recorded for all the patients and the case fatality rate at twenty-eight days was calculated. It was possible to examine this (1) for those patients treated at home and in hospital, who had been randomly allocated to place of treatment, and (2) for those who had been referred to hospital for specific reasons, or who had been deliberately treated at home. Table 7.2 presents the basic data from these comparisons. It can be seen that there was a lower case fatality in those randomly allocated to home treatment and as might be expected, a higher fatality for those who had automatically been transferred to hospital. The differences within the randomly allocated patients do not reach the conventional level of signifi-

Table 7.2   Percentage mortality at 28 days among men aged 40–65 with an acute myocardial infarction allocated at random and electively to home and hospital care

Place of treatment	Allocation of treatment	
	Random	Elective
home	10% (174)*	11% (106)*
hospital	14% (169)*	17% (754)*

Source: Mather *et al.* (1971)

*Numbers of patients in the subgroup

cance, but are most interesting because they do not support the contention that automatic admission to an intensive-care unit is beneficial.

The actual therapy provided for these two groups of patients was quite different. This immediately points to one aspect of medical-care intervention studies that differentiates them from the simpler clinical trials. There are other important considerations; treatment at home and in intensive-care units is related to major differences in the use of health-care facilities. Intensive-care units require complex equipment and a high staff : patient ratio; they are thus expensive to equip and to run. In contrast, the cost to the health service is considerably less for domiciliary treatment provided that there is adequate support in the home together with help from the domiciliary nursing service and a family doctor willing to be involved in the care of the patient.

The consideration of such trials therefore has considerable impact on the planning of care for such common problems as myocardial infarction, and for the management and deployment of staff in order to provide appropriate services. The above example indicates the basic way in which the technique can be used, the differences between a clinical trial and the medical-care intervention study being relatively slight from the point of view of method. Even in a clinical trial it is necessary to consider some of the wider issues, such as the requirement for staff and other resources in the delivery of care, and to assess in general terms the impact of the treatment of the patients. For example, in the study on diet to prevent the recurrence of coronary artery disease, due regard must be given to the acceptability of a treatment and whether it creates considerable stress within the family. The emotional impact of trying to maintain an unpleasant diet may have a considerable effect on the patient's satisfaction and a position can be reached where the majority of patients would rather not continue the 'curative diet'. Another aspect to be considered is the cost of the different treatments, and on occasion these become appreciable.

Other trials in the medical-care field have examined the effect of different lengths of stay in hospital with otherwise identical treatment. For example, the possibility of a shorter stay has been examined in the treatment of coronary artery disease (Hayes *et al.*, 1974; Boyle *et al.*, 1973), surgical treatment for hernias (Morris *et al.*, 1968) and haemorrhoids (Anscombe *et al.*, 1974). Other studies have used a combination of different locations and different treatments—for example, in a study on the surgical treatment of varicose veins, operative treatment with a conventional inpatient stay has been contrasted with injection therapy as an outpatient (Chant *et al.*, 1972). This study showed that the interval before returning to work was significantly shorter with outpatient treatment and was associated with increased patient satisfaction. Assessment of the health-service resources required for the two different forms of care showed a major saving in finance in the care of outpatient treatment. A rather unique example followed an R.C.T performed on short stay following hernia and varicose vein operations. Examination of the lengths of stay obtained from H.A.A. suggested that these changed in the trial locality compared with adjacent localities over the subsequent two years (Adler, 1978). There is a need to extend the application of such intervention studies to an examination of differences in the ways of providing community care. The future has been indicated by Bennett (1974), and by Knox and Morrell (1974) who reviewed work in this field, including an investigation of the role of the community hospital and various ways of delivering primary medical care. However, by extending the scope of the enquiry to such issues, the difficulty of arranging random allocation and bias-free assessment of outcome becomes extremely great.

7.5 Statistical Techniques

The method of deriving the numbers required in a survey has already been mentioned in subsection 4.5.4; a comparable approach is required in clinical trials and has been touched on at the beginning of this chapter. Mention has also been made in this chapter of the random allocation of individuals; the random selection of subjects has been dealt with in detail in subsection 4.2.2. However, the allocation of subjects to treatment and control groups in intervention trials poses additional problems and attention will be given to these aspects. Subsection 7.5.3 introduces the concepts of the logrank test on outcome data from an intervention study and indicates how the significance of the results may be assessed. This is followed by a brief note on the use of sequential analysis.

7.5.1 Numbers required in a fixed-size trial

Estimation of the number of subjects required for surveys has already been dealt with in subsection 4.5.4; a similar technique is used for calculating the expected numbers in an intervention trial. It requires estimates of the anticipated findings in the two comparison groups, the level of significance required to exclude chance findings and the risk that the research workers are prepared to take of reaching a negative finding by chance, when in the long run a positive finding might have been achieved. It is usual to suggest that a 5 per cent level of significance will be required and that a 1 in 10, or 1 in 20, chance of failing to observe a real difference may be justified. The smaller the difference in outcome that is expected between the two treatment groups, the higher the level of significance that is required or the smaller the chance that is considered acceptable of missing a positive finding, the larger the number of subjects required in the trial. Even in a dialogue between a research worker and a statistical advisor, clarification of the parameters to select is not straightforward. A realistic appraisal of the anticipated benefits from the new treatment is perhaps the most difficult to achieve.

The conventional calculation of the anticipated size of a trial depends on the assumption that a clear-cut measure of outcome can be defined—for example, the excess proportion relieved or cured, the proportion living without relapse or suffering from a fatal recurrence. However, it is a major assumption to consider that a single index can provide a realistic picture of the overall benefit from a treatment. The patient may be interested in pain relief, lack of distressing symptoms, a feeling of well-being, a reduction in anxiety, the ability to sleep, the lack of side effects and many other aspects, rather than a simple consideration of the reduction in fatality rate from the treatment. Organisational considerations may be important, such as the frequency with which the patient has to attend or be admitted to hospital and the length of treatment; these aspects have financial and other implications for the health service. Some treatments require rare drugs, or facilities and equipment that are expensive. All these issues have to be considered in making a transition from a judgement of effectiveness to a judgement of efficiency—and it is the latter that is really required before new treatments are introduced into the health service (with the rigid boundaries to its financial resources). A calculation depending on a simple index of outcome is forcing the clinician into a strait-jacket in his consideration of the study. This point has been stressed by Oldham (1968). These general issues require careful consideration in planning studies and are an indication of the need to avoid a too rigid adherence to a mathematical determination of sample size, based on incomplete comprehension of the issues at stake.

Many clinical studies have been based on small numbers of subjects: thus there is a possibility of an effective treatment being rejected. As with other surveys, pressures (lack of adequate numbers of patients to enter into the study, limited time, lack of staff, and lack of other resources) may be placed on the research workers to limit the size of a study. The main issue is that a result from a small trial showing a nonsignificant difference between the new and conventional treatments may often be interpreted as the new treatment is no better. However, the real interpretation should be that although there is no significant difference between the two treatments tested, the findings are compatible with an appreciable benefit in a larger series. Wulff (1973) discussed this issue in a short note and stressed the importance of quoting the confidence limits of any clinical trial. These limits can indicate the range of findings with which the study is compatible, and he provided two tables that enable the specific results of a study to be readily supplemented by an estimate of confidence intervals.

The basic method has been described with specific reference to clinical trials by Boag et al. (1971). These authors provided three graphs from which the research worker can read off the numbers required to participate in a clinical trial provided that the worker has a clear idea of (1) the anticipated percentage benefit of the two treatments, (2) the significance level required for testing the results and (3) the power of the study design that is desired. This matter has been taken further by Schork and Remington (1967), who dealt with the treatment–control comparison for chronic-disease studies in which drop out or nonadherence to one or other of the regimes is likely to create a problem. Consideration of these issues increases the sample size required. Further elaboration of the principles in estimating sample size in trials in which the patients are going to be entered over a period have been provided by Pasternak (1972), and George and Desu (1974). Both these papers provide tables that enable the research worker to identify the numbers required in particular studies.

A number of authors have stressed the inadequate size of many clinical trials; Peto *et al.* (1976) point out that a *p*-value from a large trial is usually stronger evidence of an effect than the same-sized *p*-value from a small trial (the confidence limits of the former will be narrower).

7.5.2 Random allocation

The important basis of an intervention study is that comparable groups of subjects are allocated to both the treatment and control groups. A preventive trial involves healthy subjects, while clinical-trial studies consider patients. In either case, it is usually necessary to screen subjects to check that they fall within the acceptance criteria of the study. There may be a restriction on age, or exclusion of subjects because of confounding factors, such as the presence of another disease. Confirmation of particular characteristics, such as first myocardial infarctions, is also required. Having been screened and identified as suitable for the trial, the patients should then be asked if they are willing to participate. When the subject has agreed the individual should be formally entered into the trial and allocated at random to one of the groups. This may be done by preparing a sequence of numbers, each of which is then allocated at random to the treatment or the control group. Alternatively, it may be done by using random-number tables; starting at a chosen page, and a random point on that page, numbers are then read off in turn and if the number is odd the next number on the list is allocated to the treatment group and if the number is even the next number is included in the control group. Perhaps a simpler approach to understand is the use of a coin; this is spun to allocate each of the numbers. Thus if the coin comes down 'heads', the next number may be allocated to the treatment and if 'tails', to the control group. In many trials, there may be more than two subgroups required and this means allocating the numbers to one of three or more categories. Again the random-number tables can be used. For example, if three categories are required, digits 1, 2 and 3 can be allocated to treatment A, digits 4, 5 and 6 allocated to treatment B, and digits, 7, 8 and 9 allocated to treatment C (digit 0 is ignored). Starting at a place chosen at random, the digits are again read out from the tables and consecutive numbers on the list are allocated to treatment groups according to this pattern. A little ingenuity in the use of random-number tables enables appropriate allocation to occur, however many subgroups are required.

In the past some workers have used more open methods, such as the date of admission to hospital (subjects were allocated to one treatment group on odd dates and to another on even dates). An example of a trial using this technique is that of Wright and his colleagues (1948, 1950), who studied the use of anticoagulants in the treatment of patients with myocardial infarction. The difference from a 50/50 allocation, which one would have expected if the method was random, was significant even in the initial phase of the trial involving 800 patients; this is shown in Table 7.3. A further 231 patients were entered into the trial and the discrepancy from the expected figures became even more marked. In the second phase of the study 68 per cent of

Table 7.3   Unequal distribution of patients to two treatment groups in a trial using
the day of hospital admission as the allocation method

Phase of trial	Treatment group		Number of patients
	Control	Anticoagulant	
initial phase	46%	54%	800
second phase	32%	68%	231

Source: Wright *et al.* (1948, 1950)

the patients were allocated to the treatment. Alderson (1974) suggested
that, in the initial phase of this multicentre trial, a number of consultants
were excluding patients from entry into the trial on control dates because
they wished the patient to have the anticoagulant treatment. Also, the
preliminary results of the trial were made known while the study was still in
progress and the reported benefits from anticoagulant therapy appear to
have further affected the proportion of patients entered into the control
group in the second phase of the study.

In many trials there may be a desire to balance the number of subjects
allocated to treatment and control therapy. With many centres participating
and their patients divided into subgroups, random allocation can lead to an
uneven distribution between treatment and control within the subgroups.
The technique to overcome this is to balance the number within a fixed
figure. For example, within ten subjects the allocation can be random but
ensuring that five subjects are in the treatment and five in the control group.
This adds slightly to the complexity of allocation, but means that within any
batch of ten as soon as five patients have been allocated to either treatment
or control, the remainder are automatically allocated to the other category.

In certain circumstances the preliminary screening cannot automatically
ensure that some patients are suitable for a particular subgroup in a trial. For
instance in a trial involving treatment of breast cancer by surgery, different
operations are performed for patients with stage-one disease and stage-two
disease, and within these stages there was a difference in the proposed
regime for subsidiary treatment by radiotherapy. Although the patients
were entered on clinical grounds, it was not until an operation had taken
place that it was found that some patients did not have a malignant disease,
or that they had unexpected glands in the axilla, indicating that the clinical
stage had been incorrect. Then, there is a need to exclude or reallocate some
patients, and a decision has to be made as to whether the initial allocation
number should be reused by a replacement patient.

7.5.3 The logrank test

An extension of life table analysis of clinical trial results (see subsection
6.5.2 for the method) is the logrank test of the data. The approach was
suggested by Mantel (1966) and has been clearly described by Peto *et al.*

(1977). Considering just deaths occurring in two treatment groups A and B, the logrank test compares for any particular day of follow up the observed and expected numbers of deaths in the two treatment groups. The expected number of deaths is based on the total deaths occurring for that specific day of follow up; it is divided in proportion to the numbers of survivors in each of the treatment groups on the specific day. As a very simplified example, if on day 28 after initial treatment there are 100 patients remaining in treatment group A and 75 in group B, and 14 deaths occur on that day, 8 would be expected in the A and 6 in the B group. Suppose there had actually been 7 in both treatment groups, one could compare the 'relative death rates' for the two groups: A = 7/8 = 0.875, and B = 7/6 = 1.167. (Such a calculation need only be carried out for any day on which at least one death occurs—otherwise the expected figure is zero.)

This leads on to the comparison between the two treatment groups, which can be carried out for appropriate periods of follow up (e.g. the complete span of a five-year trial, and divisions of: first year, second and third years, and fourth and fifth years). The decision about subdivisions will depend on the survival curve for the particular condition being studied, though one focus of interest will always be the comparison for the total period of the study. An important aspect of such a comparison is not 'Is there a difference in the "relative death rates"?', but 'Is there a difference unlikely to have occurred by chance?'. This can readily be tested by calculating χ^2 (as in the formula set out in 4.5.2); the number of treatment groups less one determines the degrees of freedom and the standard tables provide the figures for the probability of the observed results. Table 7.4 sets out a worked example for calculating the logrank statistics and performing the test of significance.

Table 7.4 Simplified layout of results from an hypothetical trial of two treatments, with calculation of log rank statistics and test of significance of results at end of week 52

Week	Number of Patients Group 1	Group 2	Total	Observed Deaths Group 1	Group 2	Total	Expected Deaths Group 1	Group 2
1	137	123	260	7	3	10	5.27	4.73
2	130	120	250	5	4	9	4.68	4.32
3	125	116	241	2	3	5	2.59	2.41
4	123	113	236	1	0	1	0.52	0.48
⋮	⋮	⋮	⋮	⋮	⋮	⋮	⋮	⋮
52	43	54	97	1	1	2	0.89	1.11
total				95	70	165	78.39	86.61

$$\chi^2 = \frac{(O_1 - E_1)^2}{E_1} + \frac{(O_2 - E_2)^2}{E_2}$$

$$= \frac{(16.61)^2}{78.39} + \frac{(16.61)^2}{86.61}$$

$$= 6.71$$

$p < 0.01$, on 1 degree of freedom

Though the above text and the worked example consider deaths in two treatment groups, life tables and the logrank test are applicable to all forms of intervention trial where there is a defined date of entry for each subject, and the identification of a specific outcome event on follow up. The above description is very limited, but should serve to indicate the role of this approach. Peto *et al.* (1977) provide a much more extensive explanation for the nonmathematical reader, including further worked examples where the actual computation is relatively easy.

The dangers of too small a study have already been indicated. If several trials have been reported in the literature, the results may be combined to overcome the deficiency of numbers in the individual studies; Peto *et al.* (1977) describe how this should be done.

7.5.4 Sequential analysis

Many workers involved in running clinical trials wish to obtain results as soon as possible, so that the clinicians can use the 'better' treatment on all their patients without any delay. Such an approach is, however, not directly compatible with fixed-size trials. In such trials, after due consideration of the anticipated effect of the two regimes, a decision is made about the number of cases to be entered into it. For statistical reasons, having decided on such a trial, it is then inappropriate to 'peep' at the results as these accrue. The clinicians have to wait patiently until the appropriate number of cases have been entered into the trial and follow-up data are available. Only then can definitive analysis occur. There is, however, one specific statistical technique that is appropriate to the ongoing monitoring of results as they become available; this is sequential analysis. Sequential analysis is a development of the cusum technique discussed in section 3.5.1. In the United Kingdom, Armitage (1975) has been the main proponent of this method in the medical field and has discussed the particular situations in which application of this analysis may be appropriate.

In one approach the subjects are allocated in pairs, one receiving the test treatment and the other being a control. Where there is a simple yes/no answer to the outcome (such as the case fatality within twenty-eight days), the answer for the pair can be one of three, that is both died, one lived and one died, or both lived. In cases where both lived or both died, the answers contribute nothing to a consideration of the relative effectiveness of the two treatments. Only when one of the pair survived and not the other is there any useful information (although consideration of the proportion who died is useful in assessing the result of treatment). These results can be plotted on a chart, which is designed so that with benefit from treatment a straight-line graph of slope + 1 is obtained, and with 'benefit' from the control regime a straight-line graph of slope − 1 is obtained. As each of the results comes in from the pairs entered into the trial, the line is extended. With the appropriate specification of the anticipated results it is possible to draw boundaries on the chart which indicate when a statistically significant excess of positive or negative results has occurred. An example of plotting of the preliminary results from a trial is shown in figure 7.2.

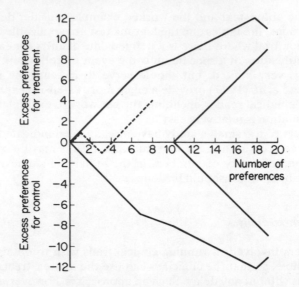

Figure 7.2 Sequential analysis plan in which a significance level of 0.05 for stopping
was required, together with a power of 0.95; the probability of a
have been entered on the chart.
Source: Aronstam and Arblaster (1974)

In many trials the clinicians involved are concerned at the thought of a
fixed-size trial continuing long after a definite result is available within the
collected material. One approach to this issue is to plan the trial as a
fixed-size trial, but to arrange for parallel sequential analysis. Such a
precaution is a useful strategy in the organisation of the trial, but it is
extremely rare for unexpected excellent results to occur with a new
treatment—the usual tendency is for the clinicians to be over-optimistic
about the anticipated benefits.

The technique is suitable where there is a clear outcome that can be
allocated into a yes/no category and where the outcome occurs relatively
soon after entry of the subject into the trial. There would be no point in
considering sequential analysis where a five-year survival rate was used as
the outcome—the whole point of the trial is to stop entering patients as soon
as a significant result is reached, and this is not compatible with a long
treatment or result interval. It must be borne in mind that the specification of
the anticipated results creates considerable difficulty. The boundaries for a
trial having been laid down, these should not be altered even if the results are
very different from those expected. The matter has been discussed by
Oldham (1968). It does appear, however, that the technique of sequential
analysis has a real, if limited, place when the appropriate conditions for its
use can be met. The technique is more suited to certain therapeutic trials
than intervention studies of prevention (with long lag to outcome), or
medical care (where a number of disparate measures of results are collected).

References

Recommended reading

Hill, A. B. (1962). *Statistical Methods in Clinical and Preventive Medicine*. Livingstone, Edinburgh
Peto, R., Pike, M. C., and Armitage, P., *et al.* (1976). *Br. J. Cancer*, **34**, 585–612
Peto, R., Pike, M. C., and Armitage, P., *et al.* (1977). *Br. J. Cancer*, **35**, 1–39

Other references

Adler, M. W. (1978). *J. Epidem.* Comm. Hlth, **32**, 143–6
Alderson, M. R. (1974). *Geront. Clin.*, **16**, 76–87
Anscombe, A. R., Hancock, B. D., and Humphreys, W. B. (1974). *Lancet*, **2**, 250–3
Armitage, P. (1975). *Sequential Medical Trials* (second edn.), Blackwell, Oxford
Aromstam, A., and Arblaster, P. (1974). Personal communication
Batterman, R. C., and Grossman, A. J. (1955). *J. Am. med. Ass.*, **159**, 1619–22
Bennett, A. E. (1974). *Br. med. Bull.*, **30**, 223–7
Boag, J. W., Haybittle, J., Fowler, J. N., and Emery, F. W. (1971). *Br. J. Radiol.*, **44**, 122–5
Bonnar, J., Goldberg, A., and Smith, J. A. (1969). *Lancet*, **1**, 457–8
Boyle, J. A., and Lorimer, A. R. (1973). *Lancet*, **2**, 346–9
Bull, J. P. (1959). *J. chron. Dis.*, **10**, 218–48
Chamberlain, J. (1982). Screening for early detection of cancer: general principles. In *Prevention of Cancer* (M. R. Alderson, ed.), Arnold, London, pp. 227–58
Chant, A. D. B., Jones, H. O., and Weddell, J. M. (1972). *Lancet*, **2**, 1188–91
Cochrane, A. L. (1972). *Effectiveness and Efficiency–Random Reflections on Health Services*. Nuffield Hospitals Provincial Trust, London
Committee of Principal Investigators (1980). *Lancet*, **2**, 379–85
Coronary Drug Project Research Group (1980). *New Engl. J. Med.*, **303**, 1038–41
Cranberg, L. (1979). *Br. med. J.*, **2**, 1265–6
Cvjetanović, B. B. (1957). *Am. J. publ. Hlth.*, **47**, 578–81
Department of Health and Social Security, Scottish Office, Welsh Office, and Ministry of Housing and Local Government (1969). *The Fluoridation Studies in the United Kingdom and the Results Achieved after 11 Years*. H.M.S.O., London
Dollery, C. (1978). *The End of an Age of Optimism*. Nuffield Provincial Hospitals Trust, London
Fisher, R. H. (1966). *The Design of Experiments*, Oliver and Boyd, Edinburgh
Gatley, M. S. (1968). *J. R. Coll. gen. Pract.*, **16**, 39–44
George, S. L., and Desu, M. H. (1974). *J. chron. Dis.*, **27**, 15–24
Hart, P. D'A. (1946). *Brit. med. J.*, **2**, 805–10
Hayes, M. J., Morris, G. A., and Hampton, J. R. (1974). *Br. Med. J.*, **2**, 8–13
Heady, J. A. (1973). *Bull. Wld Hlth Org.*, **48**, 243–56
Heaton Ward, W. A. (1962). *J. ment. Sci.*, **108**, 865–70
Hill, A. B. (1962). *Statistical Methods in Clinical and Preventive Medicine*. Livingstone, Edinburgh
Hill, M., and Armitage, P. (1978). *Br. J. clin. Pharmac.*, **8**, 7–20
Hill, L. E., Nunn, A. J., and Fox, W. (1976). *Lancet*, **1**, 352–6
Hogben, L., and Wrighton, R. (1952). *Br. J. prev. soc. Med.*, **6**, 89–117 and 205–25
Jackson, D., James, P. M. C., and Wolfe, W. B. (1975). *Br. Dent. J.*, **38**, 165–71

Knox, J. D. E., and Morrell, D. C. (1974). *Br. med. Bull.*, **30**, 209–13

Lancet (1979). *Lancet*, **1**, 534–5

Lind, J. (1753). *A Treatise on the Scurvy in Three Parts*. Millar, London

Lindley, D. V. (1975). *J. R. statist. Soc. C*, **24**, 218–28

Madsen, B. W., Woodings, T. L., Ilett, K. F. *et al.* (1978). *Br. med. J.*, **2**, 1333–5

Mantel, N. (1966). *Cancer Chem. Rep.*, **50**, 163–70

Mather, H. G., Pearson, N. G., Read, K. L. Q., *et al.* (1971). *Br. med. J.*, **3**, 334–8

Medical Research Council (1951). *Br. med. J.*, **2**, 1463–71

Ministry of Health, Scottish Office, and Ministry of Housing and Local Government (1962). *The Conduct of Fluoridation Studies in the United Kingdom and the Results Achieved After 5 Years*, H.M.S.O., London

Morris, J. N., Ball, K. P., Antonis, A., *et al.* (1968). *Lancet*, **2**, 693–700

Morris, D., Ward, A. W. M., and Handyside, A. J. (1968). *Lancet*, **1**, 681–5

Oldham, P. B. (1968). *Measurement in Medicine*. English University Press, London

Pasternak, B. S. (1972). *J. chron. Dis.*, **25**, 673–81

Pearson, K. (1904). *Br. med. J.*, **2**, 1243–6

Peto, R., Pike, M. C., Armitage, P., *et al.* (1976). *Br. J. Cancer*, **34**, 585–612

Peto, R., Pike, M. C., Armitage, P., *et al.* (1977). *Br. J. Cancer*, **35**, 1–39

Porter, A. M. W. (1969). *Br. med. J.*, **1**, 218–22

Reid, D. D., Brett, G. Z., Hamilton, P. J. S., *et al.* (1974). *Lancet*, **1**, 469–73

Reynolds, E., Jeyse, J. P. B., Swift, J. L., *et al.* (1966). *Br. J. Psychiat.*, **111**, 84–95

Rose, G. A. (1970). *Trans. Soc. occ. Med.*, **20**, 109–11

Schork, M. A., and Remington, R. D. (1967). *J. chron. Dis.*, **20**, 233–9

Schwartz, D., and Lellouch, J. (1967). *J. chron. Dis.*, **20**, 637–48

Schwartz, D., Wang, M., Zeitz, L., and Goss, M. E. W. (1962). *Am. J. publ. Hlth*, **52**, 2018–29

Shepherd, M. (1970). Evaluation of Psychotropic Drugs. In *The Principles and Practice of Clinical Trials* (E. L. Harris and J. D. Fitzgerald, eds.), Livingstone, Edinburgh, pp. 199–216

van der Linden, W. (1980). *Surgery*, **87**, 258–62

Wofinden, R. C. (1974). Personal communication

Wright, A. (1904). *Br. med. J.*, **2**, 1343–5

Wright, I. S. (1950). *Circulation*, **2**, 929–36

Wright, I. S., Markell, C. D., and Beck, D. F. (1948). *Am. Heart J.*, **36**, 801–15

Wright, P., and Haybittle, J. (1979). *Br. med. J.*, **2**, 529–30 and 590–2

Wulff, H. R. (1973). *Lancet*, **2**, 969–70

Wynne Griffith, G. (1956). *Hlth Educ. J.*, **14**, 223–30

8 Medical-care Studies

The application of epidemiological methods to a field of work rather than to one specific class of method will be described in this chapter. Medical-care studies often involve all approaches described under the very general heading of epidemiology. It must be remembered that this is only one of the disciplines involved in such work, and progress in medical-care studies usually requires the combined efforts of epidemiologists together with applied statisticians, economists, operational research scientists and sociologists.

Medical-care studies in general are carried out in an attempt to facilitate the work of managers and planners in the health service. At their simplest they may merely involve a description of one facet of the health service, although more ambitious studies may endeavour to describe the total functioning of the health and welfare services provided for a defined population. A descriptive study serves as a background to the consideration of such issues as, why is the situation like that? Are there changes that should take place? Is the health service meeting its objectives and delivering an accessible, acceptable and equitable service for those in need? Answers to these issues, provided partly by medical-care studies, are the basis of aspects of the work of administrators in the health service.

One approach to consideration of the functioning of the health service is to examine

(1) The health-care needs of the population,
(2) The demand made on the health and welfare services,
(3) The use made of the service (taking into account the workload carried by the service in relation to the staff and resources consumed),
(4) The outcome of care.

Brief examples are given of specific studies on these four topics; other examples cover planning and evaluation of services. This is intended to indicate the types of study that may be carried out.

The second section highlights the principles of medical-care studies and then the advantages and disadvantages of various types of study are discussed. Some extensions of the simpler approaches are indicated, while the final section demonstrates some of the specific aspects of statistical method that are used for medical-care studies.

8.1 Six Topics for Study

8.1.1 Assessment of Need

Before discussing studies that have been used to assess requirements, it is appropriate to define just what is meant by this concept. A health need may

221

be either perceived or unperceived by the individual. In the latter case a condition is unrecognised by an individual or his family, but may be discovered by a practitioner on careful investigation of the total physical, mental and emotional well-being of the individual. This is achieved by the use of standard techniques and accepted criteria for investigation. Such a condition, when it is thought that prevention, management or specific therapy would be of benefit, may warrant intervention, but there are also those diseases for which currently available forms of intervention are of little benefit. A health-care need is perceived when the individual or his family identifies an 'abnormality'. Subsequently they may (1) take no action whatsoever to seek medical care, (2) make use of one of the informal agencies, including self-medication or (3) contact one of the conventional branches of the health service. Not all perceived need will be accepted by the medical profession as being correctly identified—and in certain circumstances this may be labelled as over-demand or neurosis. Bradshaw (1972) attempted to provide a framework for clearer thinking about need and proposed a taxonomy of social need. Cartwright (1974) pointed out that there is still the problem of establishing criteria within the different categories.

The following example indicates how a special study may be required to identify the need for a particular facet of medical care. Some patients may be referred to the hospital in the terminal stage of cancer for specific medical needs or because the circumstances at home are unsuitable; other patients may be cared for in difficult conditions at home because of the wishes of the patient or his or her relatives. There was, however, no clear guidance about the proportion of patients who required additional facilities beyond those immediately available in the home. Alderson (1970) attempted to categorise the medical and nursing care required by patients dying from cancer in a defined population. With the permission of the hospital staff and the family doctor concerned, the relatives of a representative sample of patients dying from cancer in Manchester were approached. Information was collected from the family practitioners and the records of hospital treatment were also available.

Table 8.1 Arrangements for terminal care of 127 patients dying from cancer

Arrangements	Number of patients
hospital admission	
acute medical emergency	30
nursing care	44
home nursing	
patients' home	44
relatives' home	5
lived in nursing home	4

Source: Alderson (1970)

Table 8.1 shows the arrangements for care made for 127 terminal cancer cases. Many relatives were willing to shoulder the difficult burden of caring for a relative suffering from terminal cancer. They received great help from their family doctor, from the services provided by the local authorities and from their neighbours. There were, however, some relatives who had to contend with great difficulties; these problems included the infirmity of the relative, lack of suitable facilities in the home, such as absence of hot running water or an inside toilet, financial worries and the simultaneous caring for of young children. These factors added to the physical burden of disturbed nights and the mental stress of caring for a near relative who was suffering pain and discomfort and whose health was plainly deteriorating. In contrast, despite the home circumstances being quite satisfactory, a number of patients were admitted to hospital. These findings were based on small numbers, but do support the hypothesis that there is a certain vocal group in the community which is aware of the provisions of the N.H.S., and demands and obtains special attention. It appeared that about half the patients had been nursed in the final stage of their disease in a location (either home or hospital) which was inappropriate. It was suggested that, in a population of just over 600 000, seventy patients dying from malignant disease in one calendar month required the provision of special nursing care beyond that available in the home.

The contribution of routine data to the identification of unperceived need is marginal, but there are a few special instances where the data can be of limited value. Statistics that indicate delay in attending for medical care warrant consideration. For example, the routine returns on use of mass X-ray showed a deficient use by persons in social class V, who, at the same time, had a high prevalence of positive findings (Heasman, 1961). Alderson and Nayak (1970) examined the routine cancer-registration data to detect any delay in attending for treatment of the malignant disease in relation to age, sex, and social class. There was no appreciable social-class effect on delay, but a significant variation according to age.

The classic approach to studying unperceived need is to conduct a health-examination survey, using all the appropriate techniques to identify unmet need. More than thirty years ago, Morris (1941) carried out a survey of working males and quantified the degree to which the subjects were suffering from treatable conditions for which they had not obtained any medical advice. Sheridan (1962) discussed the advantage of routine examination in children to identify any disease or disability that could benefit from intervention. Williamson et al. (1964) showed that a disturbingly high proportion of the elderly suffered from one or more defects that warranted attention.

These three studies involved specific sections of the population. Another approach has been to search for a particular condition in the general population, such as the survey carried out in Bedford to detect diabetes (Butterfield, 1968). In the United States, a National Health Examination Survey is used, to complement the U.S. National Health Survey. Routine surveys provide a general indication of whether there is an appreciable degree of unperceived need in the population. There is considerable overlap between the consideration of unperceived need and a discussion of the value of screening examinations. The application of screening techniques to the general population, or to specific groups, will be dealt with further in subsection 8.1.6.

The General Household Survey has already been discussed (see section 3.1.4); this provided for the first time in many years information about the general health of the population. Data was collected over thirty years ago in the United Kingdom in the Survey of Sickness (Slater, 1946; Logan and Brooke, 1957). In the intervening period, several research surveys have been carried out on defined populations. Such surveys have provided very useful information about the general health of the population and the action taken to deal with identified disease. For example, there have been population surveys in south Wales (Cochrane, 1954), Southwark (Wadsworth *et al.*, 1971) and Lambeth (Holland and Waller, 1971). From these surveys it is possible to produce analyses of (1) the reported ailments of the population for which no particular care has been sought, (2) the use made of the nonhealth-service agencies (relatives, friends and welfare agencies) and (3) contact with the N.H.S. Horder and Horder (1954) first drew attention to the relative preponderance of disease for which no care was sought compared with the proportion of sick patients cared for by the family doctor and the small fraction who required hospital care.

8.1.2 Demand

A number of years ago it was suggested by Airth and Newell (1962) that demand for, and use of, hospital beds was directly related to the availability of facilities. Instead of measuring overt demand, stifled demand should be identified. The latter is perceived need that the patient, his family and even the family doctor have not translated into a demand because they believed facilities were not readily available. There is no routine information that directly throws light on this problem and it is necessary to get some general guidance from indirect sources. One approach is an examination of the disparity between estimates of anticipated need and actual demand. This will usually require an *ad hoc* study of a specific issue, such as the following example provides.

Alderson (1966) presented evidence to suggest that family doctors were less likely to refer terminal patients to hospital in the winter, when the demand for acute beds was high. This finding was derived from the examination of all available information for over 2000 deaths occurring in one year in a large county borough in England. Table 8.2 shows the percentage of patients dying from cerebrovascular accidents, who were not referred to hospital, according to period of death. The peak of 59 per cent not referred in the period January to March is a significant excess, compared with the average figure for all four quarters ($p < 0.05$).

Vaananen (1970) investigated the bed provision in relation to admission rates in each of the municipalities of the central hospital region in Finland. He produced data that indicated that whatever the bed provision the

Table 8.2 Proportion of patients dying from cerebrovascular accident who were not referred to hospital according to quarter of year

	Period of year			
	Oct.–Dec.	Jan.–Mar.	April–June	July–Sept.
not admitted*	30%	59%	43%	41%

Source: Alderson (1966)

*Based on 267 deaths

emergency admission rate was similar in each municipality. As with other studies, it was shown that there was a steady increase in nonurgent admissions in those districts with generous provision of beds.

Unmet demand may be identified for certain facets of the health service, where routine data provide evidence of long waiting lists for treatment or care. There is no routine information from primary medical care which identifies patients who are waiting for a home visit, or for other attention, nor does this issue appear to have been tackled by any special studies. Another matter that can be considered is whether the patients' expectations in their contact with the primary medical care have been met; this, however, is really a measure of outcome and will be discussed in subsection 8.1.4.

Hospitals have been encouraged to monitor the waiting time for outpatient appointments (Ministry of Health, 1964a) and it has been suggested that two weeks should be the maximum time for nonurgent cases between referral and consultation. Some hospitals on their own initiative have collected information about the waiting time for urgent and nonurgent appointments after receipt of doctors' referral letters. Stewart and Sleeman (1967) surveyed progress in thirty groups of hospitals and found that none could meet the recommended two-week requirement. Forsyth and Logan (1968) examined the time lag for over 13 000 referrals. 85 per cent of these were classed as nonurgent and three-quarters of these nonurgent referrals had been seen within one month.

Having been admitted to hospital, the patient may still have to wait for definitive treatment. Heasman and Carstairs (1971) analysed data on the period between admission and operation for patients receiving surgical treatment throughout Scotland. There are many other reasons for the prolonged stay in hospital, but no routine data are available to illustrate these. There is no clear evidence of the impact on length of stay from (1) delay in requesting or obtaining investigations, (2) lack of theatre time (which may be because of lack of nurses) or (3) delay in discharging a patient because of difficulty in arranging the return of the patient to the community or transfer to a second-line bed. This issue will be discussed further in subsection 8.1.3.3.

A special aspect of demand for care relates to that category of individuals who obtain care from resources other than the health service. This may include care provided by the individual himself, his family or other nonhealth-service agencies. Horder and Horder (1954) drew attention to the large proportion of people with minor ailments who cared for themselves; 75 per cent of all morbidity was treated by self-care and 25 per cent by the family practitioner including 5 per cent by hospitals. This general point was reinforced by the General Household Survey (O.P.C.S., 1973). A number of studies have drawn attention to the significant amount of self-medication that occurs (Jefferys *et al.*, 1960; Lader, 1965; Dunnell and Cartwright, 1972). The use of the social services as a complement to care by the health services is an extremely important aspect of the total problem of health and welfare. There are some specific categories of patients, such as the mentally subnormal, the mentally ill and those with a permanent physical handicap, who require a degree of support from the social services throughout their lives. The examination of these problems is complex and beyond the scope of this limited section. It is worth mentioning, however, the large number of people living in the community, who have reported physical or mental handicap, but who do not receive support from any agency (Harris *et al.* 1971). The estimates, based on a sample survey of persons living in private households, suggested that there were 1 130 000 persons in the United Kingdom who were handicapped. Nearly 30 per cent had not seen their doctor for at least three months, while half the severely and two-thirds of the appreciably handicapped were not receiving any ongoing care from the health or welfare services of the local authority. About 5 per cent of the handicapped had sought attention from osteopaths, a slightly smaller proportion had resorted to faith healers and a few had approached herbalists and other comparable sources of care.

An interview with over 700 Danish women aged 25–44 suggested that those living in cities or crowded homes were less likely to request medical advice for reduced fecundity than those living in rural less-crowded homes (Rachootin and Olsen, 1982). Secondary analysis of data on consultation and attendance rates in general practice in Lambeth showed an increase in these rates for those living near the practice, that was independent of social class, sex and age. This finding applied to contacts for all reasons and also to a number of specific diagnoses that were examined (Parkin, 1979).

8.1.3 Use of health-service facilities

This phrase describes the met demand (services rendered to patients), also referred to as the workload. One important point is that all segments of the health service must be considered, and not in isolation, but in relation to the staff and facilities required to cater for this use. Although the growing tendency is to consider the health service as a total organisation providing comprehensive care for all ailments of the population, the matter is simplified by separating discussion into the following groups.

(1) The community services, in particular, family practitioner and other primary care facilities.
(2) The activity of hospital outpatient departments.
(3) The use made of hospital beds and inpatient facilities.

Although for many problems the patient will require care from each of these sectors in turn, this section considers the topics in these rather artificial divisions.

As with examination of mortality and morbidity statistics, examination of 'event' data on contact with the health service may be enhanced by calculating appropriate rates. One category of denominator is estimates of staff and facilities (numbers of doctors, nurses etc.; number of hospital beds, operating theatres, X-ray plants, etc.). In addition to national publications of such material, W.H.O. collates such information and publishes this in the *World Health Statistics Annual*.

It must be emphasised that the examples provided in the following subsections are to indicate the method and no attempt can be made to cover the range of important studies that have been done on these topics in the space available.

8.1.3.1 Use of primary medical-care facilities

Although there has been little routine data collected on the activity of primary medical care in the past, a number of pioneers including the College of General Practitioners have made notable contributions in this field. Subsection 3.1.7 discussed the morbidity statistics from general practice collected by a major collaborative effort in England and Wales. The report (O.P.C.S., 1974) enabled some of the determinants of contact rates in primary medical care to be examined, such as the influence of age, sex, marital status, occupation and place of residence. Reviews of all the special studies carried out by individual, highly motivated family doctors have been produced at intervals by the Royal College of General Practitioners; the last of these was prepared by Fry (1973). This provided some interesting tables on the workload handled in family practice including: the contact rate in the surgery; the proportion of patients who are visited and the ratio of surgery attendances to home visits; the hours worked by family practitioners; the use made of ancillary services in the practice team; and the relationship between the primary-care team, hospitals and other services. These special studies have all been based on data collected by family doctors and they provide a most useful background to a consideration of the activity of general practice.

Other work has usually involved special studies of particular aspects. For example, a number of authors have examined the impact of appointment systems (e.g. Morrell and Kasap, 1972).

Another major change in the past twenty years has been the involvement of different members of a team in primary medical care; Marsh and McNay (1974) cited forty-two references and then quoted results from their own study of the contribution of the paramedical team to the total care provided by a practice.

A very different approach was chosen by Cartwright (1967) who questioned a random sample of the population about contact with their family doctor, the reason for such contact, the action taken, and their attitudes and reactions to this experience.

Limited statistics are published each year on the number of laboratory tests directly requested by general practitioners (the number has risen more steeply than those from hospital staff over the past ten years). Some special studies have been carried out, particularly an examination of whether the introduction of these facilities has had any major impact on the total workload of the laboratories or X-ray departments (Anderson, 1968). An interesting aspect of this is the question of the referral rates to hospital outpatient departments. Darmady (1964) and Fry (1971) have suggested that availability and use of direct-access facilities may reduce the referral rate to outpatients.

8.1.3.2 Use of outpatient facilities

Extremely limited information has been routinely collected about the use of outpatient departments. The basic data relate to counts of new and total outpatient attendances by speciality for each hospital in the country. Even these data, when available within regions, provide only a very crude indication of workload in outpatients. These issues have been studied in a special survey carried out by Forsyth and Logan (1968), who collected data from eighty hospitals in all parts of the United Kingdom during 1962. The report commented on the general atmosphere in different hospital outpatient departments, the trends in activity, the characteristics of the patients seen, the influence of the family doctor on referral rates, and the investigation and subsequent care of referred patients. This study drew attention to a number of facets of the outpatient system that required further detailed study. Emphasis was placed on the lack of routine information that might allow rational appraisal of the use of the service.

8.1.3.3 Use of inpatient facilities

Routine data from the Hospital Inpatient Enquiry provide regular information about the use made of hospital beds; tabulations cover characteristics of the patients, administrative particulars and diagnostic breakdown. One simple issue of importance for planning is an analysis of the relationship between sex, age, marital status and length of stay; this enables an adjustment for demographic data to be made when projecting requirements for beds in a particular locality. Figure 8.1 shows the occupied bed days in relation to these variates; the occupied bed days reflect a compound of the admission rates and lengths of stay. There is a marked rise with advancing age and a suggestion that marital status and sex independently influence the figures. It is important to determine what proportion of this additional stay associated with advancing age is because the patients must remain in an 'acute bed' because of the lack of supporting facilities for care on discharge to the community. There was, however, no evidence in a limited examination of routine data that the longer stay was particularly for those patients who ultimately required transfer to local authority residential accommodation (Alderson, 1974).

Two important issues are firstly do all patients admitted to hospital need such care and secondly what proportion of the patients currently in hospital

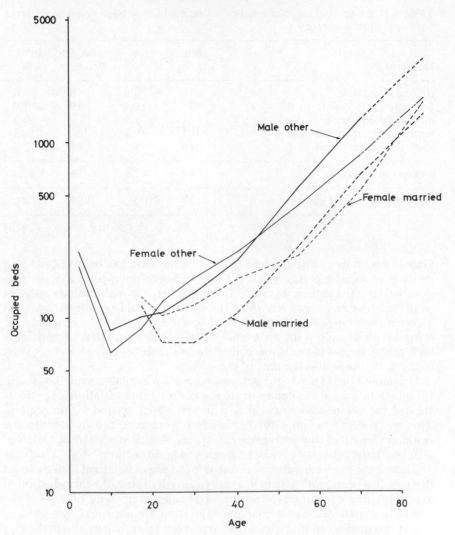

Figure 8.1 Occupied bed days per 100 000 population by age, sex and marital status
(excluding maternity and psychiatric patients) in England and Wales,
1978
Source: *Report of the Hospital Inpatient Enquiry for 1978*, D.H.S.S. and
O.P.C.S. (1981)

require other forms of care? For many years it has been recognised that a
proportion of patients is admitted to hospital because of a combination of
social and medical reasons rather than purely for acute medical care. Once
the acute episode is over, some patients remain in hospital because facilities
for their transfer either to second-line beds or back to the community are
lacking. Many studies have examined this topic since it was explored by
Amulree *et al.* (1951). Loudon (1970) reviewed a sample of inpatients in the

Table 8.3　Analysis of acute hospital days that could have been saved by different forms of care

Different care	Medical wards Bed days	%	Surgical wards Bed days	%
treatment at home	22	0.5	0	0
admission to G.P. unit	787	19.1	19	1.0
quicker investigation	232	5.6	5	0.3
earlier discharge to G.P. unit	441	10.7	368	19.1
earlier discharge home	229	5.5	47	2.4
total potential saving	1711	41.5	439	22.8
bed days occupied in survey	4127	100	1927	100

Source: Loudon (1970)

Oxford hospitals and determined whether admission had been required on medical or social grounds, whether there had been delay prior to investigation, whether the patient was suitable for discharge to a community hospital or to their own home, or even whether the patient could have been treated in a community hospital without referral to an acute teaching hospital. An abstract of his results is shown in table 8.3, which indicates that a surprisingly high proportion of patients was considered suitable for care elsewhere than in the acute hospital at the time of the survey.

Heasman (1964) used the routine information available from the Hospital Inpatient Enquiry to demonstrate the considerable variation for patients treated for comparable surgical conditions, which existed within regions. This work suggested that further studies were required to identify the optimum length of stay for certain categories of patient. Controlled trials of different lengths of stay have been discussed in subsection 7.4.3.

There have been a number of changes in the use of inpatient facilities over the past few years, with a drop in average length of stay, the introduction of short-stay and day surgery, and the increasing complexity of care of the seriously ill patients. These changes have been accompanied by a marked rise in the number of investigations carried out by radiology and pathology departments. The limited data available as a routine quantify this rise in tests performed, but do not relate investigation to medical problems, patient characteristics or even speciality in which the patient is being investigated and treated. Ashley and his colleagues (1972) abstracted data on investigations performed on patients with fifteen selected diagnoses in eight acute hospitals. They showed that diagnosis influenced the volume of investigation, but that there was also a wide variation in different hospitals.

8.1.4 Outcome

Lee and his colleagues (1957) examined the routine published data from the Hospital Inpatient Enquiry, and tabulated the case fatality for certain conditions in teaching and nonteaching hospitals. They observed an appreciable difference in these rates, with the nonteaching hospitals having a higher case fatality rate. This relationship held for a number of conditions that were examined. It was observed that there was a preponderance of elderly males treated for hyperplasia of the prostate in nonteaching hospitals and a higher proportion of emergency admissions. After standardisation of the data for age and mode of admission, there was still nearly a twofold difference in case fatality ($p < 0.03$). Further data extending the review from 1951 to 1959 showed a consistent excess mortality in patients admitted to nonteaching hospitals. Tabulation according to duration of stay showed no particular excess numbers of deaths in the first few days—as might have been expected if the patients admitted to nonteaching hospitals were more acutely ill or in poorer general health.

A prospective study was then mounted (Ashley et al., 1971) on patients treated in selected hospitals. This was an attempt to obtain detailed information about the characteristics of the patients, their general health on admission, the treatment given and the outcome, including assessment after a follow-up period. Nearly 1000 patients were included in this prospective study. It was found that the nonteaching hospitals accepted a high proportion of emergency admissions of very elderly patients who were often suffering from heart failure and with other evidence of renal failure. There was a low operative mortality for planned admissions to all the hospitals. However, there were significant variations in the residual symptoms observed at follow up linked to age and type of operation, but not to the hospital. The authors concluded that 'on the evidence, some regional board hospitals have to carry a greater burden than teaching hospitals, different services are required of them, and they have to work under greater pressure. Yet as far as resources are concerned, they are the poor relations.'

Case fatality is, however, a very limited aspect of the outcome of care. A major study examining the rehabilitation of patients discharged from hospital following treatment of an acute episode was provided by Ferguson and MacPhail (1954). Continuation of this work was then carried out in three centres in Scotland by McKenzie et al. (1962). The information from these special studies clearly indicated a need to monitor the time lag between discharge from hospital and the return to normal life, whether this is paid employment or other activity.

As part of a survey of all males under the age of seventy experiencing a myocardial infarction or sudden death from ischaemic heart disease in a defined population in 1966–7, Kinlen (1969) examined the time away from work among those men surviving a myocardial infarction for at least one month. 57 per cent had resumed work within three months of the episode, while 11 per cent were still away from work six months after the infarction. There was no obvious relationship between objective signs of organic disability and duration of absence from work.

The above discussion emphasises some of the points that have already been made in section 6.2 about the difficulty of deriving a successful measure of outcome. One approach to this, advocated by Grogono and Woodgate (1971), is the use of an index derived from the sum of scores (on a three-point scale) for ten aspects of 'well-being'. Breslow (1972) discussed the combined use of questioning an individual about his health and the objective measurement of functional reserves in order to derive a measure of health status. Rosser and Watts (1972) tested a simpler approach that required a physician to score a patient on two parameters: (1) disability by use of an eight-point scale; and (2) distress on a four-point scale. The latter incorporated a judgement of pain and/or mental disturbence and/or reaction to disability. More theoretical approaches to the measurement of health have been provided by Fanshel (1972) and Chiang and Cohen (1973). A detailed review has been provided by Fanshel and Bush (1970).

The study by Cartwright (1967), mentioned above (see subsection 8.1.3.1), provided some very useful information about patients' reactions to contact with their family doctors. An earlier study (Cartwright, 1964) had provided an equally clear picture of patients' reactions to care in hospital. Patients' opinion of their care is an important aspect of assessing outcome and one to which increasing attention has been directed over recent years. The King Edward's Hospital Fund has fostered interest in this topic and has encouraged routine collection of comments and suggestions from inpatients (Raphael, 1973). A survey in Scotland (Carstairs, 1970) showed that about 25 per cent of patients in hospital had made complaints or suggestions to someone in authority and only 40 per cent had no comments to make when interviewed about improvement in care.

8.1.5 Planning

Planning in the health field has been defined (Alderson, 1975) as the process culminating in decisions about the future of the correct balance of domiciliary, outpatient and inpatient facilities for the investigation, treatment and care of all the 'perceived health needs' of the community. A number of other definitions are available, which vary according to the viewpoint and responsibility of the individuals who have drafted them. The above wording has been deliberately phrased to emphasise that even when considering the development of a restricted facet of the health service, this will have both capital implications (buildings and plant) and revenue consequences (salaries, maintenance and replacement costs). In a service with growing demands and a finite budget, any new service implies that less money will be available to be spent on other aspects of health care. Excluded from this definition is the examination of current resources and the demand resulting in the short-term reallocation of these resources in order to meet more effectively the demand in the near future.

Bispham et al. (1971) stressed how important it is to have an adequate measure of medical need in determining a successful plan for the future. Ideally, detailed information about diseases currently affecting the population is required, and onto this one needs to build estimates of trends in the incidence of disease, possible changes in the attitude of the population to health and health care, future variation in delivery of care, impending changes of therapy, and the effect that any new therapy is likely to have on the prognosis of disease. This indicates the potential role for epidemiology. A W.H.O. report (1971) suggested that there are five basic steps in the planning process:

(1) Situational analysis
(2) Formulation of alternative tactical approaches
(3) A decision phase
(4) Discussion and implementation
(5) Evaluation.

Information is required in one form or another for at least three of these steps. Much of the routine data and special studies discussed elsewhere in the book are relevant. The following paragraphs indicate some of the specific contributions that epidemiology has made to planning.

In an attempt to measure the demand for medical care Forsyth and Logan (1960) quantified the workload for the Barrow in Furness group of hospitals. They were well aware that workload cannot indicate the extent of unmet need (services are not sought when they are not available) and seven steps were taken to improve the estimates of demand.

(1) Background information on the mortality, hospital admission rates, and prescribing statistics was examined for Barrow in Furness, the North West of England, and England and Wales.
(2) The hospital admission rates were examined for individual practices in the district (classified by urban/rural location, single/partnership practice and list size), in relation to frequency and cost of prescribing, and use of direct-access pathology and radiology.
(3) The hospital admissions due to appendicitis, tonsils and adenoids, and for other surgery, gynaecology and obstetrics were examined by practice (classified as in step 2).
(4) The clinical necessity for admission or continued stay was assessed by the epidemiologist and clinician. For surgery, medicine and paediatrics, it was estimated that there was an 8 per cent inflation of admissions.
(5) An enquiry was carried out among the general practitioners, to check whether the size of waiting lists affected their handling of individual patients. It was accepted that this was a dubious method of assessing the change in behaviour that might occur.
(6) Consideration was given to the effect on use of beds, of theatre time requirements for the surgical specialities, the availability of medical nursing and other staff, the location and size of treatment units, and the time taken to obtain an outpatient consultation.
(7) A review was made of the provision of community and welfare facilities, including preconvalescent, chronic sick and part 3 accommodation.

The report concluded by suggesting a tentative requirement for hospital beds per 1000 population and by comparing this with the findings of other surveys.

Reference has already been made to the use of data from psychiatric registers (see subsection 3.4.3) to study the trends in use of inpatient facilities for acute and long-stay patients who are mentally ill. However, for the planning of services for a new treatment the routine data will usually require to be supplemented by a special study. For example, Pendreigh and his colleagues (1972) collected data for a year about all patients in Scotland suffering from end-stage renal failure in order to derive an estimate of the need for haemodialysis and renal transplantation. Three methods of case ascertainment were used.

Badley *et al.* (1978) demonstrated the need to consider the underlying cause of disablement, the severity of the condition, and the prevalence before assessing the health-care requirements of the group of individuals. They present a reappraisal of the Harris *et al.* (1971) survey in these terms. Urquart and Ruthven (1979) examined hospital outpatients' records for referral to general medicine, surgery, gynaecology and E.N.T. clinics. Provided simple X-ray facilities were available, location of the clinic at a health centre would not impose a major constraint on the full initial consultation. Some practical problems would however arise for transferring first consultations in E.N.T. A survey of 838 elderly people (i.e. over 65) in an Oxfordshire market town indicated that 5.6 per cent had evidence of osteoarthritis of the hip; 0.7 per cent had been operated upon for this condition and a further 0.5 per cent would have benefited from total hip

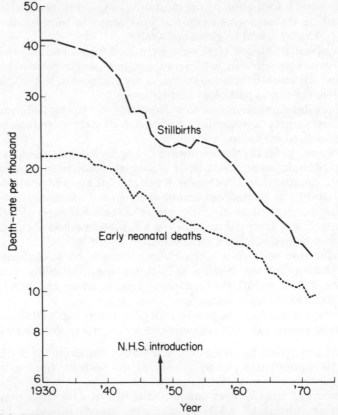

Figure 8.2 Stillbirth-rates and early neonatal death-rates in England and Wales, 1930–72.

Source: Richards and Lowe (1966); *Registrar General's Statistical Reviews for England and Wales*, Part 1, Tables Medical, H.M.S.O. (1932–74)

replacement. However, an additional 1.3 per cent, though needing the operation, were not fit for surgery (Wilcock, 1979).

Svanborg *et al.* (1982) reviewed fifteen published epidemiological studies of social and medical conditions of the elderly carried out in Canada, Japan, the Nordic countries and the United Kingdom. They indicate how surveys (with or without examination) can contribute to planning of care for the elderly and complement information from vital statistics. Grime and Whitelegg (1982) suggest that 'accessibility' is an important consideration in developing local health-plans; they demonstrate how such considerations can be incorporated (e.g. utilising survey data on travel times for visitors to inpatients).

Matthew (1971) discussed the problem of extrapolating from local findings to a wider population. He pointed out that it was unlikely that studies of samples of the population in every area of the country and on a wide range of conditions would ever be practicable. It may be possible to deduce the prevalence of disease in one population using data collected in another. This leads on to the issue of 'indicators', which is discussed further in subsection 8.5.1.

An earlier part of this section mentioned the five steps in planning. A crucial one is the decision phase. Epidemiology can indicate gaps in services and quantify trends, while modelling may indicate the repercussions following changes in provision. This factual information should be of great assistance, but it must be emphasised that future changes in medical practice are hard to predict. The planner must judge what is feasible and acceptable, and retain an element of flexibility to allow for unforeseen changes in morbidity, treatment or ways of organising services. The interrelationship between those providing data, making decisions and implementing change is discussed further in section 8.2.

8.1.6 Evaluation

Attention has already been drawn to the use of routine morbidity and mortality data to monitor the health of the population (see subsections 2.2.4 and 3.2.1). Perhaps one of the most dramatic innovations in health care has been the introduction of the N.H.S. Although no specific plans had been made to monitor the introduction of the health service in 1948, Richards and Lowe (1966) presented data on the stillbirth-rate before and after the introduction of the N.H.S. They showed that there had been a steady decline in this rate up until 1948, which then remained static for about the next ten years. Figure 8.2 shows the stillbirth- and early neonatal death-rates for England and Wales from 1930. These rates together cover the deaths that occur just before or after birth, and as Smith (1968) pointed out they should be considered together because of the variation in allocation to one or other category. There was an obvious halt in the trend of the stillbirth-rate after the introduction of the N.H.S., but no obvious change in the early neonatal deaths. Richards and Lowe suggested that this might have been due to a decline in the quality in antenatal care, when it was transferred from the local authority clinics to the general practitioners. This is a basic example of the way in which routine data may be used to monitor the major changes that can occur in the provision of health service and their impact on the health of the community. Cross (1973) suggested that concern about oxygen levels when nursing premature babies—and the risk of retrolental fibroplasia—had arrested improvement in mortality rates in the neonates. Hey (1981) described a survey in the North East of England which used many sources of information to identify all children born in 1964–79 who developed retrolental fibroplasia. He emphasised the difficulty of such a study and discussed varying ways of assessing the development of this abnormality in babies of different weight; this is only one of many indices of outcome of pregnancy. Having examined trends in perinatal mortality in Scotland in 1976–9 in relation to changes in age, parity, social class of mothers and birthweight of infants, Forbes *et al.* (1982) concluded that obstetric practice and management of the neonate were the predominant influences on improved results.

As an example of a specific service that has been introduced recently, it is appropriate to consider the screening of women for detection of pre-invasive cancer of the cervix. During the 1960s pressure was exerted on the central government to institute a national screening system. Carcinoma of the cervix is relatively common and is an extremely unpleasant disease. By screening women it was hoped that it would detect early lesions of the cervix before invasive cancer had been established and thus lead to active prevention of the invasive disease. It so happened that there was a technique for the examination of smears taken from the cervix in order to detect malignant cells. An extensive screening programme has been available in British Columbia; though there was some suggestion of an impact on mortality (Walton *et al.*, 1976), a recent review questions the contribution of the screening program (Miller, 1982).

In an attempt to gauge the impact of coronary care units, Rose (1975) noted that hospital admission rates had risen steeply and the number of hospital deaths had been stable over the period that intensive care facilities had become widespread. He suggested this was due to increasing admissions of milder cases.

Cochrane (1972) discussed some of these issues in his monograph *Effectiveness and Efficiency*. He defined effectiveness as the measure of the ability of a procedure to alter the natural history of a disease or symptom for the better. Efficiency was defined as the ratio of the minimum resources required to achieve the effect to the resource used at present. Cochrane commented on the inequality of the distribution of health-service resources within the United Kingdom and suggested that the efficiency of medical care should be examined in relation to prevention, diagnosis, including screening for disease, and treatment, including the supportive care of those with chronic disease. Clinical trials are examples of studies to test the effectiveness of new treatment; subsection 7.4.3 has indicated how such studies may be extended to the examination of medical care. Some innovations in medical care are likely to occur without definitive randomised-control trials occurring; but if this happens some procedure must be instituted for monitoring the impact of the innovation on the health of the public.

Over the past few years there has been considerable discussion about the place of evaluation of medical care. Dollery (1971) advocated a major extension of such systems to look at the quality of care in general practice and in hospital work. Doll (1973) suggested that monitoring should be restricted to the collection of information to provide a warning of the need for intervention. The definition of what that intervention should be is another matter, and advice about any consequent action is better described as control. He emphasised that this distinction between monitoring and control is not just semantic, and stressed that those who are being monitored will co-operate and have confidence in the system only if it aims to achieve a partnership between the administrator and agent and is, in itself, neutral and educational.

There are several specific attempts to evaluate medical care in the United Kingdom. Two of these are related to the provision of care in the community, one affecting general practitioners and the other affecting dentists. For about one month in twelve, data are collected centrally about the prescriptions issued for each Family Practitioner Committee (F.P.C.); this material is costed and coded to specific practitioners. It is then possible to identify those practitioners whose prescribing costs are considerably above those of their colleagues. This system not only looks at the cost of the prescriptions issued, but also is an attempt to study any variation in trends in prescribing. There has recently been an increasing emphasis on the examination of the use of drugs with known adverse side effects. Practitioners who prescribe certain drugs at much higher levels than their colleagues can be identified. Another system exists in which a sample of individuals who have had routine dental treatment under the N.H.S. is recalled for a check examination so that the quality of care can be assessed.

The cost of prescribing referred to above is only one aspect of the evaluation of the use of drugs. Reference has already been made to studies that have shown considerable variation in the consumption of prescribed treatment (see sections 4.2.6.2 and 7.3). Hulka et al. (1975) have cross-checked the medication 'misuse' among a sample of patients with chronic disease and documented the reasons for this. The greater the number of drugs being prescribed, the higher was the probability of drug omission and commission. Unrelated to the number of drugs were scheduling errors. These arose from doctor–patient miscommunication and patient noncompliance. Comparison of surveys of drug usage in 1969 and 1977, and drug prescriptions in the same years, indicated a discrepancy in increase (none in the former source, a 21 per cent increase in the latter). Anderson (1980) suggested there might be increasing noncompliance.

An example of a specific study into the quality of care was reported by Lee and his colleagues (1974), who reviewed the drug therapy that patients with rheumatoid arthritis had been receiving prior to their referral to a specialist centre. Martys (1982) tried various ways of detecting adverse reactions to antibiotics given in general practice; some patients were warned that this was to occur, others were given no indication of the impending enquiry. Half the patients were questioned by their doctor, the others by a health visitor. Difficulty in differentiating incidental symptoms from drug side effects were noted.

A confidential enquiry into maternal mortality has been ongoing since 1952, the aim of which is to encourage those concerned on a local basis to examine together the events leading up to death. Thus lessons learnt from these events may enable better care to be provided in the future. The reports of this survey have been collated and published in order to give doctors an analysis that may be of assistance (Tomkinson *et al.*, 1982). A special study was mounted in three areas in England and Wales in 1964 to enquire into deaths occurring in infants between the ages of four weeks and one year. The approach was similar to that of the confidential enquiry into maternal deaths, and a report had been published (D.H.S.S., 1970). A more recent development is the periodic visits of the Hospital Advisory Service, which have been carried out throughout the United Kingdom, to geriatric and psychiatric units. These visits by a multidisciplinary team have been followed by a report that is available to the clinicians concerned, so that they can comment on the views of the visiting team (D.H.S.S., 1973). This system is rather different from the enquiries into maternal and infant mortality, in that the team visits all units in the country and comments on the complete range of services provided. Studies have been reported of confidential enquiries into mortality after anaesthesia (Lunn and Mushin, 1982) and death in asthmatics (British Thoracic Association, 1982).

Sanazaro (1974) discussed the present experience of medical audit in the United States. He suggested that medical audit is a tool designed for a particular purpose, namely, objective documentation by doctors of how far their care conforms to their own standards of adequacy or excellence. The paper by Sanazaro was accompanied by five other papers commenting on the present situation in Britain, Sweden and Australia (Dudley, 1974; Capstick, 1974; Thould, 1974; Werkö, 1974; Howqua, 1974). Yudkin *et al.* (1980) checked general practice and hospital records and investigated all diabetic patients so identified in a defined community. This suggested that patients in social class III–V had nonoptimal surveillance and that even those attending hospital clinics did not have the ideal frequency of checks to detect complications.

Peach and Pathy (1981) examined material collected about 1274 individuals who failed to attend booked appointments at a geriatric day hospital. This represented 11 per cent of all booked attendances; particularly it was the very elderly women who on special assessment seemed more dependent than age- or sex-matched attenders but had less faith in day-care treatment. The absence of warning of nonattendance resulted in wasted ambulance journeys, domiciliary visits by community staff and deficient use of day-care facilities. The authors suggest that such material should be monitored to define a subgroup of patients for whom day-care may not be suitable.

It is important to consider the views of patients and the public in evaluating health care. At Queen Charlotte's hospital mothers were allowed to choose the method of pain relief in labour, including epidural analgesia. Morgan *et al.* (1982) interviewed 1000 women within twenty-four hours of a vaginal delivery of a live-born child, asking particularly about analgesia and satisfaction with childbirth. A year later a comparable postal questionnaire was sent to the mothers, though only 626 replied. It appeared that forceps delivery and long labour were thought to be 'bad experiences' of labour by the mothers, and they were more common in those choosing epidural anaesthesia. The authors caution against 'epidural on demand' and indicate this needs to be compared with epidural when necessary. An interview study of people living near a hostel for mentally handicapped adults showed that few of those opposed to the hostel in 1977 were still opposed in 1980. It was suggested that this was due to personal experience of the hostel, as a fresh sample also interviewed in 1980 provided similar responses (Locker et al., 1981).

One aspect of medical care omitted from the discussion so far is health education. This is one of the primary instruments of preventive medicine used to promote good health as well as to reduce behaviour-induced disease (Jones and Grahame, 1974). In the past, enthusiastic activity in this field has not been accompanied by careful investigation to determine the mechanisms for influencing attitudes and behaviour, or the evaluation of specific programmes (Ministry of Health, 1964b).

Several campaigns have been launched to try to persuade people to reduce their consumption of tobacco. A careful pre- and post-campaign survey in Edinburgh provided no evidence that people had given up smoking, nor that there was a switch to pipes or cigars (Cartwright et al., 1960). Although not a single respondent reported having given up smoking, 12 per cent claimed to know someone who had. Numbers of cigarettes smoked daily showed no change after the campaign, but 9 per cent thought that their consumption had changed. A comprehensive community prog- ramme to control cardiovascular disease in Finland in 1972–7 aimed to reduce the prevalence of smoking, serum-cholesterol concentration and raised blood-pressure. There was a reduction in those three risk factors, especially in men, in the intervention locality compared with the control county (Puska et al., 1979). Further study of the North Karelia population indicated that change in behaviour in the intervention community bore no relationship to an individual's initial risk-level (based on several factors). It was concluded that the alterations were part of a general lifestyle change in the intervention community and supported the concept that face-to-face counselling was required to specifically influence the high-risk individuals (Salonen et al., 1981).

8.2 Principles of Medical-care Studies

This section begins with consideration of the disciplines of those who might carry out medical-care studies. It then turns to the issue of the type of studies which are carried out, which leads on to the consideration of the categories of approach and the skills required to carry out such studies. The most crucial aspect of such studies is the interaction between the group carrying out the study and the professional administrator—who has to take the findings (and any positive recommendations if these are provided) and translate this into management action. As with any other class of study, an important aspect is the validity of the material used; brief comments are made about this. In a general comment about work in this field, Dollery (1978) suggested that application of research discoveries to health care is less satisfactory than in other fields of medicine and that the organisation of research in this field needs improving if the full benefits of discoveries in science and technology are to be obtained.

8.2.1 Who carries out medical-care studies?

The point has already been made (a number of times) that many very satisfactory epidemiological studies can be carried out that do not require the professional epidemiologist to be involved. The converse of this applies in the medical-care field, where the conventional epidemiological study will be only one approach that is suitable for exploring any particular issue; a very wide range of disciplines may be involved.

Knox (1975a) has suggested that such studies may be carried out by traditional epidemiological methods (including the use of retrospective and prospective observational studies); however, others that may be involved include specialists in behavioural research, computer simulation, economics, electronic data processing, operational research, social sciences, systems analysis and work study.

Engelman (1980) suggested that the contribution of economists in the N.H.S. had been overemphasised; he indicated that they were rarely involved in N.H.S. activities due to: (1) overemphasis of their potential contribution; (2) inappropriate distinction between the decision-making process and decisions involving value judgements, and (3) reluctance to acquire general training instead of specialised economic training. These points were disputed by Akehurst (1981). An analysis of health-service research proposals in the United States in 1972–5 showed little involvement of professional epidemiologists, statisticians, or sociologists (Henderson, 1976). It was suggested this was associated with poorly defined research protocols. As has already been indicated, the role of the professional administrator is crucial in any form of medical-care study. Preferably, the administrative side will be involved from the initiation of the study and whenever appropriate the clinical group whose activity may be associated with the topic of the study. The role of these groups is discussed further in subsection 8.2.4.

8.2.2 What issues should be studied?

In a brief paper on the role of D.H.S.S. in advancing medicine, Black (1974) quoted criteria for evaluating services. These can be modified to provide a checklist for considering the scope of medical care studies:

(1) What are the aims of the programme?
(2) How many people and what kinds are eligible?
(3) What proportion of people get help?

(4) What determines who gets help?
(5) Does the service make any difference and to whom?
(6) What does it cost, who pays, and how does the cost compare with potential substitutes?
(7) What does the public think about the service?
(8) What impact might the service make upon the demand for and effectiveness of other services?

This is by no means an exhaustive list, but it indicates the scope for studies on the functioning of the health service. Obviously the studies carried out will vary in complexity and scale; some will only explore relatively restricted aspects of the delivery of care (what is the need for 'out of hours' biochemistry tests?), while at the other extreme there may be the need to explore the present functioning of the complete provision of care to a community, and review alternative forms of care.

Another framework for considering studies is the one used for the subsections in the preceeding notes on types of study—from the exploration of need, to evaluation of care of a segment of the community. Very different health-care problems may be investigated, such as those of expectant mothers, the elderly or the handicapped.

8.2.3 What types of study can be carried out?

Closely linked to the consideration of the disciplines that may be involved in a medical care study is the related issue of the types of study that may be carried out. The following comments emphasise the role of epidemiology.

The simplest approach is the use of routine data; some consideration of this has already been given in earlier chapters. Descriptive statistics (both mortality and morbidity) may illuminate issues, depict variation, and suggest reasons for such differences or at least clarify the types of study that may be mounted to unravel the cause of these differences. Where there is no relevant routine data or the routine data are inadequate to examine the particular problem, then some special study is required. The technique of surveys is highly relevant here, including the search for retrievable material 'buried' within old records (that is medical and other forms of record). A simple cross-sectional survey may be inadequate, and will often be extended by questioning respondents about past events—using the methods of case–control studies (or at least the retrospective questioning techniques used in such studies). Where there is need to consider the outcome of care, the prospective type of study will often be of great value (although with care the need for follow up over lengthy periods may be avoided by the use of overlapping surveys questioning individuals about current and past events). Whenever innovations in care are to be introduced then the need for a formal controlled trial must always be considered.

Epidemiology overlaps with the skills of applied statisticians, and others who may contribute to building conceptual and simulation models that may explore medical issues; this is discussed further in subsection 8.5.2.

Further from the areas of concern of the epidemiologist is the need to carry out systems studies to examine the functioning of some aspects of the health-care system, or the contribution of behavioural scientists to the process of decision making and the implementation of change. Often it is important to consider the financial implication of differing forms of care and the true costs of care may require the economist for accurate costing. An example would be the evaluation of the screening of breast cancer, where the costs would be required of (1) the different forms of care (screening, confirmation of the diagnosis, treatment, and after-care), (2) the impact of the screening on the women (attendance at the clinics, balance of fear against relief, lives saved versus the penalty of overinvestigation and treatment).

As far as the standard techniques of epidemiology are concerned, the reader should consult the appropriate earlier chapters of this book for details of the principles involved. Medical-care studies will then require the careful application of the appropriate techniques to the specific problems; this will require an appreciation of the nuances of the particular field of work—but this is no more than the equivalent awareness that is required when moving from the study of the aetiology of perinatal death to quantification of the natural history of presenile dementia.

8.2.4 Interaction between research worker and administrator

A crucial and difficult issue is the degree of interaction that is required between the administrator and the research worker. This will obviously depend in part on the size and complexity of the problem being investigated. Study of the problem of the waiting list for a particular clinic in one hospital, or of the use of ancillary staff in a group practice, has very different implications from those of a major review for a region of the balance between hospital and home care (including support from the social and welfare services).

Obviously, because the administrator is so likely to be involved in considering the implications of any piece of work, the sooner some degree of contact has occurred the better. This is not to imply that only acceptable research findings are desirable in this general field of work. However, the instrument of change is not usually the mere writing of a research report, but its careful consideration and the discussion of all the implications of any changes advocated.

As an example of the problems that can occur, Forsyth and Varley (1981) discussed the 'Inner City Partnerships' initiative launched a few years ago. This involved collaboration between central and local govenment, and a number of different departments were involved; the health authority might provide a hospital service of national excellence but not primary-care, geriatric, and psychiatric services that were required, while financial resources may not have been allocated in relation to the present quality of service. These authors indicated that in translating some of the ideas into practice there had been difficulties due to: (1) conflicting government priorities, (2) procedural confusion, (3) conflicting local criteria, (4) distortion of local priorities, (5) conflict between inner and outer city localities and (6) financial constraints.

Some of the difficulty in establishing a good working relationship between the administrator and research worker may be failure to communicate clearly between professional groups of very different backgrounds. Rather different may be overt conflict between the different disciplines, due to misunderstanding, professional jealousies, use of different language, the failure to see issues with the view of the other, etc.

Agreement is likely to come when: the issue upon which there is a need for research is clear cut; a precise protocol is drawn up and agreed by those commissioning the study and those carrying it out; the results are produced on time in a clearly written report; and joint discussions occur over the interpretation of the results and the implementation of the findings. It must be remembered that the epidemiologist is not involved in introducing change, but may be again involved if invited to monitor the impact of any change introduced.

8.2.5 Validity

As with all the other chapters it is important to remind the reader of need for accurate data for all studies carried out on medical-care issues. When using routine or retrievable data, such as published mortality statistics, or routine data on hospital discharge, the user will have no direct control on the quality of the data; he must therefore be aware of the innate errors in the material and take steps to see that any interpretations are made with due care. When setting up some system to collect *ad hoc* data required for a particular project, the points raised in chapters 4, 5 and 6 must be borne in mind.

Illsley (1980) emphasised that self-reports may be measuring something more than 'objective' clinical assessments, and he suggested that this is borne out by the fact that subjects' health-related behaviour is more closely linked to self-perception than to assessment by medical examination.

One of the difficulties is the complex nature of the health service and the consequent difficulty in converting the relatively crude evidence that may be provided by routine data and supplemented by cross-sectional, case–control or prospective studies into a realistic and usable picture. However hard the data, change can occur for a variety of reasons that may be difficult to document. For example, Calnan *et al.* (1978) reported tonsillectomy and circumcision rates in two cohorts born in 1946 and 1958. They identified a fall of one-fifth in tonsillectomy and by half in circumcision, which were thought to reflect changing professional opinions of the worth of these operations.

An example of the way in which interpretation can create difficulty is the varying use of official statistics on perinatal mortality. People advocated diametrically opposed views 'supported' by the same set of statistics! This point is discussed by MacFarlane and Mugford (1983).

8.3 Advantages and Disadvantages of Medical-care Studies

A comparable section has appeared in chapters 2 to 7, this one serves a rather different purpose. There is no intention to contrast medical-care studies with those of another field of work; rather, the need is to discuss some of the differences in the ways that such studies may be carried out, and to elaborate on the general problems that work in this field may generate and try to indicate how some of them may be overcome.

As regards the different ways of tackling a problem, the points already made earlier apply. Routine data is of value to study a problem if relevant items have been collected in the system and especially if tabulations are already available (or can be prepared without delay). However, the routine data will often be limited in nature, and the system inflexible; some of the material may also be rather delayed when there is a desire to look at today's problems.

It is worth bearing in mind that a skilled administrator may have a very good 'feel' for a particular issue, and especially of the scope there is for change. The research worker needs therefore to do a good piece of work to improve on the judgement of such an administrator. This may be coupled with the requirement to produce the results quickly, which does not allow a definitive study to be carried out with all the care that the epidemiologist would wish (such as piloting questionnaires and validating other methods of data collection).

On the other hand the research worker may be trapped if a careful study is carried out that takes some time to complete—as the situation may have changed by the time his results are made available (much quicker changes can occur in the medical-care field than in the cause of disease).

White (1976) discussed three major attempts to plan the health services in the United States, which he indicated had been abortive: (1) acute hospitals, (2) tertiary in place of primary care and (3) comprehensive health plans. He stated that there had been lack of measures of perceived needs of the population. Knox (1976) emphasised that political attitudes affect the acceptability and applicability of medical-care studies, and that the main use of the results was via the scientific literature (this seems a distressing failure of collaboration at local level). He suggested that many studies were of local and topical interest, possibly of short-term value, with the intention to apply the results being part of the plan. If not applied, the effort is wasted. Massé (1976) emphasised that current health problems are likely to be complex, with combination of several health issues affecting subgroups of the population with an aggregation of difficulties (e.g. large families with low income, the handicapped, the unemployed, etc.). A very similar point was made by Illsley (1980), who stressed that the groups shared: lack of economic potential; behaviour not of the accepted norm; problems of multiple aetiology; and problems with low responses to curative techniques.

8.4 Extension of Medical-care Studies

This topic provides an open-ended commitment to discuss such a wide range of studies that a rather restricted approach has had to be selected, with just four special topics being chosen for discussion. None of the methods indicated are sufficiently robust or capable of the degree of variation that would make them immediately applicable to any particular situation. In general there are an unlimited number of problems that will warrant some modification of the general approaches discussed in earlier sections of this chapter.

Cohen (1981) reviewed the history of health-care research in this country. This began with work on the control of communicable disease and then clinical research; for both of these, close collaboration had been established between the government, research workers and those who would apply the findings. By the 1960s the main problem had been how to generalise the modern standards of health care throughout the regions and all specialties. The health-care problems for research that were surfacing were complex, such as the decisions needed on the topics of organ transplant or screening services. There were complex issues to evaluate and the pressures for various decisions were great. During this phase the first priority had been to establish a cadre of skilled workers throughout the country and to clarify the method for tackling some of these difficult topics, rather than to immediately obtain definitive results for specific issues. Cohen went on to identify some of the range of topics that required research: screening, evaluation, patterns of hospital care and community care, manpower studies and controlled trials.

Other stimulating lists of work in progress in other countries were provided (1) for Canada by Anderson (1976), including requirements for children's dental care, and modelling of requirements for primary/secondary/tertiary-care facilities; and (2) for Scandinavia by Mosbech (1976), including primary health-care, and accident and traffic speed planning.

8.4.1 Intervention studies in medical care

Chapter 7 has already dealt with the general issue of intervention studies and the particular problems of those in the medical-care field. This subsection just emphasises some of the relevant points for the three aspects of such work: prevention, early detection, and organisation of care.

Evans (1976) emphasised that the principal causes of death and hospitalisation in those aged 5–34 and 35–74 are not preventable by classic medical means. They all require control of obesity, smoking, lack of exercise, high-fat diets, stress and self-imposed risks (such as smoking and alcohol consumption). Their control involves far-reaching changes in personal motivation and lifestyle. The same points were evident in the government white paper (D.H.S.S. et al., 1977). This also indicated the difficulty of balancing the liberty of the individual and the possible dereliction of duty if the government adopted a noninterventionist approach. There was also the dilemma of uncertainty, and the need for the thorough assessment of appropriate evidence.

There have already been examples given of controlled trials in the fields of primary prevention of disease (such as by programmes of immunisation), early detection of disease (screening for breast cancer), and medical issues related to the organisation of services such as home versus hospital treatment, short- versus long stay in acute-care facilities, or specialist versus ancillary care (such as for attempted suicide).

For clearly defined problems the approach of a randomised controlled trial may be appropriate and carried out as indicated in chapter 7; however, for many topics the research becomes increasingly difficult as one moves from the simple innovation in one form of care to the more complex issues requiring ramified changes in the way of working of the service. Also the ideal design of randomised trial is not always practical or suitable, as for instance with the study of early detection of breast cancer. As it was not thought feasible to randomly allocate women to screening and control groups (such that neighbours may be given different forms of care), the United Kingdom trial chose to select locations and offer screening in some, offer education in self-examination in others, and keep some for comparison purposes.

8.4.2 The need for a special study

A problem to many fields of work is whether there is adequate information available or retrievable, or whether there is need for an *ad hoc* study to be mounted. The extent of available management information varies from one country to another, but an important aspect of any research team's functions should be to ensure that all the staff are familiar with the potentially available information, so that the relevance of this to any new problem can be immediately determined. In many cases, it will be possible to give some outline response to the topic from the shrewd use of retrievable data, the skill then being applied to the design of the minimal complementary field study that is required to balance this information. A number of pointers to such activity have already been given in the preceeding chapters of this book, and in the earlier sections of this chapter. It is not possible to expand further in a short space on the many ways in which such work may be pursued, but two brief examples are now given of very different reports that have combined routine with *ad hoc* data.

In order to extend the very limited information about the work of Medical Officers of Environmental Health, Waldron (1978) sent a questionnaire to all in the country, getting a response from 79 per cent. This quantified the time spent on various duties. This enabled Waldron to provide recommendations of the way in which the work might be organised locally, with some specific comments about the control of infectious disease, toxicology, and occupational health services.

Richter (1981) discussed use of data on police reports of motor-vehicle crashes involving injury, death certificates for fatalities, estimates of drivers and vehicles, estimates of distance travelled from annual fuel consumption and interurban traffic monitoring. He discussed how such material could be used to clarify lines of prevention or control of such trauma.

8.4.3 Functioning of the health service

Some very successful studies have looked at a discrete facet of the health service and have made a contribution to improving the quality (equality or effectiveness) of the service. Perhaps they have in part been successful because they were only examining a restricted issue. However, consideration of medical-care studies under specific labels, such as 'need', 'demand', 'workload', and 'outcome', provides a disjointed approach to the subject. It should be emphasised that many medical-care studies, especially those carried out for planning purposes, will not look at health needs in isolation (or one of the other aspects to which a section has been devoted). Usually need, demand, use and outcome will all have to be considered, not only as facets of the health-care system, but also in an attempt to identify the interaction between them.

A detailed survey was carried out in 1970–1 in Traralgon, a county town in Victoria with a population of 15 500 (Bridges-Webb, 1973; 1974a; 1974b). Three quite different methods were used to collect information about the illnesses suffered by the population and the treatment they received.

A random selection of families was invited to complete a diary in which they recorded all illness and medical care throughout the year.

Another source of information was a sample of individuals who were interviewed during the course of the survey—about eight families being interviewed weekly. Standard information was obtained using a questionnaire based on the American Health Interview Survey. It was decided to question subjects about illness in the two weeks preceding the interview.

The third approach was an endeavour to collect data from all health and other associated agencies. The family doctors recorded details of all morbidity seen for one week of each quarter. The age and sex of the patient, diagnosis, and length of stay were recorded for all admissions to the central hospital serving the area. The pharmacists in the district recorded details of all episodes every sixth week for which their advice was requested. In addition, data were obtained from the ambulance service, clergy, day hospital, district nurse, home helps, infant welfare clinics, Lifeline, marriage guidance council, meals-on-wheels and social workers. A careful system for collecting these data was devised. Some checks enabled an estimate to be made of the deficiency in sets of data (for example, comparison of medical records and the diaries completed by the continuously recording respondents suggested that 19 per cent of the conditions were not mentioned at their initial interview).

The three published reports provided a comprehensive account of the survey and tabulations of the principal results. There was a high reported prevalence of acute and chronic illness, injury or disability (86 per cent reporting one or more events). There was an annual consultation rate of 4.1 per person, and there were 128 hospital admissions per 1000 people per year. For the treatment of illness the doctors stood out as the major source of help, although there was a wide variety of other health and welfare agencies involved. The relationship between prevalence of illness and use of health services was examined by demographic and social factors. Although these analyses could not indicate the reasons for the wide variation in illness in relation to these factors, they provided useful information about the relationship between social factors and health care.

Only 13 per cent of all new episodes of illness were presented for medical attention; however, the majority of conditions relating to pregnancy and to cardiovascular disease came to the doctor. Half of the general-practice consultations were for new conditions, but only about one-twentieth of these required admission to hospital. Medication prescribed by doctors was taken for 25 per cent of illnesses and self-prescribed medication for an equal proportion. It was suggested that the illnesses that receive care from nonmedical sources, including self-medication, represented a vast potential demand for medical care. It was pointed out that there was no indication from the survey that medical care would bring any benefit to this category of illness.

One aim of the survey was to test the effectiveness of different methods of obtaining information on illness in a population. It was felt that the accuracy and perseverance of the continuously recording families was not enough to justify the greater effort involved for both the survey team and the participants compared with the cross-sectional interviews.

A number of studies mentioned in the preceding sections have looked at the interrelationship between community care and hospital care. It must be remembered that sometimes there will be a direct choice between home and hospital care; there may be a less direct influence when priorities are set within a rigid financial framework. More nurses in an intensive-care unit may mean fewer nurses in the community.

Subsection 8.1.3.3 has emphasised that not every patient in an acute hospital bed was admitted or retained on 'medical' grounds. Over the past ten years interest has revived in the contribution that community hospitals can make. (These are hospitals that serve a much smaller population than a district general hospital, being near to patients' homes, having no operating theatre, and being served by family practitioners but visited by consultants.) A number of studies have indicated that there is a group of patients requiring treatment beyond the resources of their own home and the community team, but who do not require the full facilities of a bed in an acute hospital. There are also a number of general practitioners who are anxious to take on the responsibility of looking after such patients in community hospitals (see Barber *et al.*, 1972; Clarke and Mulholland, 1973). A special study to evaluate the role of such hospitals has been described by Bennett (1974).

Another innovation in general practice has been the use of deputising services to provide on-call cover in the evenings and at weekends. Williams and his colleagues (1973a; 1973b; 1973c; 1974) looked at the development and use of these services throughout the country, and in particular in cities around Sheffield. They looked at the use of accident and emergency departments, and suggested that the deputising service did not add to the workload of these departments either through direct referral or due to a tendency for patients to use these departments in preference to the service. Another study by Williams and his colleagues (1973c) found no influence of emergency admissions referred by these services on patient characteristics, speciality, diagnoses, operations performed, length of stay or case fatality, when compared with a control group of emergency admissions.

The above examples indicate the need to examine the interrelationship of the various segments of the health service in order to obtain a comprehensive picture of its functioning. Alderson and Dowie (1979) discussed how information on (1) demography and environment, (2) mortality and morbidity, (3) health-care needs, (4) health resources, (5) health facilities, (6) utilisation and (7) outcome must be blended together. This is a difficult task and it may seem 'pie in the sky' to expect a routine information system to provide such a global picture, but it should be noted that Florence Nightingale (1863) advocated the analysis of a comparable set of statistics. A balance has to be struck between extensive collection of routine data (which can be analysed automatically or processed in response to specific queries), the organisation of special surveys, and mathematical modelling, which can provide a description of the present and permits examination of hypothetical situations.

8.4.4 Resource allocation

An important general issue in considering the use of the health-care services is an assessment of whether there is a uniform provision of facilities throughout the country and whether there are any barriers to use of the service. Reference has already been briefly made (see subsection 4.2.3.4) to the inverse relationship between need for and use of preventive and screening programmes. Cartwright and O'Brien (1976) recently reviewed this issue and also presented some information about the variation in the nature of general practitioner consultations in relation to the social class of the patient. This complex problem requires careful consideration in assessment of the functioning of the service. Hart (1971) suggested that there is an inverse care law, with a comprehensive provision of facilities in those parts of the country where the need is least. In addition, there is evidence that demand for and use of services are not directly linked to objective measures of need (see subsection 8.1.1).

Ashford et al. (1973) investigated some of the techniques used in industry and commerce, in an attempt to move towards a formal process of resource allocation in the N.H.S. They quantified some of the costs and output measures, but identified a series of problems with the method: (1) doctors were a major determinant of the use of resources, (2) doctors differed in their use of resources for the same clinical problem, (3) there were differences (historical and other) in the resources available, (4) market forces did not apply, (5) the traditional Pareto criterion for economic welfare did not apply. They examined in detail the complex real-life aspects of maternity care, constructing a conceptual model of the health-care system and using mathematical programming to look at the possible consequences of different management policies.

Opit and Day (1975) selected ophthalmic services for study because of the circumscribed nature of the workload and the likelihood that there was little difference in selection for treatment, method of treatment, and results across the country. For each of eleven regions they examined: bed availability; consultant staffing; a social index for the region; the ratio of the costs for diagnostic, therapeutic and nursing services to the expenditure on clinical salaries; bed occupancy in relation to waiting lists; 'productivity' in terms of discharges, day cases and new outpatients related to clinical provision; paramedical workload at outpatients; and hospital discharges for specific conditions. They identified various indications of appreciable imbalance in the regions between the treatment load and the staff and facilities provided.

A major innovation in the United Kingdom was the introduction of a scheme for adjusting the annual funding of the health authorities, so that the sums made available year by year moved towards amounts that were thought to represent equitable funding for the populations served (rather than being based on historical provision). A committee in England and Wales (D.H.S.S., 1976) indicated that 'needs' for authorities should be based on the population served, weighted to reflect age, sex, fertility, mortality and marital status, with further adjustment for patient flow across boundaries, cost differences and teaching load. The intention was that funding should move towards the equitable allocation 'as fast as is consistent with practical constraints on the pace of change.' A comparable approach was advocated for Scotland (S.H.H.D., 1977), with some variations in the way mortality was used as an indicator of morbidity (the S.M.R.s in Scotland were based on ages 0–64 rather than all ages).

Barnard and Ham (1976) emphasised the importance of 'Political constraints' in reallocation of resources. Dyson (1978) and Jeffries (1978) discussed the difficulties created for those regional authorities where funding was being pared down. A number of authors have commented about the method used in determining equitable resource-allocation (see Snaith, 1978; Geary, 1977; Senn and Shaw, 1978; Palmer *et al.*, 1980). Knox (1982) suggested adaptation of the method so that it could be more readily applied at local level; he advocated an approach based on estimates of lifetime consumption of health-care resources for those that die ('terminal accounting').

8.5 Statistical Aspects of Medical-care Studies

This section uses a much broader approach to statistics than did comparable ones in previous chapters. It deals with two applied issues: (1) the development of indicators of health status of individuals and health needs of populations, and (2) the application of modelling techniques to the medical-care field.

8.5.1 Indicators

Many planners now dream of having a single index of the health status of the community, which would serve as a guide to a range of health problems.

However, it is extremely unlikely that such an index could be calculated, as it can in the economic field, where monetary units can be derived from a number of highly diverse components.

In a major review of this topic Murnaghan (1981) indicated that the set of indicators might reflect the key objectives of national- or community-health policies. It was suggested that a variety of contrasting viewpoints could be obtained on the measurement of levels of health: (1) politicians and civil servants drawing up budgets versus providers/managers at local level, (2) researchers interested in specific topics versus statisticians in central government looking at broad trends, (3) disease-orientated clinicians versus population-orientated epidemiologists, (4) those responsible for health services generally versus those in charge of specific programmes, (5) those from developing countries versus those with more data than they can digest. Fenton Lewis and Modle (1982) have discussed the use of indicators, with examples of their application to various aspects of the health-care field.

Black and Pole (1975) demonstrated how the burden from different diseases could be quantified, using available data on inpatient days, outpatient referrals, consultations in general practice, sickness benefit and loss of expectation of life. Heasman (1979) discussed the use of statistics on hospital discharge, sickness absence, morbidity seen in general practice and population surveys. He pointed out that these would not readily produce an optimum measure of community morbidity, but further work on the development of this was warranted. Goldberg *et al.* (1979) reviewed the classic concepts of health indexes based on mortality and morbidity statistics; they emphasised that these may underestimate morbidity with appreciable social or economic impact, and fail to reflect the effects of health-care delivery. They indicated the potential improvement from measuring disability and assessing positive health.

The use of census and other data to classify small areas into similar socio-economic groups was discussed by Scott-Samuel (1977), with examples of application in health-care planning and research. Carstairs (1981a) used census variates to classify the 37 Glasgow and 23 Edinburgh wards for degree of 'deprivation'; this was then related to: mortality for all and selected causes, perinatal deaths, infant deaths, discharges and bed days in general hospitals for all and selected causes, admissions to mental hospitals and low birth-weight. There were fairly strong associations with mortality, hospital discharges and bed days, and low birth-weight; perinatal and infant deaths were not related and this could not be explained by small numbers of events. There was no evidence of variable availability of hospital beds influencing use of such facilities. The general aspects of small-area analysis of health and associated data have been discussed by Carstairs (1981b). She emphasised: the advantage of more homogenous populations; the ability of allocating some events to areas; the ability to study aetiology and health-care issues; the difficulty of allocating some events to areas, unless postcodes are used; the lack of population estimates, which can be overcome in studying infant mortality, with births as the denominator; the need for age-adjustment, and the distorting effect of long-stay institutions; the variation from use of events based on small numbers, which can be partly overcome by aggregation over several years; and the difficulty of aligning some of the environmental data to the selected small areas.

Another approach to this was used by Cochrane *et al.* (1978), who examined the relationship between age-specific mortality rates and a range of health input-variables (health-service provision, dietary indices, economic and demographic factors) for eighteen developed countries. They found a strong negative association with per capita gross national product, and a marked positive association between provision of doctors and mortality in the younger age-groups (i.e. perinatal up to 25–34).

Another issue is the validity of the denominator for health localities. Pinder (1982) compared various methods of estimating the catchment population of health districts; he suggested that a method of net flow was the most accurate, but other methods (such as proportionate flow) were suitable when there was high cross-boundary flow and low variation in admission rates.

Comparison of scores for the health indicators of Grogono and Rosser showed poor correlation, when data were collected by persons unfamiliar with the patients (Coles *et al.*, 1976). Items with good concordance being retained, additional items were constructed to provide further information; it was found that improved results were obtained by staff who knew the patients and used data from problem-orientated medical records. Kalimo and Rabin (1976) obtained survey data in twelve areas in seven countries on: disability data in days in the past two weeks, other health problems in the past two weeks, chronic illness, specific symptoms, vision problems, dental problems and anxiety. There was a low level of relationship among the specific indicators in all study areas. Hunt *et al.* (1980) compared aspects of perceived health status with four small groups of elderly with different health statuses; they suggested that the perceived status accorded well with the objective assessment of health.

There are a number of statistical aspects to the handling of such data. Bertrand *et al.* (1979) discussed ways in which data could be analysed to identify 'environmental' indicators relevant to community health. They advocated principal-component analysis of ridits; the data they used related child/household/neighbourhood factors to mortality under five years of age. Often the measures of morbidity will involve components of differing 'seriousness'; McKenna *et al.* (1981) describe a method of allocating appropriately scaled weights to the different components.

8.5.2 Mathematical models in medical-care studies

It has already been mentioned that epidemiology is only one of the disciplines involved in the examination of medical problems. Common to several of these approaches is the use of mathematical models. Reference to models has already been made in an implicit way when considering the use of multivariate techniques in prediction. Another approach, however, is used in medical-care studies, which involves simulation and other techniques to provide a dynamic picture of the functioning of a facet of the health service.

This may be used to facilitate examination of the present situation, to extrapolate the future workload and to study the repercussions of change of inputs into the system.

In 1972 there was growing concern about the pressure placed or the obstetric services in the Basingstoke district. This is an overspill town for London, and the new housing estates incorporate a large number of young married couples, who often arrive in the area with the wife pregnant. There were conflicting views as to whether the birth-rate was high in this district, and there was clear evidence of the pressure on the obstetric services. An examination of this situation was undertaken (Slattery, 1974); the first step was to look at the birth-rate. Taking into account the age, sex and marital status of the population, it was found that the birth-rate was no higher in Basingstoke than one would have expected. The crude birth-rate was certainly high, but this was merely a reflection of the structure of the population. Estimates were available of the anticipated build up of the population over the coming decade, with some indication of the likely age structure of this population. This enabled a projection to be made of the number of births per year in the district. When the study was initiated, a considerable proportion of the pregnant women were receiving obstetric care at hospitals outside the catchment area. An estimate was made of the increasing proportion of mothers in the district, who would be cared for by the local facilities, using Hospital Inpatient Enquiry data and local discussion. An estimate was also made of the proportion of mothers who would be cared for in general practitioner units and in consultants' units; a very small percentage had a home confinement.

In order to project future requirements for the various obstetric facilities, an estimate was made of the proportion of women requiring antenatal admission and the distribution of antenatal length of stay. In addition, a breakdown was provided of the distribution by type of delivery, associated stay in the first and second stages of labour, the proportion requiring theatre facilities, and the postnatal stay for each category of delivery. These data incorporated estimates of the proportion of mothers requiring an induction, having a normal vaginal delivery, a forceps delivery, a planned Caesarian section, an emergency Caesarian section and those being sterilised in the postnatal period. Assuming random arrival of mothers requiring antenatal stay and in labour, the data were converted into a distribution of the daily requirements for beds in antenatal and postnatal wards and the number of mothers expected to be in the labour suites. It was a relatively simple matter to re-examine these data for variation in the birth-rate and alterations in the parameters, such as the proportion of pregnant women in the district being delivered in the district general hospital, the proportion being cared for in the consultant unit, or the variation in the distribution of types of delivery and associated lengths of stay.

A computer simulation of this material was carried out and the graph shown in figure 8.3 was generated. This graph is for an estimate of 1180 births *per annum*. The distribution of bed occupancy in relation to the number of beds provided is shown and also a curve of the risk of 'overflow' in relation to beds provided. For example, with forty beds provided there

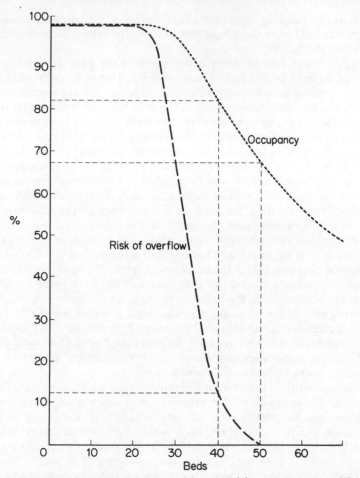

Figure 8.3 Relationship between bed provision and (1) occupancy, and (2) risk of overflow in an obstetric unit.
Source: Slattery (1974)

would be an average bed occupancy of 82 per cent, but on about 11 per cent of days there would be a risk of overflow. Overflow is currently catered for in obstetric units either by unplanned early discharge of some of the mothers or by putting up additional beds in the wards; both practices create difficulties. The chart indicates that with an additional ten beds the average bed occupancy would drop to approximately 67 per cent and it would be rare (less than one day per 100) for the number of beds to be inadequate for the demand. Providing additional beds means that the average occupancy drops and a balance has to be struck between providing adequate facilities and overproviding in order to safeguard against very occasional peak demand. The clinicians and planners can examine material such as this and decide on the optimum provision.

A general discussion of the application of this type of approach to medical-care studies is provided by Luck *et al.* (1971), while Lilienfeld (1976) has indicated the various uses of models in studying cause of disease. Knox (1973, 1975b) described the value of models in investigating screening programmes for cervix and breast cancer. Adaptation of the Kermack and McKendrick infectious-disease model was used to indicate how heroin use spreads in 'epidemic' fashion. MacKintosh and Stewart (1979) indicate how this model might be used to clarify a strategy for intervention. A simulation model was developed by Hakulinen and Pukkala (1981) to forecast incidence of lung cancer on the basis of hypothetical changes in the smoking habits of males. They indicate how this can be utilised to direct health education to the groups where change in smoking habits would have the greatest effect. Woodward (1982) presented a model to predict the changes in total size and age structure of a long-stay mental-hospital population.

References

Recommended reading

McCarthy, M. (1982). *Epidemiology and Policies for Health Care Planning.* King Edward's Hospital Fund, London
Nuffield Provincial Hospital Trust. Publications on a wide range of topics
Yates, J. (1982). *Hospital Beds: A Problem for Diagnosis and Management?* Heinemann Medical, London

Other references

Airth, A. B., and Newell, D. J. (1962). *The Demand for Hospital Beds.* University of Durham, Newcastle
Akehurst, R. L. (1981). *Comm. Med.*, **3**, 149–53
Alderson, M. R. (1966). *Proc. R. Soc. Med.*, **59**, 719–21
Alderson, M. R. (1970). *Br. J. prev. soc. Med.*, **24**, 120–3
Alderson, M. R. (1974). Unpublished
Alderson, M. R. (1975). In *The Theory and Practice of Public Health* (W. Hobson, ed.), Oxford University Press, London, ch. 3
Alderson, M. R., and Dowie, R. (1979). *Health Surveys and Related Studies.* Pergamon, Oxford
Alderson, M. R., and Nayak, R. (1970). *Med. Offr*, **124**, 313–5
Amulree, Lord, Exton-Smith, A. N., and Crockett, E. S. (1951). *Lancet*, **1**, 123–6
Anderson, D. O. (1976). In *Epidemiology as a Fundamental Science* (K. L. White and M. M. Henderson, eds.), Oxford University Press, New York, pp. 17–43
Anderson, J. A. D. (1968). *Lancet*, **2**, 97
Anderson, P. (1980). *J. Epidem. Comm. Hlth*, **34**, 299–304
Ashford, J. R., Ferster, G., and Makuc, D. M. (1973). In *The Future and Present Indicatives* (G. McLachlan, ed.), Oxford University Press, London, pp. 57–90
Ashley, J. S. A., Howlett, A., and Morris, J. N. (1971). *Lancet*, **2**, 1308–11
Ashley, J. S. A., Pasker, P., and Beresford, J. C. (1972). *Lancet*, **1**, 890–2

Badley, E. M., Thompson, R. P., and Wood, P. H. N. (1978). *Int. J. Epidem.*, **7,** 145–51

Barber, J. H., Bain, D. J. C., Bassett, W. J., and Haines, A. J. (1972). *Br. med. J.*, **4,** 27–30

Barnard, K., and Ham, C. (1976). *Lancet*, **1,** 1399–400

Bennett, A. E. (1974). *Br. Med. Bull.*, **30,** 223–7

Bertrand, W. E., Brockett, P. L., and Levine, A. (1979). *Int. J. Epidem.*, **8,** 161–6

Bispham, K., Holland, W. W., and Stringer, J. (1971). *Hospital*, **67,** 82–7

Black, D. (1974). *Proc. R. Soc. Med.*, **67,** 1306–8

Black, D., and Pole, J. D. (1975). *Br. J. prev. soc. Med.*, **29,** 222–7

Bradshaw, J. (1972). In *Problems and Progress in Medical Care*, 7th Series (G. McLachlan, ed.), Oxford University Press, London, pp. 69–82

Breslow, L. (1972). *Int. J. Epidem.*, **1,** 347–55

Bridges-Webb, C. (1973). *Int. J. Epidem.*, **2,** 63–72

Bridges-Webb, C. (1974a). *Int. J. Epidem.*, **3,** 37–46

Bridges-Webb, C. (1974b). *Int. J. Epidem.*, **3,** 233–46

British Thoracic Association (1982). *Br. Med. J.*, **285,** 1251–6

Butterfield, W. J. H. (1968). In *Screening in Medical Care*, Oxford University Press, London, pp. 65–80

Calnan, M., Douglas, J. W. B., and Goldstein, H. (1978). *Int. J. Epidem.*, **7,** 79–85

Capstick, I. (1974). *Br. med. J.*, **1,** 278–9

Carstairs, V. (1970). *Channels of Communication.* Scottish Home and Health Department, Edinburgh

Carstairs, V. (1981a). *Comm. Med.*, **3,** 4–13

Carstairs, V. (1981b). *Comm. Med.*, **3,** 131–9

Cartwright, A. (1964). *Human Relations and Hospital Care.* Routledge Kegan Paul, London

Cartwright, A. (1967). *Patients and Their Doctors.* Routledge Kegan Paul, London

Cartwright, A. (1974). *Br. med. Bull.*, **30,** 218–22

Cartwright, A., Martin, F. M., and Thompson, J. H. (1960). *Lancet*, **1,** 327–9

Cartwright, A., and O'Brien, M. (1976). *Sociol. Rev. Monogr.*, **22,** 77–98

Chiang, C. L., and Cohen, R. B. (1973). *Int. J. Epidem.*, **2,** 7–14

Clarke, M., and Mulholland, A. (1973). *J. R. Coll. gen. Pract.*, **23,** 273–9

Cochrane, A. L. (1954). *Br. med. Bull.*, **10,** 91–5

Cochrane, A. L. (1972). *Effectiveness and Efficiency: Random Reflections on the Health Service.* Nuffield Provincial Hospitals Trust, London

Cochrane, A. L., Leger, A. S. St., and Moore, F. (1978). *J. Epidem. Comm. Hlth*, **32,** 200–5

Cohen, R. H. L. (1981). In *Matters of Moment.* (G. McLachlan, ed.), Oxford University Press, London, pp. 1–24

Coles, J. M., Davison, A. J., Neal, D. M., and Wickings, H. I. (1976). *Int. J. Epidem.*, **5,** 237–46

Cross, K. W. (1973). *Lancet*, **2,** 954–6

Darmady, E. M. (1964). *J. clin. Path.*, **17,** 477–81

Department of Health and Social Security (1970). *Confidential Enquiry into Post-neonatal Deaths, 1964–66.* H.M.S.O., London

Department of Health and Social Security (1973). *Annual Report of the Hospital Advisory Service to the Secretary of State for Social Services and Secretary of State for Wales for 1972.* H.M.S.O., London

Department of Health and Social Security (1976). *Sharing Resources for Health in England.* H.M.S.O., London

Department of Health and Social Security, Department of Science, Scottish Office, and Welsh Office (1977). *Prevention and Health.* H.M.S.O., London

Doll, R. (1973). *Proc. R. Soc. Med.*, **66,** 729–40

Dollery, C. T. (1971). In *Challenges for Change* (G. McLachlan, ed.), Oxford University Press, London, pp. 3–32

Dollery, C. (1978). *The End of an Age of Optimism*, Nuffield Provincial Hospitals Trust, London

Dudley, H. A. F. (1974). *Br. Med. J.*, **1**, 275–7

Dunnell, K., and Cartwright, A. (1972). *Medicine Takers, Prescribers and Hoarders.* Routledge Kegan Paul, London

Dyson, R. (1978). *Br. med. J.*, **1**, 383

Engelman, S. R. (1980). *Comm. Med.*, **2**, 126–34

Evans, J. R. (1976). In *Epidemiology as a Fundamental Science* (K. L. White, and M. M. Henderson, eds), Oxford University Press, London, pp. 3–10

Fanshel, S. (1972). *Int. J. Epidem.*, **1**, 3319–38

Fanshel, S., and Bush, J. W. (1970). *Ops. Res.*, **18**, 1021–66

Fenton Lewis, A., and Modle, W. J. (1982). *Health Trends*, **14**, 3–8

Ferguson, T., and MacPhail, A. N. (1954). *Hospital and Community*. Oxford University Press, London

Forbes, J. F., Boddy, F. A., Pickering, R., and Wyllie, M. M. (1982). *J. Epidem. Comm. Hlth*, **36**, 282–8

Forsyth, G., and Logan, R. F. L. (1960). *Demand for Medical Care*. Oxford University Press, London

Forsyth, G., and Logan, R. F. L. (1968). *Gateway or Dividing Line?*, Oxford University Press, London

Forsyth, G., and Varley, R. (1981). In *Matters of Moment* (G. McLachlan, ed.), Oxford University Press, London, pp. 39–70

Fry, J. (1971). *Lancet*, **1**, 148

Fry, J. (1973). *Present State and Future Needs of General Practice*. Royal College of General Practitioners, London

Geary, K. (1977). *Br. med. J.*, **1**, 1367

Goldberg, M., Dab, W., Chaperon, J., Fuhrer, R., and Gremy, F. (1979). *Rev. Epidem. Santé Publ.*, **27**, 51–68; 133–52

Grime, L. P., and Whitelegg, J. (1982). *Comm. Med.*, **4**, 201–8

Grogono, A. W., and Woodgate, D. J. (1971). *Lancet*, **2**, 1024–6

Hakulinen, T., and Pukkala, E. (1981). *Int. J. Epidem.*, **10**, 233–40

Harris, A. I., Cox, E., Smith, C. R. W. (1971). *Handicapped and Impaired in Great Britain*, H.M.S.O., London

Hart, J. T. (1971). *Lancet*, **1**, 405–12

Heasman, M. A. (1961). *Mass Miniature Radiography*, H.M.S.O., London

Heasman, M. A. (1964). *Lancet*, **2**, 539–41

Heasman, M. A. (1979). *Health Bull.*, **37**, 103–7

Heasman, M. A., and Carstairs, V. (1971). *Br. med. J.*, **1**, 495–8

Henderson, M. M. (1976). In *Epidemiology as a Fundamental Science*, (K. L. White, and M. M. Henderson, eds). Oxford University Press, London, pp. 84–96

Hey, E. (1981). In *Perinatal Audit and Surveillance* (I. Chalmers and G. McIlwaine, eds), Royal College of Obstetricians and Gynaecologists, London, pp. 188–97

Holland, W. W., and Waller, J. (1971). *Comm. Med.*, **126**, 153–6

Horder, J., and Horder, E. (1954). *Practitioner*, **173**, 177–85

Howqua, J. (1974). *Br. med. J.*, **1**, 281–2

Hulka, B. S., Kupper, L. L., Cassell, J. C. *et al.* (1975). *J. chron. Dis.*, **28**, 2–21

Hunt, S. M., McKenna, S. P., McEwen, J. *et al.* (1980). *J. Epidem. Comm. Hlth*, **34**, 281–6

Illsley, R. (1980). *Professional or Public Health*. Nuffield Provincial Hospitals Trust, London

Jefferys, M., Brotherston, J. H. F., and Cartwright, A. (1960). *Br. J. prev. soc. Med.*, **14**, 64–76

Jeffries, M. (1978). *Br. med. J.*, **1,** 426–7; 495–6; 638–9
Jones, W. T., and Grahame, H. (1974). *Br. med. Bull.*, **30,** 276–81
Kalimo, E., and Rabin, D. L. (1976). *J. chron. Dis.*, **29,** 1–14
Kinlen, L. J. (1969). Thesis accepted for D.Phil., Oxford
Knox, E. G. (1973). In *The Future and Present Indicatives* (G. McLachlan, ed.), Oxford University Press, London, pp. 17–29 and 30–56.
Knox, E. G. (1982). *Comm. Med.*, **4,** 209–16
Knox, G. (1975a). In *Probes for Health* (G. McLachlan, ed.), Oxford University Press, London, pp. 1–12
Knox, G. (1975b). In *Probes for Health* (G. McLachlan, ed.), Oxford University Press, London, pp. 13–44
Knox, G. (1976). In *Epidemiology as a Fundamental Science* (K. L. White and M. M. Henderson, eds), Oxford University Press, New York, pp. 181–9
Lader, S. (1965). *Practitioner*, **194,** 132–6
Lee, J. A. H., Morrison, S. L., and Morris, J. N. (1957). *Lancet*, **2,** 785
Lee, P., Ahola, S. J., Grennan, D., *et al.* (1974). *Br. med. J.*, **1,** 424–6
Lilienfeld, A. M. (1976). *Foundations of Epidemiology*. Oxford University Press, London
Locker, D., Rao, B., and Weddell, J. M. (1981). *Comm. Med.*, **3,** 98–107
Logan, W. P. D., and Brooke, E. M. (1957). *Survey of Sickness 1943–52.* H.M.S.O., London
Loudon, I. S. L. (1970). *The Demand for Hospital Care: Inpatient Care Alternatives and Delays*, United Oxford Hospitals, Oxford
Luck, G. N., Luckman, J., Smith, B. W., and Stringer, J. (1971). *Patients, Hospitals, and Operational Research*. Tavistock, London
Lunn, J. N., and Mushin, W. W. (1982). *Mortality Associated with Anaethesia*. Nuffield Hospitals Provincial Trust, London
MacFarlane, A., and Mugford, M. (1983). *Birth Counts—Statistics of Pregnancy and Childbirth*. H.M.S.O., London
McKenna, S. P., Hunt, S. M., and McEwen, J. (1981). *Int. J. Epidem.*, **10,** 93–7
McKenzie, M., Weir, R. D., Richardson, I. M., *et al.* (1962). *Further Studies in Hospital and Community*. Oxford University Press, London
MacKintosh, D. R., and Stewart, G. T. (1979). *J. Epidem. Comm. Hlth*, **33,** 299–304
Marsh, G. N., and McNay, R. A. (1974). *Br. med. J.*, **1,** 315–8
Martys, C. R. (1982). *J. Epidem. Comm. Hlth*, **36,** 224–7
Massé, L. M. F. (1976). In *Epidemiology as a Fundamental Science* (K. L. White and M. M. Henderson, eds), Oxford University Press, New York, pp. 181–9
Matthew, G. K. (1971). In *Portfolio for Health* (G. McLachlan, ed.), Oxford University Press, London, pp. 27–46
Ministry of Health. (1964a). *Management Problems of Outpatients Departments*, HM (64) 102. Ministry of Health
Ministry of Health (1964b). *Health Education—Report of a Joint Committee of the Central and Scottish Health Services Council*. H.M.S.O., London
Miller, A. B. (1982). In *Trends in Cancer Incidence* (K. Magnus, ed.), Hemisphere, Washington, pp. 311–20
Morgan, B. M., Bulpitt, C. J., Clifton, P., and Lewis, P. J. (1982). *Lancet*, **2,** 808–10
Morrell, D. C., and Kasap, H. S. (1972). *Int. J. Epidem.*, **2,** 143–51
Morris, J. N. (1941). *Lancet*, **1,** 51–3
Mosbech, J. (1976). In *Epidemiology as a Fundamental Science* (K. L. White and M. M. Henderson, eds), Oxford University Press, New York, pp. 114–23
Murnaghan, J. H. (1981). *Ann. Rev. publ. Hlth.*, **2,** 299–361
Nightingale, F. (1863). *Notes on Hospitals*. Longman Green, London
Office of Population Censuses and Surveys (1973). *The General Household Survey—Introductory Report*. H.M.S.O., London

Office of Population Censuses and Surveys (1974). *Morbidity Statistics from General Practice*. H.M.S.O., London

Opit, L. J., and Day, P. R. (1975). In *Probes for Health*. (G. McLachlan, ed.), Oxford University Press, London, pp. 85–106

Palmer, S. R., West, P. A., and Dodd, P. (1980). *J. Epidem. Comm. Hlth*, **34,** 212–6

Parkin, D. (1979). *J. Epidem. Comm. Hlth*, **33,** 96–99

Peach, H., and Pathy, M. S. (1981). *Comm. Med.*, **3,** 123–30

Pendreigh, D. M., Howitt, L. F., MacDougall, A. I. *et al.* (1972). *Lancet*, **1,** 304–7

Pinder, D. C. (1982). *Comm. Med.*, **4,** 188–95

Puska, P., Tuomilehto, J., Salonen, J., *et al.* (1979). *Br. med. J.*, **2,** 1173–8

Rachootin, P., and Olsen, J. (1981). *J. Epidem. Comm. Hlth*, **35,** 262–4

Raphael, W. (1973). *Patients and Their Hospitals*, 2nd edn, Kings Fund, London, p. 1073

Richards, I. D. G., and Lowe, C. R. (1966). *Lancet*, **1,** 1169–73

Richter, E. D. (1981). *Int. J. Epidem.*, **10,** 145–53

Rose, G. (1975). *Br. J. prev. soc. Med.*, **29,** 147–50

Rosser, R. M., and Watts, V. C. (1972). *Int. J. Epidem.*, **1,** 361–8

Salonen, J. T., Puska, P., Kottle, T. E., *et al.* (1981). *Am. J. Epidem.*, **114,** 81–94

Sanazaro, P. J. (1974). *Br. med. J.*, **1,** 271–4

Scott-Samuel, A. (1977). *Br. J. prev. soc. Med.*, **31,** 199–204

Scottish Home and Health Department (1977). *Scottish Health Authorities Revenue Equalization*. H.M.S.O., Edinburgh

Senn, S. J., Shaw, H. (1978). *J. Epidem. Comm. Hlth*, **32,** 22–7

Sheridan, M. D. (1962). *Mon. Bull. Minist. Hlth*, **21,** 238–45

Slater, D. (1946). *Survey of Sickness, October 1943–December 1945*. H.M.S.O., London

Slattery, M. (1974). Personal communication

Smith, A. (1968). *The Science of Social Medicine*. Staples, London

Snaith, A. H. (1978). *J. Epidem. Comm. Hlth*, **32,** 16–21

Stewart, R., and Sleeman, J. (1967). *Continuously Under Review*. Bell, London

Svanborg, A., Bergstrom, G., and Mellstrom, D. (1982). *Epidemiological Studies on Social and Medical Conditions of the Elderly*. W.H.O. Regional Office, Copenhagen

Thould, A. K. (1974). *Br. med. J.*, **1,** 279–80

Tomkinson, J., Turnbull, A., Robson, G., *et al.* (1982). *Report of Confidential Enquiries into Maternal Deaths in England and Wales 1976–78*. H.M.S.O., London

Urquart, J., and Ruthven, H. (1979). *Comm. Med.*, **1,** 199–205

Vaananen, I. (1970). In *Information Processing of Medical Records* (J. Anderson and J. M. Forsyth, eds), North Holland, Amsterdam, pp. 160–8

Wadsworth, M. E. J., Butterfield, W. J. H., and Blaney, R. (1971). *Health and Sickness: the Choice of Treatment*. Tavistock, London

Waldron, H. A. (1978). *The Medical Role in Environmental Health*. Oxford University Press, London

Walton, R. J., Blanchet, M., Boyes, D. A., *et al.* (1976). *Can. med. Ass. J.*, **114,** 1–28

Waterhouse, J. A. H. (1950). *Br. J. prev. soc. Med.*, **4,** 197–216

Werkö, L. (1974). *Br. med. J.*, **1,** 280–1

White, K. L. (1976). In *Epidemiology as a Fundamental Science* (K. L. White and M. M. Henderson, eds), Oxford University Press, New York, pp. 66–77

Wilcock, G. K. (1979). *Int. J. Epidem.*, **8,** 247–50

Williams, B. T., Dixon, R. A., and Knowelden, J. (1973a). *Br. med. J.*, **1,** 593–9

Williams, B. T., Dixon, R. A., and Knowelden, J. (1973b). *Br. J. prev. soc. Med.*, **27,** 126–8

Williams, B. T., Dixon, R. A., and Knowelden, J. (1973c). *J. R. Coll. gen. Pract.*, **23**, 642–6

Williams, B. T., and Knowelden, J. (1974). *Br. med. J.*, **1**, 9–12

Williamson, J., Stokoe, I. H., Gray, S., *et al.* (1964). *Lancet*, **1**, 1117–20

Woodward, M. (1982). *Comm. Med.*, **4**, 217–30

World Health Organisation (1971). *Statistical Indicators for the Planning and Evaluation of Public Health Programmes.* W.H.O. Technical Report Series No. 472, W.H.O., Geneva

Yudkin, J.S., Boucher, B. J., Schopflin, K. E., *et al.* (1980). *J. Epidem. Comm. Hlth*, **34**, 277–80

9 Genetic Studies

Murphy (1978), after suggesting that epidemiology was the recognition and interpretation of nonrandom distribution of characteristics in the population, indicated that substantive genetics was precisely that area of epidemiology which deals with heredity and that it was a fruitful area for development. This reference can be taken as a specific example of the overlap between genetics and epidemiology. There are two rather different aspects of the relevance of genetics to epidemiology: (1) the need to quantify the influence of genetic factors in the aetiology of various diseases; (2), where the role of genetics has been quantified, a wide range of medical-care issues, such as genetic counselling, or determining the suitability of screening techniques to detect abnormality. Wyatt (1982) has recently stressed the need for accurate, complete, and up-to-date information upon which to base estimates of the risk prior to genetic counselling.

The format of this chapter is similar to the basic structure of the earlier ones. However, because there are several quite different types of study that may be carried out by the epidemiologist, the second section on principles concentrates in the cardinal features of four different types of study. These are discussed in section 9.3, while some indication of the way in which such studies can be extended is given in section 9.4. A brief introduction to the relevant statistical techniques is given in the final section.

9.1 Basic Example of a Genetic Study

In 1948 Dean emigrated from England to South Africa, where he practised as a physician. He soon noticed a marked difference in the frequency of certain diseases there, as compared with in England; for example, he was called in consultation to see a series of patients who appeared to be hysterical and who then developed generalised paralysis (see Dean, 1972). One such patient had had abdominal pain for years, for which sedative drugs had been prescribed, but they only appeared to make the condition worse. Dean saw her after her second abdominal operation, for which she had had pentothal given as part of the anaesthetic. She was very emotional and complained of abdominal and limb pains; her muscles seemed weak and she had small sores on her hands and arms. Her urine was reddish-brown and showed the absorption bands of porphyrin on spectroscopy. The patient rapidly deteriorated and died. Three weeks later a similar but younger patient was seen; despite treatment, she also deteriorated and died. The father of this second patient had had ten children and three of his daughters had already died with the same symptoms. The father, who was one of fourteen children, had a sensitive skin, which abraided easily. Three of the father's brothers, the grandfather, the great-grandfather and a number of cousins had similar skin; this skin abnormality was more marked on the male side of the family. One sister and a number of cousins had died of illness similar to that of the two patients just described.

This information set Dean upon a thorough search for members of the family; the great-grandfather, Gerit Renier van Rooyen, was born in 1814 and had 10 children. All of these were traced by 1951; of 478 descendants, 434 were still living. These individuals were contacted, a history taken, and their urine tested for excess porphyrin. Of those who were over 18 at the time of the survey, in the second generation of those with a porphyrin-positive parent, 5 out of 10 also had porphyria; in the third generation, 16 out of 37 children; in the fourth generation, 32 out of 59 children; in the fifth generation (the majority of whom were under 18 and thus excluded), 7 out of 19 children. Thus in the family as a whole, of the 125 with a porphyric parent, 60 (48 per cent) had inherited the condition. This is very nearly the 50 per cent expected from the Mendelian law for a dominant, non-sex-linked characteristic.

Further study of 13 families in South Africa showed by 1951 that 53.4 per cent of patients' descendants were affected (51.3 per cent of males and 48.7 per cent of females). Eventually Dean had studied 174 families, all of whom demonstrated dominant inheritance of porphyria. This appeared in an acute form, as a cutaneous disease, or in quiescent form; Dean and Barnes (1959) subsequently named this type of porphyria, porphyria variageta, as it could present in a variety of ways.

Whenever Dean saw an affected patient he traced the genealogical tree and tried to interview all the relatives. A history of a sensitive skin on the back of the hands that blistered easily was a useful clue to the affected side of the family. All the families studied came from Afrikaner (Boer) stock, although many had married English settlers; often the farm or district in which the family lived was known and the baptismal registers of the Dutch Reformed Church were used to trace members. There was also a standard way of naming children; the first son of each family was named after the father's father, the second son after the mother's father, the third son after the father. The daughters were similarly named. In addition to the baptismal registers, a register of old Cape families had been published in 1893, tracing the Boer families back to the seventeenth century. (There was the usual problem of some liaisons resulting in offspring whom deliberate attempts were made to hide.) Tracing these families was done with the help of an archivist and the use of wills and inventories left by the early families and stored in the archives. Several thousand letters were written over five years in this painstaking search; at last a master family-tree was drawn up which showed how the first twenty-eight major groups of porphyric families studied were themselves descended from one original forebear. This involved the tenth-, eleventh-, twelfth-, thirteenth-, fourteenth- and fifteenth-generation descendants of the original forebear—Gerrit the son of Jan, who married Ariantje the daughter of Jacob in Capetown in 1688. Four of the eight children of this marriage were forebears of the porphyric families, but it was not possible to tell if this was inherited from the mother or father—Ariantje or Gerrit the son of Jan. All of the first thirty-two families traced back to the one main stem; in one family it was not certain which was the connection to the main stem, as there are two possible routes. Since this work, many other family groups have been traced back to the original family.

The studies show that until recently the gene responsible did not have a particularly deleterious effect, as the porphyric families seemed to have the same number of children on average as the other immigrant Boer families. In South Africa as a whole, twenty original settlers and their wives have about seven hundred thousand descendants—a very great increase in numbers compared with the much more slowly growing populations such as those of England. This great increase partly accounts for the large number of porphyria subjects in South Africa; an early settler was affected and his descendants multiplied very rapidly. It is possible that, apart from the side effects with certain modern medicines (e.g. barbiturates and sulphonamides), the gene for porphyria might bring certain advantages to the phenotype.

In 1959 routine testing of urine commenced for all patients admitted to the hospitals in which Dean worked. This identified a number of affected individuals and unexpected attacks of acute porphyria largely ceased. This routine testing showed an incidence in the Eastern Cape of about 1 in 250 tests performed. It was estimated that the overall incidence was about 3 per 1000 of the white population, with about 13 000 ± 2000 affected individuals in South Africa as a whole (based on the 1981 population). By alerting the medical profession to the hazard of drug use in these subjects, this work of Dean led to the reduction of the severe and often fatal complications of the condition. A review of the diagnosis and treatment of the condition appears in Dean (1978).

9.2 Principles of Genetic Studies

The example chosen for the begining of the chapter indicated how a major health problem may be recognised and investigated. Once the syndrome had been recognised and the ability to record the prior history of disease in family members confirmed then a painstaking inquiry was required. Difficult as this was, the condition happened to be a dominant trait, which could fairly readily be picked up in the family history. It would probably have been much more difficult to produce an equivalent pedigree for a recessive trait, or an autosomal dominant with poor penetrance.

A number of factors may have contributed to this fascinating story; the work was carried out by a doctor new to the country, who may have been more conscious of the difference in the patterns of disease than others; there may have been a very special pattern of migration and breeding in the original immigrants; the genetic disorder was accompanied by an emerging medical problem due to the atypical reaction to a new range of drugs; the original syndrome had an overt skin marker which was recognised by the forebears in the family.

There are now over 120 known specific genetic enzyme defects—only three of these are autosomal dominants (with such easily recognised positives in every generation). The remainder are chiefly autosomal recessives, with a few X-linked recessives. It must be remembered that the majority of diseases which are inherited in a simple manner are very rare, while common familial diseases usually follow no simple pattern of inheritance.

Unlike the other chapters, this one is concerned with a whole range of studies; it therefore discusses first general principles in relation to the studies that involve genetic concepts, then turns to those that may be carried out by the epidemiologist.

9.2.1 Issues covered by genetic studies

The main interest is with the aetiological studies that can be mounted; these cover the aspects: Is there a dominant genetic inheritance of the trait being studied? Is there a recessive inheritance? What does the familial (genetic) factor contribute to the overall multifactorial aetiology of the condition being studied? Very different work may then follow such aetiological studies, investigating the various steps that may be taken to control the condition through prevention or early detection; these medical care aspects are not explored in this chapter. This is the general field of chapter 8, while the contribution of genetic registers to this aspect of control has been indicated in subsection 3.4.3.

Four different types of study can be used, which are described below; these are dealt with from the simplest to the most complex. As will be appreciated, there is variation in the difficulty of studying the above three aspects; in particular, the interpretation of the contribution of genetic factors to multifactorial aetiology will be incorrectly estimated with too simple a study design. Smith (1966) has emphasised that when genes and the environment interact in the aetiology of a condition, it is important to be able to correctly apportion the contribution from each different factor, as when planning intervention it will usually be much easier to influence the subsequent effect of the environment than alter marriage and procreation habits through genetic counselling.

It is assumed that the reader is familiar with some of the basic biological concepts that are relevant to the study of genetics; discussion of these is beyond the scope of this presentation, but the recommended reading at the end of the chapter indicates where further guidance can be obtained on the subject. However, there are three points worth indicating at this stage, as they influence the interpretation of results from some of the studies.

(1) Some conditions are thought to be autosomal dominants, yet they occur more frequently in the population than might be expected from the prognosis of the condition itself and the impact of this upon fertility. This is thought to be due to some other selective advantage of the much more common heterozygous condition. For example, in phenyl-ketonuria, an increase in fertility of 1 per cent in the heterozygote would outweigh the loss of the genes in the affected children who die (Emery, 1979). This phenomenon is known as genetic polymorphism and is thought also to exist in conditons such as sickle-cell trait, fibrocystic disease and perhaps schizophrenia.

(2) Some conditions may be genetically determined, but not through the effect of a single gene. For example, characteristics that exhibit continuous variation such as height may depend on the concerted effect of alleles at many loci (i.e. a polygenic system of inheritance).

(3) A condition of known genetic origin may appear in a family without previous cases being recognised in the earlier generations. There may be four quite different explanations for this, each of which needs to be considered when interpreting familial studies: illegitimacy; one of the parents is affected, but only with a very mild form of the disease and thus not recognised (i.e. there may be incomplete penetrance of the gene); there may have been a mutation (this is the usual explanation of the appearance of a case of achondroplasia); the environment may have affected the expression of the gene (i.e. there is an overt difference between the genotype and the phenotype).

9.2.2 Pedigree studies

The general method has already been indicated in the lead example for this chapter. This indicated how the investigator can set about tracing the members of the families; the opportunities for such work will depend upon the vital-statistics and health-records systems existing in the country, the degree of internal and external migration that has occurred in previous generations, the various records that are retained by families and other bodies (such as the church, other clubs and societies). There are recognised techniques for assembling a pedigree of a family, which have been clarified by those carrying out genealogical work (see Colwell, 1980).

A rather different issue is the ease with which the condition being studied can be recognised from the family histories; this will be chiefly dependant on the cardinal symptoms of the condition and whether these are quite distinct from other diseases. It is assumed that for this kind of study the investigator is trying to cover a very wide span of years and there is no possibility of cross-checking the diagnostic information given for the members of the families before the previous generation (unlike the slightly more restricted family-studies of the next section). The analysis of this type of study is fairly simple, as it will chiefly be checking the relative frequency of the abnormality in the blood relatives in accordance with the basic Mendelian laws.

Obviously there are problems about the validity of the material from this type of study; in addition, interpretation will be more difficult when unexpected events occur. (Reasons for this have already been given at the beginning of this section.) The opposite is the deficit of expected cases. For example, if a mother with Down's syndrome has children, approximately half of her ova will have two chromosomes 21, but about half of the conceptions will abort, thus only one-quarter of her children will be affected. This indicates how the expected proportions of affected children can be markedly different from the observed. It is now very unlikely that much effort will be spent in the future on this kind of study; the problems that remain for further research require the more sophisticated types of study discussed in the following subsections.

9.2.3 Familial studies

These are similar to pedigree studies, but usually cover a much more restricted span of generations (usually the three generations of a nuclear family, i.e. probands, siblings, grandparents and children, together with the nonblood relatives through marriage of the proband). Though there is this restriction on the number of generations included in the studies, there is often more detail collected about the disease patterns in the families; this is often supplemented by obtaining documentary evidence of medical diagnosis from the treating hospitals. It is usual to classify the first-degree relatives as parents, siblings and children of the index subjects; second-degree relatives are grandparents, aunts and uncles, half-siblings, nieces and nephews, and grandchildren. The distinction is based on the proportion of genes shared.

There are three quite different approaches that can be implemented to collect data for such studies, based on the traditional methods of epidemiology—cross-sectional, 'retrospective', and prospective studies. The following three examples indicate each of these different ways.

Tager *et al.* (1978) studied 430 propositi aged 45–54 and 1340 first-, second- and third-order relatives. They identified subjects with chronic bronchitis and obstructive airways disease and demonstrated a higher prevalence in first-order relatives, which was independent of risk factors (sex, smoking history of respiratory illness, residence in a common household, geographical distribution, or alpha-antitrypsin pi-typing).

Fraser *et al.* (1982) reviewed data from a number of their own and other published series of the frequency of various abnormalities in sibships where malformations had been reported. There was disagreement in the literature whether the familial risk was restricted to repeat of the same malformation, or a more general risk of any malformation. They suggested that there was a general risk of neural tube defect in siblings of children with various malformations; they emphasised that this requires further quantification in order to appropriately identify mothers at high risk of having a baby with a neural tube defect.

Albano *et al.* (1981) described their method for identifying cancer families; a trained nurse takes an initial history, which excludes those respondents with less than two primary relatives with cancer. A physician then reviews the history and where appropriate requests verification of an extended pedigree. Using various criteria, 'cancer' families are then identified—about 4 per cent of all patients developing cancer. The authors do not indicate how they distinguish the influence of nongenetic behaviour and the similarity of the environment in causing a positive history.

Because of the difficulty of obtaining an unbiased history of previous diseases in family members, which is discussed further in subsection 9.2.6, the prospective approach has been used for studying this. Having identified a patient with a particular disease, there is the need to follow up all members of the family to see which subsequently develop the disease of interest. Some of the usual techniques of prospective studies are involved, and either the incidence or the mortality of the other members of the family will be recorded. The aim is to obtain an unbiased estimate of the frequency of disease in blood relatives and nonblood relatives; as with the other approaches of collecting data, the material may then be examined for internal differences, as well as permitting comparison with population data. There are a number of problems about such comparisons:

(1) Ascertainment in many classes of the family structure may be incomplete, e.g. for grandparents.
(2) What is the validity of the diagnoses reported by relatives or is documentary evidence of the diagnosis required?
(3) How representative are the probands and other study members, compared with the general population whose rates are used to calculate expected figures?
(4) Some studies have compared the site-specific cancer ratio with that for all cancers; this is a relatively crude measure as it takes no account of the age distribution of the families.

In this type of study a rather different type of analysis is carried out, contrasting the incidence or mortality from the disease of interest between the families and the general population, or the difference in the rates for blood and nonblood relatives within the families. From questioning of relatives of cases and controls, it has been frequently suggested that there is only a two-fold excess of cancer in first-degree relatives of patients. Peto (1980) pointed out that this inference is incorrect, as the point of interest is the ratio of risk in susceptibles to that in nonsusceptibles; this is only weakly reflected by the risk in patients' relatives compared with that in the population as this is diluted by (1) cancers occurring in nonsusceptibles, (2) the lower proportion of patients' relatives being susceptible, and (3) the population containing both susceptibles and nonsusceptibles. He demonstrated that if susceptibles are a frequent or infrequent occurrence in the population then the overall risk in monozygous twins was only from 1.5 to 2 times that of the general population.

9.2.4 Twin studies

Monozygous twins have 100 per cent of their genes in common, while dizygous twins share only 50 per cent of their genes (as any other siblings). In the nineteenth century, Galton argued that since identical twins have the same genetic constitution, any differences between them must be due to the environment (see Emery, 1979). As usual, if the study shows reasonable control of all measured variables, there is still the possibility that the apparent verification of the causal hypothesis is false, because of an unknown and unevaluated competing environmental risk factor correlated to the exposure under study. However, with care, it is possible to distinguish the independent effects of (1) genes and (2) environment—including facets of behaviour in causing disease—such studies providing a valuable opportunity to determine the degree to which patterns of behaviour are associated with genetic influence and thus to unravel the confounding of such relationships.

The rate of twinning varies with different populations. While the rate of dizygotic twinning in the Caucasian race is on average 6.6 per 1000 pregnancies, it is much higher in Nigeria, with a rate of about 40 per 1000 and lower in Japan at about 2 to 3 per 1000. Crude rates for twins are provided in the United Nations *Demographic Year Book*. There is an appreciable effect of parity and maternal age on the dizygous twinning rate. There is a higher overall rate in Ireland than in England and Wales; Dean and Keane (1972) suggested that this was due to both a higher maternal age-specific twinning rate, and the tendency for Irish mothers to have a higher proportion of their babies at older ages.

9.2.4.1 *Sources of identifiable twins*

The epidemiological approach required that the twin pair is unbroken at the start of the study; relatively high early mortality thus reduces the numbers available. If the research also requires same-sexed twins, or ones with discordant environmental exposure, then the numbers available for study are markedly reduced.

It is possible to establish contact with twins through the recognition of disease in members of twin pairs attending hospital. This approach has been used in the past, though warning is given about starting from patients in hospital in the next section.

To carry out a population census, and ask each respondent if he is a twin, is possible but time-consuming—with only about one in fifty of those questioned being suitable for subsequent study. A better start point is individual birth records, noting the twins and then trying to locate them in the population. An important point is the need to obtain information about all individuals, and there is therefore need to trace those for whom there is no initial information on follow up. This may require tracing from initial birth registration by painstaking search for movement from place to place; the ease of this will depend upon the national system for population registers.

Advertising in the media for twins is of unknown merit—but probably relatively unreliable with regard to completeness. There seems to be lack of information about bias in response from this approach; this is discussed further in subsection 9.2.6.5.

9.2.4.2 *Zygosity determination*

The resemblance between the partners of a pair can be judged by inspecting photographs of the twins as children; Cederlof *et al.* (1977) asked whether the twins regarded themselves as being very alike as children. Those agreeing with the expression 'as like as two peas in a pod' were classed as monozygous. If the respondents marked such items that they were only of 'family likeness', the pair were regarded as dizygous. These responses had been validated in a sample of 200 pairs using serological analysis; of the 72 coded as monozygous on the questions, 71 were agreed by the serology. Of the 114 coded as dizygous by questions, 104 were recorded as the same on testing sera. (14 subjects could not be coded from the questionnaire.) It was considered that the high costs of the serological investigations could not justify their use for all subjects in an epidemiological study.

9.2.4.3 Data recording

Obviously, after the twin pairs are identified for the study, appropriate information must be recorded to determine zygosity. The next issue to be resolved is the quantification of exposure to the environmental factor that it is desired to study. Standard methods will usually apply, with use of interview (or postal questionnaires), plus check of any retrievable records—such as those giving details of previous occupation of the subjects.

A W.H.O. meeting on collaborative twin registers in 1969 (quoted by Cederlof et al., 1977) suggested that 'to interpret the role of smoking and disease it will be essential to collect data on other living patterns and environmental factors, as well as personality type, behaviour, and the more commonly recognised risk factors.'

9.2.4.4 Use of twin studies

A study by the W.H.O. (1966) identified thirty-nine twin registers, but many were small and of the selected type. Large population-registers appear to be available only in Denmark (Hauge et al., 1968), Sweden (Cederlof et al., 1977), and the United States (Jablon et al., 1967). These registers have been used for a range of studies of chronic diseases, including chronic bronchitis, hypertension, ischaemic heart disease, psychiatric disease and various malignant conditions. The Swedish and Finnish registers have recently been described by Cederlof et al. (1982).

Knox (1974) used data on dizygous twinning rates to test his hypothesis of a foetus–foetus interaction in the aetiology of anencephalus. This hypothesis had been based upon evidence of discordance and excess like-sexed pairs among affected twins.

9.2.5 Case–control studies

A rather different type of study as far as this chapter is concerned is the use of a case–control study to explore the influence of familial as well as other factors in the aetiology of a particular disease. The technique of case–control studies has already been fully described in chapter 5; as far as genetic studies are concerned, there is only need to consider the addition of questions about disease in families to the range of material in earlier sections of chapter 5. The points already indicated in earlier sections of this chapter are relevant to the consideration of the validity of the material and the best way of obtaining unbiased information about the disease prevalence in blood and nonblood relatives.

The principle is that the start point of the study is a group of patients with the disease being studied, and an appropriately matched number of controls. The information about familial disease will usually be only one minor aspect of the total data collected; this provides the opportunity to collect detail about all the relevant environmental confounding factors. This will permit consideration of whether there is a familial excess risk of the disease independent of the known environmental and behavioural factors; if this is so, the issue then to be resolved is whether there is likely to be confounding between the families in other nonmeasurable aetiological factors, or whether there is really a genetic component in the aetiology.

It is particularly in case–control studies that the use of various markers of genetic traits have been used, such as H.L.A. typing. A rather different approach is to investigate the degree to which there is aggregation of disease in families in relation to time, to space, to birth order, or to maternal and paternal age. These issues are discussed further in section 9.4.

9.2.6 Validity of genetic studies

The general points covered in earlier chapters apply equally to genetic studies as to surveys, case–control studies or prospective studies. This section deals with those issues that are more specific to genetic studies. The first two issues are of the validity of the material, while the next two deal with aspects of potential bias in the work. The final subsection is somewhat longer and deals with a number of the difficulties of twin studies.

9.2.6.1 Undeclared marital conceptions

This raises no particular new point of principle, but must always be borne in mind when trying to interpret either pedigree or familial studies. It is an issue where tact in data collection is obviously important, but there are cytological and enzyme tests that can be applied to living respondents, which provide an independent check upon the validity of the subject's responses.

9.2.6.2 Illness in the relatives

Again it is not a new concept, that there is error in the information given about past disease in the subjects in a study. However, because of the crucial effect this can have upon the interpretation of genetic studies, there is need to consider if the material can be independently cross-checked; if not, due allowance for error in the material must be made in the analysis.

9.2.6.3 Bias in identification of respondents

In those subjects who carry a deleterious gene, it is possible for increased 'wastage' to occur in the path from conception, in early infancy or through-out life. If the genetic trait being studied was also accompanied by a predisposition to high mortality in childhood, then its influence would be greatly underestimated in any conventional study. In a comparable example, Altman (1982) pointed out that a study of longevity that used only living index-patients and pairs with dead parents introduced two biases (excluding index deaths in youth, and long-lived parents).

9.2.6.4 Confounding of behaviour and environment

One of the great difficulties with family studies is to disentangle the confounding between genetic influences, and a whole host of other factors that may be associated within families, such as facets of behaviour, the 'micro-environment' of the home, or the more general environment, including the locality and the tendency for individuals in families to work in the same jobs. This can be tackled partly by trying to distinguish between the risk in blood and nonblood relatives of the disease being studied. However, this is only a partial solution to the problem, as there is confounding between behaviour before and after the age of twenty in the risk of various diseases. For example, diet patterns may be established in childhood, and also the level of physical activity; smoking and drinking habits are often initiated in late adolescence, while the selection of a job and some of the consequences of mobility may have major influences on patterns of exposure to harmful environmental agents, chiefly in adult life. There is therefore a different degree in confounding between these different external factors on sibs and upon marriage partners.

It was to resolve the above problem that twin studies were advocated, as the simpler studies had presented difficulty in interpretation. An intermediate is to consider the use of data on half-sibs, or to examine the degree of consanguinity in persons developing certain diseases. Particular problems can occur in certain communities where there is variation in the degree to which relatives marry; for example, in certain Moslem countries it may be the usual pattern in rural areas that men should first search for a cousin as a marriage partner, and only consider marriage with others having failed to find a family partner.

9.2.6.5 Twin studies

Because of the higher mortality of twins compared with singleton births the subjects in twin studies are often selected by virtue of surviving through to adult life. They thus may be selected for qualities associated with withstanding increased risk of death. This may have biased the past exposure of the surviving twins to various external agents.

Some reports have been based on an aggregation of cases trawled from the literature, especially from isolated case-reports. This is a highly dubious way of collecting such material; if there was a tendency for case reports of like twins with a disease to be reported preferentially then the aggregated material would be impossible to interpret.

The identification of twins through the chance contact in hospital of an affected member of a twin pair may lead to a biased study. By definition, at least one member of the pair will be affected with this method of entry. There is also the possibility of increased collaboration when the second member of the pair suffers from the disease being studied (thus artificially inflating the concordance rate).

Advertising for twins has been one method of ascertainment. Using national and local press and radio, volunteer twins were contacted and full information was obtained from 1415 out of about 1600 twin pairs

(Waterhouse, 1950). The bias in respondents was shown by the relative excess of like-sexed female pairs (48 per cent compared with 31 per cent expected on national figures) and the relative deficiency of mixed-sex pairs (22 per cent compared with 36 per cent expected).

Allen (1965) reviewed various problems of twin research, including:

(1) The existence of a third type of twin intermediate between monozygous and dizygous
(2) Exchange of blood through the placental anastomosis in dizygous twins, leading to chimerism with potential effect on haematological and immunological systems
(3) Possible effects of aetiological factors responsible for twinning
(4) The effects of twinning during gestation and early infant life
(5) The difficulty of identifying all twins, especially of survivors who lost a partner in infancy
(6) Correct estimation of zygosity
(7) Need to adjust for confounding factors influencing twinning rates, when considering comparison with population figures
(8) Possible bias in diagnosis of certain diseases in second twins (stimulated by the remembrance of the first member of the pair)
(9) Difficulty of calculating heritability and estimating penetrance.

9.3 Advantages and Disadvantages of Genetic Studies

This section compares the four approaches to genetic studies discussed in the previous section (i.e. pedigree, familial, twin, and case–control). If an epidemiological study of an analytic type is to be mounted, probing genetic issues, one of these approaches will be required. The comparison is between the four different methods discussed in this chapter, and not with any different form of epidemiological study. Therefore the focus of this section is very different from that of many of the equivalent sections in earlier chapters, which were concerned with a weighing of the techniques in one chapter against those in another; here the contrast is within the chapter. A different aspect is whether the study should be population-based or laboratory-based; this is rather beyond the scope of this section, and will require discussion with those familiar with the range of laboratory techniques so that the relative role can be defined of population versus laboratory studies.

The problems of the four different types of study have already been described in subsections 9.2.2–5; a brief distillation of those points follows.

(1) Pedigree studies are suitable for the examination of simple patterns of inheritance (i.e. those that are dominant, autosomal recessive, or sex-linked recessive). Where there is a clear-cut 'marker' of the condition, the investigation is greatly simplified. Work is facilitated by studying relatively isolated communities, with good records about earlier generations; in the absence of written records, the work will be facilitated if the community has a strong oral tradition for passing on family histories.

Particularly where there is need to distinguish the transmission of disease from the sporadic occurrence of mutation, the larger the numbers of generations available for study the easier the interpretation. However, the most important factor in the analysis is the number of subjects for whom complete data are available. If the disease is of fairly late onset, there is no point investigating subjects who are relatively young; thus third-generation members in a three-generation study may not contribute any useful information.

The difficulty of studying some conditions was illustrated by Polani and Berry (1982), who suggested that perhaps half the various forms of blindness of genetic origin are due to about 50–70 different mutations at the gene loci, about half of which are of autosomal recessive type. Such conditions would be very difficult to investigate by multigeneration pedigree studies.

(2) Family studies suffer from severe difficulty in obtaining unbiased information about the earlier generations; this can be obviated by carrying out a prospective study of index patients, but unless the incidence is fairly high there will be great difficulty in obtaining enough patients for analysis. As with pedigree studies, the work is simplified if there is an easily recognised marker of the disease being studied. Tracing the medical history of people who died many years ago is not very fruitful, unless the certified cause of death is thought to be a good indicator of the occurrence of the disease. The work may be facilitated if large numbers of living members of the families can be contacted and some clinical or laboratory tests carried out.

One particular method of improving the analysis of the study will be a comparison of the incidence (or mortality) of the condition in first- and second-degree relatives with that in unrelated marriage partners, as well as in controls or in general population. This will be suitable only for those conditions that develop late in life, where it thought unlikely that there is an environmental factor that operates early in life. Though there are some advantages in this approach, there may be difficulty in obtaining sufficient marriage partners for analysis (there being about five first- and eighteen second-degree relatives for any proband who is married).

(3) Twin studies are difficult to mount, if the condition being studied is relatively rare. For example, Draper *et al.* (1977) reported on the occurrence of all tumours in children occurring throughout Britain in the period 1953–74. About half of these children suffered from leukaemia, and yet there were insufficient data on twins from which to calculate concordance rates. When studying the much commoner problem of lung cancer, even the national registries of the Scandinavian countries find difficulty in accumulating enough patients for analysis. This can rule out the appropriateness of twin studies, even without considering the problem of determining zygosity.

There is a simple pitfall that should be avoided when looking at the proportion of twins in any particular study. For example, Stevenson *et al.* (1950), in a study of 677 children with congenital malformations, had 16 twin pairs; as there were twins in the population at the rate of 1 in 83 births, it was concluded that the risk of malformation was doubled in the twins. Among the 16 twin pairs there were 20 affected children; it must also be remembered that there are 2 twins in every 84 births. Thus, where O = observed malformed twins and E = expected ones,

$$O = 20$$

$$E = \frac{677 \times 2}{84}$$

$$= 16.1$$

$O/E = 1.24$, i.e. an excess of 24 per cent

(4) Case–control studies are easily mounted, but have the major problem of difficulty in checking the validity of the reported events in the family histories, let alone determining the effect of various confounding factors. The difficulties of obtaining unbiased data has been discussed in subsection 5.2.5; one variation to be remembered is the possibility of mounting some form of prospective study, so that events occurring can be verified by the research worker.

9.4 Extension of Method of Genetic Studies

This brief section just hints at some of the ways in which the types of studies already described can be extended. This is from the point of the epidemiologist, though the opportunity is taken to indicate the fields in which laboratory scientists play a crucial part and collaboration would be essential for a satisfactory study. The section begins with those minor extensions that are possible using conventional epidemiological approaches, and then moves on to consideration of the studies using more complex laboratory techniques.

9.4.1 Investigation of additional epidemiological items

9.4.1.1 Clustering of disease, birth order and parental age

MacMahon and Pugh (1970) point out that one would expect parental genes to be distributed to offspring independently of the order of birth in the sibship. Any evidence that risk of a disease varies with birth order is evidence that environmental factors play a part. They show how the distribution by birth order can be calculated, and, as an example, demonstrate an increasing risk of a subject being diagnosed as having a neurosis with higher birth-order (with an excess risk of about 22 per cent in the sixth rank compared with the firstborn).

Other examples of appreciable birth-order difference are perinatal mortality, pyloric stenosis and twinning. These raise questions about a wide variety of environmental factors, the discussion of which is beyond the scope of this brief note. Barker and Record (1967) have emphasised the scope for misinterpretation of such data, where sibships of different size are being compared. Unless this is taken into account there is likely to be difficulty due to the confounding with other characteristics of small and large families.

A condition with a very clear association with maternal age is Down's syndrome. The information has been used to determine the optimum age for screening in the antenatal period; an affected foetus can be detected by chromosome studies following amniocentesis. This screening test is offered to pregnant women over the age of thirty-seven, who may then consider having an abortion if a positive result is obtained (Weatherall, 1982).

9.4.1.2 Consanguinous marriages

Such marriages must increase the frequency of homozygous individuals in the population and increase the genetic variance in the absence of selection. A small but significant increase in malignancies might go undetected if the coefficient of inbreeding is low relative to the frequency of the gene of interest, and the increase of homozygotes is small. With rare recessive traits, parents of affected individuals are more often related than couples in the general population. This is because cousins are more likely to carry the same genes and thus have children homozygous for the specific gene. For example, only about 1 in 200 marriages are between cousins in the population, but about 1 in 4 parents are cousins for children with alkaptonuria (Emery, 1979).

9.4.1.3 Clustering of events

MacMahon and Pugh (1970) discuss the contribution from the investigation of 'time-clustering' in family studies. They examined the interval between consecutive births, following a child born with a neural tube defect; they studied the relation of the interval to risk of abnormality in the subsequent child. The risk decreased with increasing interval, which suggested an environmental rather than a genetic factor. Other studies of this nature have looked at the temporal relationship in familial cases of Hodgkin's disease, leukaemia, multiple sclerosis and suicide.

There is an important point of method that must be considered in such studies. There may be quite a different type of family in which there is a short compared with a long interval between births. This confounding must be considered; if it is thought that the short interval is only a marker of other differences, then attempts should be made to identify the underlying influences.

9.4.1.4 Teratogens and genetic effects

A number of studies have shown that radiation, drugs and infection to which the mother is exposed may affect the ovum before conception, or the foetus during the pregnancy. This is really considering the full circle of genetic effects, where the environment influences the genetic make-up of the new child, and this leads to a genotype that manifests itself by the congenital abnormality (rather than the genotype being influenced by the environment and the phenotype then reflecting that influence).

To study this particular category of aetiological factor, a classic case–control approach can be used, provided there is some check on the influence of the abnormality on the recall of the mothers. Some studies of this nature have already been described in earlier parts of this book (see 5.1 and 5.5.1).

9.4.2 Studies of multifactorial aetiology

This issue has already been referred to, but a few additional points are required, particularly as the major unsolved aetiological problems that now remain are probably of this nature. There is now evidence for a genetic component in a wide range of conditions, including ankylosing spondilitis, asthma, bronchitis, cancer of various sites, congenital malformations, diabetes, hypertension, immune deficiency, ischaemic heart disease, multiple sclerosis, peptic ulcer, schizophrenia and virus infections. An example of the complexity of factors influencing various diseases is the recorded sex-difference in psychiatric disorders. *The Lancet* (1982) suggested that there may be: dominant X-linked inheritance of depression; endocrine factors (such as precipitation of psychotic and neurotic illness by childbirth, or the influence of puberty in the two sexes); differential experience of life events; variation in patterns of behaviour of men and women; the traditional 'learned helplessness' of women; differential frequency in consulting in response to symptoms; differential referral-rates from practitioner to specialist; variation in labelling of women by the male-dominated medical profession.

It is particularly with twin studies that multifactorial issues will be explored, as indicated in the following example. Carefully controlled studies have suggested that there might be heritable factors acting independently and synergistically with smoking in the cause of lung cancer (Schimke, 1978). There is also evidence that smoking is related to various personality variables (Cherry and Kiernan, 1976). Using data from the Swedish and Finnish twin registers, Kaprio *et al.* (1982) suggested there was evidence of significant genetic and familial influence on cigarette smoking. Eysenck (1980) has suggested that genetic variation is responsible for the association between smoking and lung cancer (through independent contributions of genetic factors to personality, smoking, and lung cancer risk). There is laboratory evidence for a genetic component in susceptibility to lung cancer (through variation in ability to metabolise potential carcinogens). Various studies have confirmed that there are a range of discrete occupational hazards that contribute to risk of lung cancer (see Alderson, 1982). The above brief comments suggest a set of models which may represent the aetiological pathways in causation of lung cancer. It must be emphasised that the following are: (1) highly schematic, (2) only indicative of some of the possible pathways, (3) ordered from simple to complex, rather than in order of plausibility, (4) not indicative of the relative frequency of the various paths in any model.

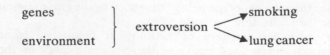

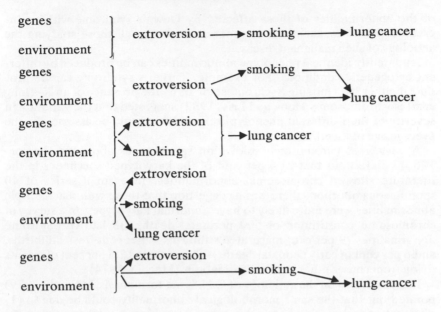

Whichever is the actual mechanism will have very different implications for correct research design to quantify the relationships, and also for subsequent preventive campaigns. There are problems in studying the interrelation of these variables, as regards both data collection and analysis. A way ahead has been suggested by Haley and Last (1981), using adult twins (identical and nonidentical), their spouses and offspring, and juvenile twins and their parents. Methods of fitting genotype environmental models to appropriate multivariate data have been developed by Eaves *et al.* (1978).

9.4.3 Chromosome studies

These have been dependent on the development of technical aspects, such as the culture of fibroblasts, culture of bone-marrow tissue, stimulation of division of peripheral blood lyphocytes, culture of amniotic cells, autoradiography, and application of various banding techniques. These developments lead to: recognition of the correct number of chromosomes in man; the identification of individual chromosomes; association of abnormal autosome- or sex-chromosomes with certain disorders (e.g. Down's and Klinefelter's syndromes); quantification of the incidence of congenital abnormalities, or acquisition of premalignant and malignant disease; gene mapping; the study of chromosomal breakage after exposure to various agents, or in certain diseases; clarification of the role of chromosomes in neoplasia. These issues have been reviewed by Lawler and Reeves (1976).

The above points are only indirectly relevant to many of the fields of work of the epidemiologist. Particular interest can occur when the chromosome abnormality is also associated with some other disease. Thus the association of the abnormalities of those affected by Down's syndrome with an increased risk of leukaemia is of general interest to all those studying the aetiology of such malignant disease.

Apparently identical phenotype abnormalities can be produced by different cytogenetic conditions. For example, Turner's syndrome can be produced either by a missing X-chromosome or by the presence of an X- (long arm) isochromosome. Hook and Liss (1982) suggested that the variation in severity of their different phenotypic expressions could be assessed by the average age of ascertainment.

A review of chromosome studies on spontaneous abortions (Larson, 1969) pointed out that 21.4 per cent of the karyotyped specimens in the literature showed chromosomal abnormalities. In a small series of 40 spontaneous abortions there was a suggestion that those with macroscopic abnormalities were more likely to have abnormal karyotypes. In a survey of chromosome constitution of 500 perinatal deaths, 38 had chromosome abnormalities (9 per cent macerated stillbirths, 4 per cent fresh stillbirths, and 6 per cent of early neonatal deaths). This included 2.5 per cent of infants dying from causes other than malformations (Machin, 1974).

In a discussion on the aetiology of C.N.S. malformations, Melnick (1979) pointed out that the same morphological abnormality could be due to (1) different genetic aetiologies, (2) a range of environmental factors or (3) genetic or environmental factors.

9.4.4 Markers of genetic effects

It is possible to detect genetic effects associated with some diseases through the phenomenon of genetic linkage, where the genes are carried on the same chromosome and there is linkage of the respective loci. This can occur with the study of blood-group differences, H.L.A. types, or certain defects of enzymes. Such studies need to be interpreted with caution. Clarke *et al.* (1955) reported an excess of blood group O in patients with duodenal ulcer compared with population data on blood-group distribution. However, Penrose had pointed out that to assess the causality it was necessary to study the blood groups of the patients' relatives rather than use blood donors or other hospital patients as controls (see Clarke *et al.*, 1956). When this was done, there was no evidence that the individuals with blood group O were more likely to have a duodenal ulcer than their A, B or AB siblings.

As far as H.L.A. types are concerned, there is strong association between risk of ankylosing spondylitis and H.L.A. antigen B27. There is conflicting evidence of a single multiple-sclerosis gene linked closely to H.L.A. type (Ebers *et al.*, 1982). Sivak *et al.* (1981) reported a kindred in which every affected member had at least one carcinoma of the colon; the average age of onset was 38 years, and multiple primaries occurred in 23 per cent of the patients. H.L.A. typing suggested a genetic linkage, but it was emphasised that a large amount of data must be assembled from unrelated kindreds for verification of such an effect. These examples just indicate a very small proportion of the diseases where a relation to H.L.A. has been suggested.

9.5 Statistical Techniques

This section shows how zygosity may be estimated from counts of the number of like- and unlike-sexed twins, and then indicates how concordance rates may be calculated.

9.5.1 Zygosity rates in twins

A relatively simple method exists for estimating the zygosity of twins if the number of like- and unlike-sexed pairs is known. This follows from the fact that it is assumed that there is an equal chance of each twin in dizygous pairs being a boy or a girl; the twin pairs may thus be: boy + boy, boy + girl, girl + boy, girl + girl. From this it may be seen that half these twins will be like-sexed, thus the total number of dizygous twins will be twice the number of unlike-sexed twins. The remainder will therefore be monozygous. Table 9.1 sets out the calculations for some recent data for England and Wales.

Table 9.1   Calculation of zygosity rates by maternal age for twins born in England and Wales, 1980

	Maternal age				
	< 20	20 –	25 –	30 –	35 – 39
total twins	342	1 558	2 281	1 572	479
like-sexed twins	63	396	709	539	149
dizygous twins	126	792	1 418	1 078	298
monozygous twins	216	766	863	494	181
maternities	60 914	201 342	222 547	129 211	33 741
twin rate per 1000 maternities					
dizygous	2.07	3.93	6.37	8.34	8.83
monozygous	3.55	3.80	3.88	3.82	5.36

Source: *Birth Statistics, England and Wales, 1980*, FM 1, No.7; O.P.C.S. (1982)

9.5.2 Concordance rates in twins

One measure of resemblance is the concordance rate; the proband concordance is the most general index, and is defined as the proportion of affected individuals among co-twins of previously defined index twins (Allen *et al.*, 1967):

$$\text{proband concordance} = \frac{d}{t}$$

where d = number of diseased twins and t = total number of twins.

However, where the investigator encounters an 'affected' twin among hospital patients and collects further information about the second twin, the sample has at least one member affected and this makes the estimate of concordance biased. The 'pairwise' concordance is therefore calculated, which is the proportion where both twins are affected out of all pairs with at least one affected.

$$\text{pairwise concordance} = \frac{C}{C + D}$$

where C = number of concordant affected pairs and D = number of discordant pairs.

If some of the twins are entered into the study because one member was known to be affected, while others were initially healthy, the proband concordance may be calculated by adjusting the formula as follows:

$$\text{proband concordance} = \frac{C + C'}{C + D + C'}$$

where C' = number of pairs independently entered through both affected twins.

In a cautionary note, Marshall and Knox (1980) emphasised some of the difficulties in quantifying disease concordance in twins. They suggested that Weinberg's method was unsatisfactory owing to bias when twins were selected on the basis of disease, and that a combination of environmental and genetic determinants introduces further complications. They developed a model framework which permitted investigation of empirical data in relation to timing of causative events before and after cleavage in monozygous twins. Examples were given of the application of this model to reported data for five conditions where genetic influences had been previously postulated. Some of the assumptions of this approach were questioned by Hutchinson (1982).

There are other statistics that may be calculated from twin data, but they are beyond the scope of this limited introduction.

9.5.3 Hereditability

Where a disorder is of multifactorial aetiology, hereditability is that proportion of the total variation of the phenotype due to genetic factors; the greater the value, the more important the genetic role. It may be calculated from the incidence or mortality of a condition in various categories of relatives on the one hand and in the general population (or in a control sample) on the other. It is a rough but useful estimate but the calculation may be distorted by a number of biases:

(1) If a dominant gene plays a part in determining risk of disease then the calculated value may be 100 per cent.
(2) If a recessive gene plays a part in determining risk of the disease then the calculated value will be greater in the siblings of the proband than for parents or children.
(3) Shared environment is likely to cause a greater effect on the calculated value for siblings than for parents or children.

As is so often the situation, unless a shrewd idea of the biological situation exists at the time of the study, interpretation may be difficult. The calculation of these values is discussed by Emery (1976).

References

Recommended reading

Emery, A. E. H. (1976). *Methodology in Medical Genetics: an Introduction to Statistical Methods.* Churchill Livingstone, Edinburgh
Emery, A. E. H. (1979). *Elements of Medical Genetics.* Churchill Livingstone, Edinburgh
Nora, J. J., and Fraser, F. C. (1981). *Medical Genetics: Principles and Practice.* Lea and Fibiger, Philadelphia

Other references

Albano, W. A., Lynch, H. T., Recabaren, J. A., *et al.* (1981). *Cancer,* **47,** 2113–8
Alderson, M. R. (1982). *Prevention of Cancer,* Arnold, London, 33–4
Allen, G. (1965). *Prog. med. Genet.,* **4,** 242–69
Allen, G., Harvard, B., and Shields, J. (1967). *Acta Genet.,* **17,** 475–81
Altman, D. G. (1982). *J. chron. Dis.,* **35,** 411
Barker, D. J. P., and Record, R. G. (1967). *Appl. Statist.,* **16,** 13–16
Cederlof, R., Friberg, L., and Lundman, T. (1977). *Acta med. Scand. Suppl. 612*
Cederlof, R., Rantaslald, I., and Floderus-Myred, J., *et al.* (1982). *Int. J. Epidem.,* **11,** 387–90
Cherry, N., and Kiernan, N. (1976). *Br. J. prev. soc. Med.,* **30,** 121–31
Clarke, C. A., Cowan, W. K., Edwards, J. W. *et al.* (1955). *Br. med. J.,* **2,** 643–6
Clarke, C. A., Edwards, J. W., Haddock, R. D., *et al.* (1956). *Br. med. J.,* **2,** 725–31
Colwell, S. (1980). *The Family History Book: a Guide to Tracing Your Ancestors.* Phaidon, Oxford
Dean, G. (1972). *The Porphyrias: a Story of Inheritance and Environment.* Pitman, London
Dean, G. (1978). *Practitioner,* **221,** 219–27
Dean, G., and Barnes, H. D. (1959). *S. Afr. med. J.,* **33,** 246
Dean, G., and Keane, T. (1972). *Br. J. prev. soc. Med.,* **26,** 186–92
Draper, G. J., Heaf, M. M., and Kinnier Wilson, L. M. (1977). *J. med. Genet.,* **14,** 81–90
Eaves, L. J., Last, K. A., Young, P. A., and Martin, N. G. (1978). *Heredity,* **41,** 249–320
Ebers, G. C., Paty, D. W., Stiller, C. R., *et al.* (1982). *Lancet,* **2,** 88–91
Emery, A. E. H. (1976). *Methodology in Medical Genetics: an Introduction to Statistical Methods.* Churchill Livingstone, Edinburgh
Emery, A. E. H. (1979). *Elements of Medical Genetics.* Churchill Livingstone, Edinburgh
Eysenck, H. J. (1980). *The Causes and Effects of Smoking.* Temple Smith, London
Fraser, F. C., Cziezel, A., and Hanson, C. (1982). *Lancet,* **2,** 144–5
Haley, C. S., and Last, K. A. (1981). *Hereditary,* **247,** 221–36
Hauge, M., Harvald, B., Fisher, M., *et al.* (1968). *Acta, genet. med. Gemellol.,* **17,** 315–33
Hook, E. B., and Liss, S. M. (1982). *J. chron. Dis.,* **35,** 207–9
Hutchinson, T. P. (1982). *J. Epidem. Comm. Hlth,* **36,** 155–6
Jablon, S., Neel, J. V., Gershowitz, H., and Atkinson, G. F. (1967). *Am. J. hum. Genet.,* **19,** 133–61
Kaprio, J., Hammar, N., Koskenvuo, M., *et al.* (1982). *Int. J. Epidem.,* **11,** 378–86

Knox, E. G. (1974). *Br. J. prev. soc. Med.*, **28**, 73–80

Lancet (1982). **2**, 194–5

Larson, S. L. (1969). *Int. Surg.*, **51**, 124–31

Lawler, S. D., and Reeves, B. R. (1976). *J. clin. Path.*, **29**, 569–82

Machin, G. A. (1974). *Lancet*, **1**, 549–51

MacMahon, B., and Pugh, T. E. (1970). *Epidemiology: Principles and Methods*. Little Brown, Boston

Marshall, T., and Knox, E. G. (1980). *J. Epidem. Comm. Hlth*, **34**, 1–8

Melnick, K. (1979). *Birth Defects*, **15**, (3), 19–41

Murphy, E. A. (1978). *Int. J. Epidem.*, **7**, 7–14

Peto, J. (1980). In Banbury Report 4: *Cancer Incidence in Defined Populations*. Cold Spring Harbour Laboratory, Cold Spring Harbour, pp. 203–13

Polani, P. E., and Berry, A. C. (1982). *Lancet*, **2**, 106–7

Schimke, R. N. (1978). *Genetics and Cancer in Man*. Churchill Livingstone, Edinburgh

Sivak, M. V., Schleutermann, D., Braun, W. A., and Sullivan, B. H. (1981). *Cancer*, **48**, 76–81

Smith, A. (1966). *Genetics in Medicine*. Livingstone, Edinburgh

Stevenson, S. S., Worcester, J., and Rice, R. G. (1950). *Pediatrics*, **6**, 37–50

Tager, I., Tischler, P. V., Rosner, B., *et al.* (1978). *Int. J. Epidem.*, **7**, 55–62

Waterhouse, J. A. H. (1950). *Br. J. Soc. Med.*, **4**, 197–216

Weatherall, J. A. C. (1982). *Hlth Trends*, **14**, 85–8

World Health Organisation (1966). *W.H.O. Chron.*, **20**, 121

Wyatt, P. R. (1982). *Lancet*, **2**, 1051

10 Studies of Occupational Hazards

Epidemiology is one of the disciplines that can help in the investigation of occupationally induced disease; it can contribute to identifying possible hazards, quantifying dose–response relationships, and evaluating preventive measures. The types of epidemiological study are based upon the methods described in earlier chapters but they warrant further discussion in the present chapter to emphasise the adjustment in method required to suit them to the occupational field. Obviously, when reading a section in the present chapter, for example on case–control studies, the points included in the main chapter on this method should be considered.

This chapter begins with an example of one particular type of study, an historical prospective study. This is followed by brief notes on the eight main methods that may be used to study occupational disease. The section on principles identifies some common themes relevant to the different types of study; the section on advantages and disadvantages contrasts points relevant to the selection of different methods and the assessment of results.

10.1 Basic Example

Three interrelated studies have been carried out to examine the patterns of mortality of oil-refinery and distribution-centre workers, and maintenance men employed by the London Transport Executive (Rushton and Alderson, 1981a, 1982a, 1982b). The first study involved eight refineries which had been on stream at least since the early 1950s. Entry was restricted to men who had had a minimum of one year's continuous service in the period from 1 January 1950 to 31 December 1975. The second study involved all the distribution centres, including airports and blending plants, that belonged to three companies in Great Britain, with entry restricted as in the refinery study. The third study involved all maintenance men at London Transport Executive (L.T.E.) bus garages and the Chiswick works who had had at least one continuous year's service between 1 January 1967 and 31 December 1975.

Details were abstracted from personnel records at the locations or head offices about the present job of each worker in the industry, or the last job of those who had left. The standard approach was used to identify the study population, tracing leavers, calculating person-years at risk, estimating expected deaths based on national mortality rates, and testing the difference between the observed (O) and expected (E) deaths.

There were 34 781 men eligible for the refinery study, 23 358 for the distribution study, and 8684 men in the London Transport study. The overall trace-rate was over 99.5 per cent for all men in the studies. The average length of follow up was 16.6 years for the refinery study and 17.1 years for the distribution study, but in the London Transport study it was

Table 10.1 Observed deaths, ratio of observed to expected deaths, and *p*-values for various causes of death in a prospective study of the oil industry

	Refinery study			Distribution study			L.T.E. study		
	Observed deaths	O/E	p*	Observed deaths	O/E	p*	Observed deaths	O/E	p*
all causes	4406	0.84	xxx	3926	0.85	xxx	705	0.84	xxx
all neoplasms	1147	0.89	xxx	1002	0.87	xxx	216	0.95	
ca. stomach	167	1.04	xxx	123	0.85		26	1.02	
ca. intestine	84	1.07		57	0.79	x			
ca. rectum	58	1.03		57	1.06				
ca. pancreas	50	0.97		39	0.83				
ca. lung	416	0.78	xxx	384	0.80	xxx	102	1.01	
ca. prostate	47	1.02		53	1.09				
ca. bladder	34	0.77		32	0.75	x			
ca. brain	36	0.80		39	1.07				
leukaemia	30	0.94		28	1.04				
vascular lesion C.N.S.	408	0.90	x	374	0.87	xx	58	0.78	x
arteriosclerotic heart disease	1428	0.90	xxx	1377	0.99		244	0.88	x
other diseases of heart	85	0.75	xx	71	0.64	xxx			
hypertensive disease	76	0.72	xx	65	0.71	xx			
diseases of arteries	92	1.03		81	0.91				
pneumonia	157	0.86	x	133	0.72	xxx	28	0.87	
bronchitis	253	0.64	xxx	240	0.67	xxx	50	0.77	x
motor-vehicle accident	110	1.08		75	1.07				

p-values: xxx = < 0.001; xx = < 0.01; x = < 0.05

Source: Rushton and Alderson (1981, 1982a, 1982b)

only 5.9 years. Table 10.1 shows the main comparisons of observed and expected deaths for those causes of death where there were at least 25 deaths. Before attempting to interpret the findings from a study such as this, it is important to consider a number of points that impinge on the validity and biases inherent in the material. These points are discussed in section 10.2 and subsection 10.3.7.

The overall level of mortality was reduced in all three studies compared with the national standard, giving O/E ratios of 0.84, 0.85, and 0.84. This reduced ratio is typical of many studies of this nature; it is known as the 'healthy-worker effect' and is discussed in section 10.3.9. As far as the non-malignant causes of death were concerned, most of those causes for which there were large numbers of deaths had considerably reduced observed deaths.

A point of interest is the consideration of smoking-related diseases (e.g. lung cancer, ischaemic heart disease and bronchitis). Lung cancer was reduced in the refinery and distribution workers, but not in the London Transport men. Bronchitis was reduced in all three studies, ($O/E = 0.64$, 0.67 and 0.77). It was suggested that the reduced risk of lung cancer, ischaemic heart disease and bronchitis in some of these workers might be due to reduced smoking compared with the general population. In contrast, for distribution workers, ischaemic heart disease was not reduced and no obvious explanation could be provided; it was suggested that further study of this issue was required.

The total number of deaths from all neoplasms was significantly reduced in both the refinery and distribution studies, whilst there was a nonsignificant reduction for London Transport ($O/E = 0.95$, $p = 0.46$). Lung cancer showed a highly significant reduction in both the refinery and distribution workers; the lack of difference between observed and expected deaths from lung cancer in the London Transport study is partly a reflection of the use of national mortality rates. The refinery workers showed a significant excess of cancer of the nasal cavities and sinuses, and of melanoma (the latter at two refineries in particular). Interpretation of these results was difficult owing to the small numbers of deaths involved.

10.1.1 Different types of study

The following subsections briefly indicate the way various epidemiological methods can be adapted to study occupational disease.

10.1.1.1 Occupational mortality statistics

At each census questions have been asked about the occupations of the individuals listed in each household and this information can provide a denominator for the calculation of occupational mortality rates. It was a major advance when the Registrar General (1855) first collated such information from the 1851 census with the mortality returns for that year. He wrote:

The previous investigations of the various rates of mortality in the districts of the Kingdom have shown how much the health and life of the population are affected by fixed local influence. The professions and occupations of men open a new field of enquiry on which we are now prepared to enter, not unconscious, however, of peculiar difficulties that beset all enquiries into the mortality of limited, fluctuating, and sometimes ill-defined sections of the population.

Subsequent analyses of occupational mortality have been produced following each decennial census. In recent decennial reports the mortality data have been based on deaths in five or three years around the time of the census in order to provide a larger number of deaths in any individual occupation. The occupation used for the numerator in calculating the rates is the final occupation recorded at death registration. Enhancement of the method has been by the following:

(1) Selection of well-defined jobs for examination
(2) Combination of allied or easily confused occupations
(3) Cross-classification of job by geographical region
(4) Use of occupation and industry to provide increased specificity.

A number of authors have drawn attention to the fact that the onset of an occupationally induced disease might be associated with the decline in the ability to work, and that this could result in an individual changing his job. Alderson (1972) concluded that occupational-mortality data provided an extremely useful background to the study and understanding of occupational disease and mortality, despite doubt about the accuracy of the data. Although the material has rarely been used in generating hunches in the case of specific occupationally induced disease, it serves as a ready means of testing hypotheses derived from other sources and for monitoring the general and specific mortality-rates in various occupations.

The latest report on occupational mortality (Registrar General, 1978) provided data which showed the age-standardised stomach-cancer mortality in England and Wales in 1970–2 for various occupational orders. Table 10.2 shows excerpts from this indicating the occupational orders where the

Table 10.2 Occupational orders showing high stomach-cancer mortality in England and Wales, 1972

Occupation	Proportional mortality ratio	
	15–64	65–74
miners and quarrymen*	141	127
glass and ceramic makers	108	73
labourers*	113	108
warehouseman*	107	108

Source: Registrar General (1978)

* Cancer registrations were also significantly high in 1966–7 and 1968–70.

S.M.R. was significantly raised. An asterisk against three of these orders indicates those where the cancer incidence was also high in 1966–7 and 1968–70. Such material can only serve as a pointer to a topic for study, rather than any suggestion of action required. In this particular example, the common thread between these different occupations might be the fact that they all involve exposure to dust. If this is the common factor, it is dust of quite varying nature, sometimes being organic and sometimes inorganic.

Alderson (1972) indicated the following problems with using such data:

(1) The validity of the cause of death—does knowledge of the job bias the wording on the certificate?
(2) Validity of occupation recorded at death registration—does the information inflate the importance of job of the deceased?
(3) Use of denominator from a different source—how is someone temporarily out-of-work from sickness or redundancy or prematurely retired classified?
(4) Selection biases—into and out of certain occupations in relation to physique, mental stamina, health?
(5) Use of last-held occupation, instead of job held longest.
(6) Relation of occupation to work environment—is there dilution due to aggregation of very different types of work?
(7) Confounding with nonoccupational factors—do individuals in certain jobs smoke more, eat foods with high fat content, etc?

Where there are major problems with providing a valid denominator, use can be made of proportional mortality ratios. For example, the Registrar General's supplement has used this approach for persons dying aged 65–74 (because of the major discrepancy in occupation recorded at census and death registration for this age group). The statistical method is described in subsection 10.5.1.

10.1.1.2 Record linkage

A more powerful probe of an occupational influence may be provided by record linkage. One example is the longitudinal study carried out in England and Wales, which permits linkage of job details provided at census to subsequent patterns of mortality through national record linkage (O.P.C.S., 1973). A recent report (Fox and Goldblatt, 1982) presented a wide range of results from mortality of the 1971 cohort over the period 1971–5. Chapter 12 provided results by occupational order; there are marked overall differences from the decennial supplement, with the linked study showing relatively low rates for all occupational orders and a high S.M.R. for men unoccupied at the time of the census. The relatively low S.M.R.s for the occupational orders is due to the 'selection' of those fit for work and is another aspect of the 'healthy-worker effect' (see subsection 10.3.9). Comparison between occupational orders showed some with relatively high S.M.R.s, which were in agreement with the direction of the differences found in the decennial supplement. Though the longitudinal study overcomes the numerator/denominator biases, it will be many years before sufficient deaths have accummulated to permit examination by occupational unit or by individual cause of death.

Instead of organising record linkage as a routine, and then periodically using the linked file for special studies, an alternative approach is to carry out a specific record-linkage study in order to probe a particular problem. Alderson (1980) arranged for O.P.C.S. staff to link records from the 1961 census with subsequent mortality. The census files were searched for codes compatible with an occupation as hairdresser. This enabled the census staff to identify the original census schedules, check the occupation and abstract full identification particulars for each individual. About 2000 men were identified (a 10 per cent sample of the occupation for 1961); the identification particulars were used to trace each individual on the National Health Service Central Register, and thus find the death entries for those who had died. The record-linkage exercise was carried out in 1979; 92 per cent of the men were traced and all deaths occurring in the period to the end of 1979 identified. These data were used to calculate expected mortality and contrast this with observed numbers of deaths for five malignancies which other studies had suggested might be associated with exposure to hair dyes. The overall mortality was significantly lower than expected, but there was no evidence of an excess for all malignancies or any of the specific ones studied.

The main conceptual difference of an *ad hoc* study of this nature is that the effort of linkage is devoted solely to the individuals of particular interest, rather than using routine record-linkage for the total population. Also it was possible to go back to the 1961 census, because the computer records that still existed for this could provide the cross-index to the hard-copy original schedules for all hairdressers.

10.1.1.3 Collation studies

A less precise probe but one more readily carried out is a range of collation studies; the general method has already been described (see subsection 2.4.2). American counties have been classified by industrial activity, and variation in particular industries in relation to cancer incidence or mortality examined. As part of this study, Blot *et al.* (1977) compared 39 'petroleum industry' counties with 117 counties matched for geographic region, population size and various demographic indicators. The definition of a petroleum county was one where (1) at least 100 persons were employed in the industry, and (2) at least 1 per cent of the county's population were estimated to be petroleum employees. Age-adjusted mortality-rates during 1950–69 for 23 cancer sites were calculated for white residents. Males in the petroleum industry counties experienced significantly more cancer for seven sites of malignancy; these sites with the ratios of the mortality rates and p-values are shown in table 10.3. The excesses for cancer of the stomach, rectum and testis occurred in the more highly populated petroleum industry counties. The paper commented that other industries are generally to be found in the same location as the petroleum industry, but no attempt was made to define which other industry, if any, might have contributed to the high mortality from various disease groups.

Table 10.3 Ratios of age-adjusted mortality-rates for white males in petroleum-industry counties to those in control counties in the United States by cancer site, for 1950–69

Site	Ratio	p
stomach	1.09	< 0.01
rectum	1.07	< 0.05
nasal cavity & sinuses	1.48	< 0.01
lung	1.15	< 0.01
testis	1.10	< 0.05
skin including melanoma	1.10	< 0.05
brain	0.94	< 0.05

After Blot *et al.* (1977)

10.1.1.4 Proportional-mortality analysis

A relatively simple check of an issue can be carried out where records are available that identify the cause of death in a group of workers. The analysis merely requires for each individual who has died: sex, date of birth, date and cause of death. The technique tests whether the proportion of deaths from the cause of interest is greater or less than one would expect in relation to deaths from all causes. The expected figure is usually calculated by applying the death-rates for the country as a whole to the distribution of actual deaths, taking age, sex and calendar period into account.

Boyd and his colleagues (1970) cross-checked the initial observation of a pathologist in Cumberland that ferrite miners appeared to have a higher prevalence of lung cancer at autopsy than one would expect (bearing in mind the relative frequency of this as a cause of death in males in England and Wales). They had access to the death certificates issued for all males dying in Cumberland in 1948–67. These were sorted to identify all decedents recorded as being iron-ore miners; the deaths of all other individuals were used as the comparison group. Taking age and calendar period into account, the relative proportion of deaths from lung cancer, other cancers, respiratory disease and all other causes were examined. The results, shown in table

Table 10.4 Proportional mortality analysis of deaths in iron-ore miners in Cumberland, 1948–67

	Lung cancer	Other cancers	Respiratory disease	Other causes
observed deaths	42	74	174	306
expected deaths				
national data	27.7	71.3	59.8	527.2
local data	28.8	75.3	75.8	506.1

Source: Boyd *et al.* (1970)

10.4, demonstrated a significantly higher proportion of observed deaths from lung cancer than expected either on the basis of the comparison population from Cumberland or the death-rate for England and Wales. Their results thus supported the initial observation of the pathologist, though no definitive cause of the malignancy was identified. (A suggestion was made that the atmosphere in the mine was contaminated with radon, which might have accounted for the enhanced risk, rather than this being due to the dust from the iron ore.)

For a condition that is relatively common it may be possible to use local rather than national statistics in order to estimate the expected distribution of deaths; this may have an advantage of correcting for any regional, social class, or other local factor that influences the pattern of mortality other than that possible due to the specific occupation.

A brief description of the statistical technique for handling such data is provided in subsection 10.5.1.

10.1.1.5 Cross-sectional studies

The prevalence of respiratory disease was investigated in miners and millers of talc in the United States (Wegman *et al.*, 1982). Out of 174 approached, only 142 collaborated (82 per cent), of whom 116 were 25 years or older. A full medical history was obtained, pulmonary function assessed, and chest radiographs taken; long-term dust exposure was quantified from periodic surveys measuring dust levels combined with histories of the plants and past working practices. Pulmonary function values were less than predicted; there was evidence of an exposure effect after adjusting for cigarette smoking, but no evidence of interaction between talc and smoking.

Such cross-sectional studies are only of value where there is a sensitive measure of minor changes in function, the prevalence of the disease being studied is 'relatively' high, or there is an identifiable precursor of a chronic disease.

It is a relatively simple matter to identify subgroups of workers in industries where irradiation or benzene exposure is possible, and to classify the groups by extent of exposure. Samples of the men may then be approached and in addition to collecting data on other possible influences of chromosome abnormality the men may be requested to give an appropriate sample so that detailed chromosome analyses may be carried out. Such a study was carried out on workers exposed to benzene, though the initial findings of a highly significant excess of abnormalities in the benzene workers was not confirmed in a follow-up study, which showed an even higher abnormality rate in the control population selected (Tough and Court Brown, 1965; Tough *et al.*, 1970). The prevalence of chromosome aberrations was determined in the peripheral blood lymphocytes of dockyard workers exposed to mixed neutron–γ radiation when refuelling nuclear submarines. Exposures were mostly below the accepted permissible level of 0.05 Gy per year, but a significant increase in chromosome damage was noted with increased exposure (Evans *et al.*, 1979).

10.1.1.6 Case–control studies

Conventional case–control studies may be used to probe for occupational associations with risk for particular disease. As with more generally aimed case–control studies (see chapter 5), these may be used either as a source of a fresh hypothesis ('fishing' for variation that stimulates some line of thought about possible aetiology) or else to explore specific hypotheses.

In the United States Third National Cancer Survey interviews were obtained from 7518 persons with cancer in 8 areas (a response of only 57 per cent). Information was collected on alcohol and tobacco use as well as an employment history. The analyses consisted of two-times-two tables of counts of persons with/without a particular cancer against having/not having a specific employment; with 29 sites and 202 employment categories, this generated 5858 comparisons. This use of 'intercancer comparisons' has the problem that a cancer in the control group may be exposure-biased (under- or over-represented); unless this cancer was more than a small proportion of the total, this effect would be minimal. Williams *et al.* (1977) suggested that a major advantage of the study was that it permitted use of smoking, alcohol and socio-economic status as control variables. In addition, the recent industries reported by the patients were compared with data from the 1970 census; this provided a large body of comparitive data, but it could be used only for the cancer patients who were not retired and lacked information on smoking, alcohol and socio-economic status.

Despite the above statement on one of the advantages of this study, the authors noted less confounding than anticipated from tobacco and alcohol. As compared with the Registrar General's material, this study obtained a full history of all occupations and industries of the subjects with the subjects time spent in each. It is not clear to what extent the poor response affected the results; the study was restricted to predominantly urban areas with only a restricted range of industries present. It was emphasised that the results from such multiple comparisons should be treated with caution when used as a source for forming hypotheses and planning studies.

Siemiatycki *et al.* (1981) described their case–control system to 'fish' for occupational hazards. They advocated use of several hospitals as source of cases, and controls with other cancers. It appears that they recommended several sites, so that even if an agent causes multiple-site cancer, this may still be identified from the site having the greatest relative risk. They stressed the advantage of using chemists and/or engineers to review the job histories and identify agents to which each subject is likely to have been exposed.

10.1.1.7 Historical prospective studies

The basic example of this chapter was a study of this nature. Where there are available records of individuals' work histories, with a complete file of data on mortality that has occurred among these individuals, it should be possible to relate the data on the 'population at risk' to the identifiable outcome (i.e. mortality). The occupational records are used to identify each individual in the study. It is essential to know: each individual's date of birth (or age at starting work); the date of entry to the occupation; some indication of potential environmental exposure; the follow-up status. The latest date known to be alive should be obtained for all individuals, including those still in the workforce or retired. Individuals who have left the industry should be traced such that their status can be obtained. Such leavers are likely to be different in a number of ways from those staying in the industry; without follow-up information on such individuals, the statistics may produce an incomplete or biased result. Rushton (1982) compared the results from a study which included tracing all those leaving the industry prior to retirement with results excluding this group. There were no appreciable differences and it was pointed out that avoidance of the lengthy and costly tracing should be considered, bearing in mind the age of these premature leavers, their length of service, and the proportion of deaths they are likely to contribute to the study results. For all deaths that have occurred in the study population the date of death and cause of death is required. This material can be manipulated in a standard fashion to generate 'person years at risk', which are tabulated by age and calendar period (see subsection 3.5.2). By applying national age, sex and calendar period cause-specific mortality rates, the expected numbers of deaths by cause may be calculated. A comparison is then made between the respective numbers of observed and expected deaths for particular causes; the statistical aspects of this comparison are discussed in subsection 10.5.2.

This approach can be used to explore the risk of a specific cause of death, or to examine patterns of mortality of the workers in more general terms.

Occasionally, full details of each member of the workforce are not available, but company records may be able to provide estimates of the numbers of employees and pensioners by age-group over the period for which death details are available. Using such material, Dean *et al.* (1979) were able to calculate expected deaths by cause and compare these with observed deaths for the blue-collar workers at a Dublin brewery in 1954–73. This technique is less precise than using the calculated person years at risk based on data for each individual, but provided a sounder statistic than proportional-mortality analysis.

10.1.1.8 Prospective studies

In 1961–2 a survey of flax-mill workers was carried out in Northern Ireland; a questionnaire on respiratory symptoms was completed and lung-function tests done on 2528 workers (82 per cent of all those aged over 35 in the industry). At the same time measurements were made of dust levels in 147 workrooms in 17 mills. Subsequent follow-up to 1978 showed no evidence that either respiratory disability or initial dust levels had any effect on the survival experience of the men. Elwood *et al.* (1982) point out that it is difficult to envisage any chronic lung disease severe enough to cause disability that does not also impair survival, though most of the evidence on this topic stems from studies of chronic bronchitis.

10.2 Principles of Occupational Studies

The following subsections discuss some of the general aspects of occupational studies. In addition to the points made here, attention must also be paid to the earlier chapters discussing the wider aspects of these epidemiological methods.

10.2.1 Who is at risk of an occupational hazard?

It is not only workers involved in primary production who may be at risk of cancer from exposure to carcinogens. An obvious example of the chain is that associated with asbestos; this involves those working in the mines, handling the 'raw' asbestos in factories, applying asbestos as in lagging and insulating, even stripping insulation out of various articles at breakers' yards, etc. In addition to this chain of exposures it has been shown that the families of workers and those living in the vicinity of an asbestos factory had an increased mortality from mesothelioma (Newhouse and Thompson, 1965). This was thought to be due to (1) contamination of the workers' clothes which then exposed the wives who washed these, and (2) contamination of the locality surrounding the factory with fibres transmitted in the air. This indicates the expanding ring of contacts who need to be considered when assessing any hazard from a particular industrial process. Rather more difficult to investigate is the possibility that the next generation may be at risk—from foetal loss, excess stillbirths or congenital malformations. A number of studies have been carried out on the reproductive abilities of anaesthetists and other operating-room staff; for example, Axelsson and Rylander (1982) found a raised (but not significant) excess of first-trimester miscarriages in women with high exposure to anaesthetic gases compared with unexposed women. Using data from hospital discharge statistics, Hemminki et al. (1980) found that spontaneous abortion was more common in the manual social classes, and women who worked in industrial and construction work, forestry, agriculture, fishing, sales, transport, communication and services. These findings were not thought to reflect bias in hospitalisation, inaccuracies in the hospital data, or confounding with parity.

Beyond the scope of the present considerations are the potential hazards to purchasers of industrial products. Investigation of the safety of products by chemical-toxicological and other means raises issues very different from the study of the health hazards of the work environment.

10.2.2 Which individuals are eligible for inclusion in a study?

A number of points of eligibility need to be considered in planning a study. It is often desirable to exclude workers with a minimum duration of employment (to restrict those transients with limited relevant exposure). This may be excluding those who have worked for only one month, three months, one year or perhaps five years. It is recommended that individuals with employment over the minimum (such as a year) should be included, even though their exposure is relatively limited, as they help provide estimates of a dose–response relationship. Also, those who have been employed for under ten years may be used after a complete follow-up as a data base from which to calculate occupation- or industry-specific expected figures. (The assumption being that such individuals have a more comparable basic mortality pattern than that obtained from the national data.)

If a hazardous agent is extremely potent and the latent interval for generating the hazard is less than twenty years then an adequate indication of this may come by studying just those in employment. However, if the condition is rare, and the latest interval is long, then it is unlikely that the hazard will be clearly identified in those under the age of sixty-five. If the turnover in the occupation is high then it is even more important that not only pensioners, but also those leaving prior to retirement are followed up. It is usually possible to organise retrieval of vital status for pensioners, but it is much more expensive to trace the leavers. However, if the number who have worked on a particular plant or process is small, it may be crucial to trace these individuals in order to obtain enough numbers of events for statistical analysis. Rather different is the point that if the workers who leave the industry are a biased group of those who have been exposed to risk it is extremely important to trace them—for example, were they the dirty workers who had a higher than average exposure? Were they individuals who were in some way sensitive to the environment? In the past, many studies of occupational hazards have excluded women, because of the small numbers involved. However, with the advent of legislation against sexual discrimination the inclusion of women becomes more appropriate. It is also possible that the exposure and reaction to exposure differs between the sexes and again this argues for the inclusion of women. One particular aspect of this is if the hazard influences the risk, not to the exposed person, but to the next generation; ionising radiation may, for example, have an effect on the pregnant woman which it cannot have on the exposed male.

In many industries contractors may come onto the site and have an environmental exposure entirely different from that of the normal plant operators. However, because the organisation of their employment records are different, it is often difficult to include contractors' personnel in an occupational study. Rather different are 'visitors'—for instance in some fields of work it may be customary to have individuals coming from abroad to work for a limited period of months or years. It is an important issue to consider whether such individuals also need inclusion in the study.

10.2.3 Factors influencing initiation of a study

With finite resources and the likelihood of a stream of fresh leads to consider, it is not possible to launch a definitive study on each 'hunch'. Less tangible issues may be critical to the decision, such as the enthusiasm of the research workers, the degree of collaboration available for the project, or even the very implausibility of a new and previously unsuspected health hazard. Having selected the appropriate research topic, there is then need to ensure that appropriate research facilities are available; these may be the techniques, the ideas, the equipment, and other facilities required. Providing the facilities are available, there must be access for the study to be carried out. The specific points requiring clearance will depend upon the design of the study, but many require access to retrievable records, or the investigation of individuals. As far as retrievable records are concerned, this may need access to (1) personnel records, (2) environmental data and (3) follow-up data on individuals who have left the industry. Such access requires the approval of management and union, with permission to disclose the identity and release information required to trace individuals who have left the industry. The tracing of leavers raises the issue of confidentiality of personal records; the Medical Research Council (1973) has provided guidelines for research in this field. The Faculty of Occupational Medicine (1982) has also produced notes of guidance on the ethics for occupational physicians, which include comments about data on computers, biological monitoring, clinical research and informing safety representatives of various issues.

10.2.4 Validity

The general aspects of validity of data have already been dealt with in each of the earlier chapters; for example, points raised in the chapter on mortality statistics (see 2.2.5) should be considered when handling occupational mortality statistics. This section covers additional points that are particularly relevant to the field of occupational studies. The issues have been separated into those dealing with (1) bias in subjects studied, (2) dilution of environmental effect, (3) validity of exposure and (4) validity of outcome.

10.2.4.1 Bias in subjects studied

A preliminary consideration is whether all employees 'at risk' were covered in the study. Marsh and Enterline (1979) stressed the importance of independent check of the completeness of occupational cohorts. In a validation of records for six plants in the United States, additional records for 21 per cent further subjects were found by cross-checking against Inland Revenue records.

Rather different is the consideration of the selection process involved; Ogle (1885) gave a clear description of some of the biases associated with selection into and out of occupations. For example, some jobs can only be done by the physically strong and active; these characteristics of the workforce may determine their patterns of morbidity and mortality, rather than any aspect of the work environment. An associated aspect is the influence of nonoccupational factors on risk of disease that may also be linked to work. For example, many occupational studies have involved examination of the (potential) hazard of lung cancer—a cancer for which there is a known major behavioural risk factor (smoking). If smoking habits have not been recorded for the employees in a specific occupation, it is always questionable whether variation in smoking could account for any difference in lung-cancer mortality in the workers. Of course, if information is available on intensity and duration of chemical exposure and a dose–response relationship is found with lung cancer, this is less likely to be due to confounding with smoking; however, such results do not rule out a multiplicative or interactive effect between the smoking habits of the workers and their occupational environment.

10.2.4.2 Dilution of environmental effects

When a work hazard only directly effects a restricted group of individuals, the impact of this may be diluted or lost by studying a broader group of the workforce. In general terms this was well recognised over a hundred years ago (Registrar General, 1855); it is a point that warrants consideration whenever it is not known precisely what is the specific hazard responsible for the health problem being studied. Without clear definition of the discrete group of workers 'exposed to risk', there may be loss of precision in the study; this may also be an inevitable consequence of those studies using routine or retrievable data, when job titles cover broad categories of worker (see Alderson, 1983).

10.2.4.3 Validity of exposure data

With a process involving a single suspect-agent it may be satisfactory merely to document whether or not exposure was likely to have occurred. More-suitable data for analysis are provided by the quantification of the intensity of exposure and the duration of exposure. It may be difficult to gauge in which broad category of exposure-level individual workers should be placed; in many industries, no records exist of environmental or personal monitoring for specific chemicals. This difficulty is exacerbated where a complex chemical-works has many plants and workers move from one plant to another. Sometimes the range of chemicals involved in some of the plants and processes might not be known, let alone their levels in the environment monitored. Indirect assessment of potential exposure of process workers may be possible. This becomes much more difficult, if not impossible, for maintenance staff who move throughout a site; often, because of the nature of their work, exposure may be very difficult to gauge and very different from that of the normal working of the plants. Smith *et al.* (1980) developed a method which calculated the expected yearly exposure for each case from the work histories of controls matched on year of birth and year of hire. They suggested that this permitted exploration of exposure level, latency and interaction in such studies.

Obviously, the scope for the research worker to handle valid data will depend on the type of study being carried out. Where routine or retrievable data are used, the issue has to be dealt with by cautious interpretation of available material. In a planned survey or prospective study, steps should be taken to ensure the data collected are of adequate validity.

10.2.4.4 Validity of 'outcome' data

In surveys and case–control studies the researcher should be able to control the quality of the diagnostic information. In prospective studies an important primary task is to check that all the study group are correctly followed up and the 'end-points' identified (i.e. development of disease, death or emigration). Providing complete ascertainment can be achieved, the next step is to consider the validity of the diagnostic information. Obviously when using some form of record linkage, and calculating expected events, thought must be given to possible biases and confounding factors that can account for the differences between observed and expected deaths (e.g. differences in social class, region, behaviour, non-work environment, etc. that could be responsible).

10.3 Advantages and Disadvantages of Occupational Studies

This section is concerned with the relative advantages and disadvantages of the various ways of studying occupationally induced disease; the following comments therefore apply only within the context of such work.

It is important to bear in mind the different types of occupational study. Initially routine data (for example, the decennial supplement on occupational mortality) and cross-sectional studies may be used for descriptive purposes, to indicate the number of deaths and the patterns of morbidity and mortality for different categories of worker. The material may also be used to look at variation from one occupation to another, or variation in one occupation from earlier periods of time. An extension of the simple descriptive use of statistics is their use as a source of a fresh hypothesis ('fishing'—see 10.1.1.6 above). In general, descriptive studies and hypothesis-generating ones will involve relatively broad categories of occupation. Occasionally routine statistics may be used to examine the disease-specific incidence or mortality for a particular occupation in hypothesis testing. However, hypothesis testing will be predominantly by *ad hoc* studies of specific groups of workers—wherever possible identifying those exposed to a specific environmental agent, and distinguishing categories of worker with variation in degree of exposure (both intensity or level and duration of exposure).

The factors affecting detection of risk should be borne in mind. It has been suggested (Alderson, 1979) that these are: the size of the relative and absolute risks; the specificity of the risk; the number of individuals exposed; the degree of job stability; the latent period for generation of disease; the contribution of confounding factors. These points affect the relative efficiency of different methods of studying the same problem.

10.3.1 Routine data

The ready availability of routine data and low cost to the user are the principal advantages, which have to be balanced against lack of precision of environmental exposure and inflexibility. In general terms, as in other fields, routine data are primarily a tool of descriptive studies, to be followed by analytical work using other approaches.

10.3.2 Record linkage

The power of record-linkage studies, including historical prospective studies, may be relatively greater than in other fields of work, as there may be data on potential aetiological exposure that is of higher quality than for other behavioural and environmental agents.

10.3.3 Collation studies

Collation studies have the same advantages of other studies that use routinely available data—the material should be immediately available for the proposed use (providing that any relevant data are collected in the national or other systems). However, as indicated in subsection 2.4.2, collation studies depend upon the available information, which may not readily permit the exclusion of confounding effects (e.g. the production of organic chemicals may be a marker of affluence rather than a specific environmental hazard). Also, when the studies are carried out without any prior hypothesis in mind, the results have to be interpreted with caution; the vast number of comparisons that can be made permit the research worker to fully probe so many permutations of the material that the chance of a number of intriguing hypotheses being generated is high.

Siemiatycki *et al.* (1981) suggested that such studies were suitable for identifying those isolated localities where there was a single-process industry with a particular health-hazard.

10.3.4 Proportional-mortality analyses

The basic drawback, on finding an excess proportion of deaths, is that one does not know if the overall mortality from other causes is low, or if the actual death-rate from the disease being studied is high. The approach can only be used as a pointer to further work, rather than as a definitive examination of a particular issue.

A proportional-mortality analysis is very simple to carry out, provided the basic records on the deaths exist; such records may be available through the pension fund or union records, or obtainable from the system for registering mortality in the population. The ease of carrying out such a study is obviously an advantage, but must be balanced against the difficulty in interpreting the data (see subsection 10.5.1). Such a study may therefore be used to explore a preliminary suggestion of a hazard, but will usually require confirmation from a definitive study using other techniques.

10.3.5 Cross-sectional studies

These are suitable for studying disease where there is a high prevalence of the condition in the workforce, and a clear-cut method of identifying early abnormality or disease. The advantage will be enhanced if this information can readily be associated with information about 'present' exposure, and this is thought to reflect variation in the potential hazard of the environment. Obviously the converse will apply, so that the method will not be any use to study disease that is rare, or only occurs after a long latent interval.

10.3.6 Case–control studies

The distinction from the cross-sectional surveys is that the case–control studies are usually concerned with aetiological factors that operated in the past. The validity will therefore depend to a great extent on the degree to which it is found possible to quantify the past exposure of the individuals in the study and also assess the influence of confounding factors.

The relative advantage is that the studies can be quite quickly mounted and they do not require even as large numbers as the cross-sectional surveys, let alone prospective studies. The data collection is usually dependent upon questioning the subjects, rather than examination or investigation; the costs of data collection are thus usually low.

10.3.7 Historical prospective studies

Such studies depend upon the quality of the retrievable data on past exposure, and then the efficiency of the linkage process that determines the outcome in the cohort. These are problems of such studies, whether they are exploring occupational factors or not. The other crucial issue is the appropriateness of the outcome data and the comparison statistics used. Case and Lea (1955) acknowledged that an external standard may not be applicable to men in a particular study, and demonstrated how 'industrial comparisons' could be made. In a series of papers Mancuso and his colleagues (e.g. see 1968) raised a number of topics: dilution due to imprecise job descriptions; bias in follow up with loss of deaths in some categories of individuals; the advantages of cross-checking the death details; multiple-cause coding; the use of morbidity as an alternative end-point; the 'healthy-worker effect' and use of workers' rates to calculate expected figures; the influence of age at entry, length of follow up, age at death, and latent interval in the results. A number of other authors have discussed the advantages of internally based expected deaths (Redmond and Breslin, 1975; Enterline, 1976; Ott *et al.*,

1976). This issue is further discussed in subsection 10.5.3.

Many historical prospective studies commence with a list of all employees engaged at a point in time, to which are linked recruits over the ensuing years. Person-years are only accumulated from the start date, but there may be some information about the initial cross-section of employees prior to the date of the study start—such as the date of joining the company or jobs performed. Care must be taken in analysing such material, as those subjects may not be typical of all those who had previously been employed; some of those who had left may have suffered from ailments (whether or not caused by their occupation) making them unfit to continue in the industry, or else may have left on promotion to other more mentally challenging or physically demanding work. In the absence of information about all employed prior to the start date of the study, it is difficult to interpret any analyses for those who remained.

10.3.8 Prospective studies

These are usually reserved for the definitive study of a known hazard, when it is important to quantify the dose–response effect of the agent, and examine other specific points about the aetiology. The method is suitable for a stable industry, where facilities exist for assessing the changes that occur in the work environment over time. Usually the method will be reserved for those conditions that have a relatively high incidence.

Such studies are not lightly undertaken, and the expenditure of time and effort may be justified when there is some hope that early recognition of the disease in the workforce will result in medical intervention that is of benefit to the individuals concerned.

A historical prospective study will give a relatively quick probe of a topic, but with limited specificity, while a genuine prospective study will explore the problem slowly, but with much greater power to quantify the exact aetiological relationships.

10.3.9 The healthy-worker effect

An issue that is of particular relevance to historical prospective studies, but that should be borne in mind when trying to interpret other types of study, is now commonly referred to as the healthy-worker effect. Seltzer and Jablon (1974) analysed the 5345 deaths of 85 491 Second World War white male veterans followed from 1946–9; expected mortality was calculated from United States national death-rates. In particular, they looked at the trend in deficiency of deaths over time; malignant-disease deaths were about 55 per cent of the expected in the first 5 years and then rose to about 90 per cent (no difference for 6, 10, 16 or 21–23 years of follow up was significant). There were even more prolonged effects for other main causes of death. They emphasised the protracted effect of selection on any subsequent mortality and stressed that many subgroups of the population might differ in both known and unknown ways. Passage of a few years would not overcome the unwanted confounding effects.

There has been increasing disquiet about the suitability of national rates to generate a valid expected number of deaths. In many studies this has resulted in a ratio of O/E considerably less than one; often, the all-cause figure is about 0.75 and some recent studies have reported even lower figures. This creates confusion in the interpretation of the data, because the lower figure should not automatically be interpreted as indicating absence of a health hazard. Also, when specific causes of death are examined, it has been suggested that the all-cause ratio may be used as a yardstick against which to measure results from specific causes. Thus with an all-cause figure of 0.75, it has been claimed that a ratio of 1.0 for cancers is raised (i.e. represents an increment of one-third over the expected figure of 0.75). This can produce considerable argument over the interpretation of the data, especially where the results are based upon large numbers of deaths and such differences are statistically significant. A number of authors have discussed this topic (Goldsmith, 1975; Enterline, 1975; Gaffey, 1975; McMichael *et al.*, 1975; McMichael, 1976).

Ogle (1885) had indicated that occupational cohorts demonstrate properties of selection, survival and length of follow up. Fox and Collier (1976) presented data for workers engaged in vinyl-chloride manufacture and demonstrated that the reduced risk of death compared with the general population diminished with the lapse of time after entry to the industry. There was also an indication that those who left the industry had a relatively higher risk of death compared with those who remained.

Vinni and Hakama (1980) linked 1960 and 1970 census records for 20 000 Finnish workers and then followed the individuals to 1976. This enabled them to quantify the selection and survival effects. They suggested that the mortality of those who stayed within the same industry was 60 per cent of those who retired prior to age 65, while the mortality of those who changed their job was 90 per cent of those who stayed in the same job. There were also differences in this 'survivor' effect in various occupational categories.

An integral part of the analysis is the adjustment for the age of the study population. Liddell (1960) reviewed the application of four methods of age standardisation and commented that no mortality index should be used without a knowledge of the inherent inadequacy due to variation in the relative death-rates. Cook (1979) drew attention to the age dependence of the S.M.R. and the inability to compare rates for samples where the age distribution is different. There followed a dispute between Harnes (1980) and Cook (1980), in which various manipulations were suggested for trying to overcome this problem. Neither appeared to provide a generally acceptable solution to the problem. Alderson (1981) has suggested that an alternative to comparison of the ratio of observed to expected deaths might be more-detailed analyses based on the difference between the observed and expected deaths. This calculation provides something akin to an attributable risk (see subsections 5.5.5 and 6.5.1); this may then be examined in relation to various estimates of 'exposure' (intensity of exposure and duration of exposure), and latent interval between first exposure and generation of the hazard.

Gilbert (1982) examined the influence of various biases on mortality of men employed at Hanford nuclear facility in the period 1947–76. This confirmed that reduced mortality occurred in the early years of follow up and for those with higher socio-economic status. Elevated mortality was present in those employed for less than two years and those who gave up work below retirement age.

10.4 Extension of Method of Occupational Studies

This section provides brief notes on four ways of extending the basic methods described in section 10.1. The first is a different approach to collecting detailed information in a case–control study, which warrants a different statistical analysis. The second topic suggests a different approach to using routine data, while the final two subsections indicate steps now being taken to enhance the availability of information within industry.

10.4.1 Case–control within a cohort study

A very different approach is to perform a case–control study within a historical prospective study. The mortality study of oil refineries described in the first section of this chapter identified 30 deaths from leukaemia. There were 31.96 expected, with no indication therefore of a hazard from leukaemia. However, in order to explore the possible association with benzene exposure the 30 deaths from leukaemia, together with 6 where leukaemia was a contributory cause, were used for a case–control study (Rushton and Alderson, 1981a). Each of these 36 deaths was matched with two sets of controls; the first set of three controls being matched for refinery and year of birth, and the second set of three controls being matched for refinery, year of birth and length of service. The detailed job-histories of each individual were abstracted; in the absence of measurement of benzene in the work environment the job histories were used to allocate each man to one of three categories of benzene exposure ('low', 'medium' or 'high'). Logistic models were fitted to the cases and controls matched on year of birth; the results are set out in table 10.5. The risk for those men identified as having had 'medium' or 'high' exposure relative to the risk of those with 'low' exposure reached the formal level of significance when length of service was taken into account, either in the matching of cases and controls, or in the analysis. It was suggested that if there was an increased risk of leukaemia due to benzene exposure, it could have only been one that affected a very small proportion of the men within the total refinery workforce. It must be emphasised that the estimation of benzene exposure was not based on environmental or personal measurements.

Further discussion of this approach can be found in Liddell et al. (1977), McDonald et al. (1980) and Darby and Reissland (1981).

Table 10.5 Relative risks and 95 per cent confidence limits of death from leukaemia with logistic model fitted to year of entry and degree of benzene exposure in oil refinery workers

	Benzene exposure relative risk	Year of entry relative risk	Length of service relative risk	χ^2	d.f.
benzene exposure	2.01 (0.94, 4.28)			3.32	1
benzene exposure and year of entry	2.26 (1.01, 5.01)	1.43 (0.86, 2.39)		5.24	2
benzene exposure and length of service	2.99 (1.24, 7.20)		0.71 (0.51, 0.98)	8.01	2

Source: Rushton and Alderson (1981)

10.4.2 Job titles indexed to chemical exposure

An American list which catalogued different occupations exposed to specific chemicals was used to identify fourteen occupations thought to involve benzene exposure (Vianna and Polan, 1979). Deaths in the period 1950–69 in males in New York State were classified and the relative risk of lymphomas in these workers examined. A significant excess of deaths was found; though the possible importance of aromatic hydrocarbons could not be excluded, benzene was the only chemical used by all the occupational groups studied.

Though there were some questions about the method of the above study, it does indicate the way in which a cross-index of job titles to potential chemical exposure may be used to probe an issue. It would provide a preliminary cross-check of any hypothesis where (1) the chemical in question was identified in the chemical–job listing, and (2) the outcome data such as cancer incidence or mortality recorded jobs in sufficient detail.

10.4.3 An historical data-base

Many industries are paying increasing attention to the practicality of carrying out various forms of prospective study. The identification of exposed individuals from 'old' occupational records is a time-consuming task and the validity of this material is questionable. Where (1) such records exist for a large workforce, (2) they contain details of chronological job histories and (3) the industry is relatively complex, then it is appropriate to consider the suitability of making such historical records more easily retrievable. Conceptually this is in order to carry out a series of historical prospective studies; having once established the file of relevant data, it can be used to explore subsequent queries as they arise. This will avoid having to go back to the manual records every time a specific query is raised about the mortality of past employees in relation to particular chemicals. Providing follow-up status is available, including the cause of death for those who have died, the observed and expected mortality should be readily examined (see Hoar *et al.*, 1980). A system for recording, storing and retrieving occupational exposure data and linkage with medical information for individuals working in the chemical plants in Europe and the United States was described by Baxter and Henshaw (1982).

A rather different use of such material is where there is need to cross-check on past exposure of workers dying from a specific and relatively rare disease. If the historical file incorporates a mechanism for accumulating the cause of death for each decedent, it is a relatively simple matter to identify those dying from the particular cause of interest (for example, brain tumours). A sample of control subjects can be obtained from the occupational data-base. Using this material as a starting point, much more detailed enquiry could be made about the occupational histories of the small sample of subjects dying from brain tumours and the controls. Such a case–control approach has been discussed in the previous section; the historical data-base merely facilitates such a study.

10.4.4 Occupational monitoring systems

An important issue to consider is whether industrial health-records can be so organised that they can assist in the establishment of monitoring schemes to detect environmental hazards. The expression 'monitoring' is used to indicate the collection and regular analysis of information in an attempt to identify fresh hazards, not previously recognised. This should be distinguished from 'surveillance', which involves the regular review of material on a known hazard to check on the functioning of control measures. Support for the introduction of monitoring systems comes from the World Health Organisation (1974) and the Council of European Communities (1979). Their reports indicated the need to collect data on environment, on the population classified by exposure to agents, and on follow up of the health of employees. In order to set up a monitoring system one requires an enlightened management, a labour force which appreciates the value of such an approach, and the availability of a sound industrial-hygiene service. These elements are essential prerequisites; then comes the need to collect, analyse and interpret relevant data.

It does not follow automatically that because more sophisticated data are being fed into a monitoring system that it will automatically provide valuable fresh leads. There are major statistical problems in the analysis and interpretation of such data; when more complex material is fed in (even assuming it is accurate data and up to date) there may be greater difficulty in interpretation. This is because the number of separate analyses and the range of factors that have to be taken into account increase geometrically; with this increase in complexity of the data base, there is increase in the difficulty of distinguishing between false and genuine positive leads of equal statistical significance. The greater the number of separate comparisons that are carried out, the greater the number of results that will be 'statistically significant' at any chosen level. It may be possible to identify fresh leads and distinguish them from false leads by replication and comparison of subsets of data, taking into account the relationship between risk and dose, and time trends. It is important to remember that relative risk, absolute risk, specificity of risk, number of men exposed, job stability, latent period, and the influence of confounding factors are important in determining whether hazards can be readily identified. In planning such systems consideration needs to be given to the availability of data, the feasibility of data collection, the interpretation of data, the process of 'decision making' on results from the system, costs and benefits, and confidentiality.

Though there have been frequent suggestions that monitoring of workers should occur in order to identify fresh leads, there have yet to be published definitive studies that demonstrate the value of this approach. Table 10.6 sets out the range of items that one report indicated might be collected (Epidemiological Project Study Group, 1979). The range of items is very comprehensive, when one considers the material presently available for the majority of workers in this country in any form of retrievable record system.

Table 10.6 Items suggested for data collection system on health and working conditions

---

1 EMPLOYEE HISTORY
1.1   *Personal data*

Name	Sex
Personnel No.	Date of birth
National registration No.	Marital status
Address	Ethnic origin

1.2   *Work history*
        Company/Location/Department/Workplace
        Job title and position for every job
        Date starting and ending each job
        Day/Shift worker

1.3   *Reason for leaving*

2 MEDICAL EVENTS
2.1   *Morbidity*
        Record of all absences for illness
        Confirmed diagnosis for all spells over 21 consecutive days
        Review of diagnoses for cumulative absence over 21 days in a year

2.2   *Medical history*
        Smoking
        Use of medicines   Revised every 2 years

2.3   *Mortality*
        Date of death
        Causes of death (up to 4 on certificate)
        Method of diagnosis

(*continued overleaf*)

Table 10.6 (*continued*)

3   ENVIRONMENTAL EXPOSURE
3.1   *Potential exposure*
        Chemicals used listed by workplace

3.2   *Area monitoring*
        Measurement in various work areas to give derived exposure level

3.3   *Individual exposure*
        Actual environmental measurements on sample of workers to provide
            group personal exposure

4   BIOMEDICAL DATA
        Haematology
        haematocrit
        haemoglobin
        platelets
        R.B.C. count
        W.B.C. count

        Urinanalysis
        albumin
        glucose
        haemoglobin
        ketones
        pH
        sediment

        Biochemistry
        cholesterol
        creatinine
        gamma G.T.
        glucose
        S.G.O.T.
        S.G.P.T.
        triglycerides
        uric acid

        Medical review
        history
        examination
          B.P.
          height
          weight
        investigations
          audiogram
          E.C.G.
          F.E.V$_1$.
          F.M.F. 25 : 75
          F.V.L.
          X-ray chest

Based on Epidemiological Project Study Group (1979)

A recent supplement of the *Journal of Occupational Medicine* (1982; **24,** 781–866) provides a description of the use of various medical information systems in fourteen American companies. Some of the method issues have been discussed by Paddle (1981). Because of the complexity of work in this field, it is suggested that further research is still required in order to clarify the optimum approach. This needs to look at the two rather different aspects of (1) the desirable level of detail on environment, potential exposure, and morbidity; (2) improved techniques for analysis of such complex files.

10.5 Statistical Techniques in Occupational Studies

This section provides a guide to proportional mortality analysis, and the testing of differences between the observed and expected number of deaths; these are two frequent procedures in occupational studies. This is followed by an introduction to other forms of analysis that are suitable for prospective studies.

10.5.1 Proportional-mortality analysis

The application of this technique has already been discussed (see 10.1.1.4). The method of calculation requires, for the 'standard population', the number of deaths from all causes and from the cause of interest within appropriate age-groups. The proportion of specific-causes to all-causes deaths is then applied to the number of deaths from all causes in the study population, to give the expected deaths. This is repeated for all the age-groups involved. The proportional-mortality ratio is then given by:

$$\frac{\text{sum of observed deaths}}{\text{sum of expected deaths}} \times 100$$

The calculation is set out in table 10.7, for the relatively simple data handled in this way in the decennial supplement on occupational mortality for 1959–63 (Registrar General, 1971).

This method can be used for national data, where the denominator is not readily available (in the example used in table 10.7, there is appreciable variation in recording of occupation between census and death registration for persons 65–74 and indirect standardisation using rates is not appropriate). The example in section 10.1.1.4 used national and local data to calculate the proportional mortality of miners in Cumberland from various causes. The national cancer registration scheme records occupation, where known, for each patient registered with cancer. As the information is not recorded for an appreciable number of patients and there are not readily available figures of the population at risk, proportional registration rates (P.R.R.s) by occupation unit are calculated. The method is essentially the same as indicated in table 10.7, but involves calculations for twelve five-year age-groups from fifteen to seventy-four.

The principal drawback to this technique is that as rates are not available,

Table 10.7 Calculation of proportional mortality ratio (P.M.R.) for coronary artery disease in two occupational orders in England and Wales, 1959–63

Occupation	Cause	Age			
		65–69	70–74	65–74	P.M.R.
all men	all causes	181 288	205 604		
	coronary deaths observed	47 311	48 954		
	proportion of coronary deaths	0.2610	0.2381		
professional and technical	all causes	7 613	9 346		
	coronary deaths observed	2 598	2 781	5 379	
	coronary deaths expected*	1 987.0	2 225.3	4 212.3	128
miners and quarrymen	all causes	9 318	11 190		
	coronary deaths observed	2 047	2 251	4 298	
	coronary deaths expected*	2 432.0	2 664.3	5 096.3	84

Source: Registrar General (1971)

*expected deaths = all-causes × proportion of coronary deaths
e.g. = 7613 × 0.2610
= 1987.0

one does not know if the overall mortality is low or high in the study population. Thus when a specific cause has a low proportional mortality ratio, this may be genuinely low, or 'apparently low' due to an actual excess from another cause. This dilemma in interpretation of the material means that the approach can only be used as a pointer to further work. Sartor (1982) discussed some of the problems of interpreting P.M.R.s, and stressed that the P.M.R. will only be equal to the S.M.R. if the overall death-rates are equal in the study and 'comparison' group.

10.5.2 Is the observed mortality significantly raised?

A very common requirement in occupational studies is to check whether the observed number of deaths is significantly increased. This involves the concept of 'person years at risk' (described in 3.5.2), which is used to calculate an expected number of deaths. Case and Lea (1955) set out the method for such studies, in the occupational field. The following note indicates how the results may be tested.

Table 10.1 presented data from an historical prospective study, which generated observed and expected numbers of deaths from various categories of workers. This was the result of a very common form of study; where no specific hypothesis is being tested, many comparisons within the data may be explored, looking at subsets of the workforce and also many different causes of death. There is need for some relatively simple system for checking the probability of obtaining the observed (or a greater) number of deaths in comparison with the expected deaths.

The actual technique will depend upon the numbers of events involved; if at least five deaths were expected, then the difference can be simply probed as follows:

$$\chi^2 = \frac{(O-E)^2}{E}$$

Substituting the values found for hypertensive disease in the refinery study,

$$\chi^2 = \frac{(76-105.56)^2}{105.56}$$

$$= \frac{(-29.56)^2}{105.56}$$

$$= 8.28$$

Check of the appropriate tables for the χ^2-distribution for one degree of freedom shows this value is very unlikely to be obtained by chance (i.e. $p < 0.01$).

Another way to probe the same data is to examine the confidence limits of the ratio O/E; this is done by using the approach advocated by Bailar and Ederer (1964). For any given value of observed events, the factors for the comparison O/E can be read from a table they provide; these are then used as divisors to generate the 95 per cent or 99 per cent confidence limits for the particular ratio. For 70 observed events (76 is not tabulated), the factors are 0.791 and 1.28 for 95 per cent significance; these are used to divide the original ratio of O/E thus:

$$95 \text{ per cent confidence limits} = \frac{0.72}{0.791} \text{ to } \frac{0.72}{1.28}$$

$$= 0.91 \text{ to } 0.56$$

It can be seen that these results are asymmetrical about the original value of 0.72, but they do not encompass the value of 1.0; this agrees with the test of significance that the results are unlikely to be due to chance.

Instead of using the tables of Bailar and Ederer, an approximate formula for the 95 per cent confidence limits may be used:

$$95 \text{ per cent confidence limits} = \frac{(O-2\sqrt{E})}{E} \text{ to } \frac{(O+2\sqrt{E})}{E}$$

$$= \frac{(76-2\sqrt{105.56})}{105.56} \text{ to } \frac{(76+\sqrt{105.56})}{105.56}$$

$$= 0.525 \text{ to } 0.915$$

Again, these values do not encompass 1.00 and support the contention that the results are statistically significant.

Where the expected number of events is less than five, the data are treated as a Poisson variate. The test then examines the probability of obtaining the observed or a more extreme number of events, given that the expected value represents the mean value for the events in the parent population. The simplest way to examine this is to consult published tables, such as those of

Pearson and Hartley (1970). Volume 1 of this work includes a table giving the probability of each increment in observed events for a given mean figure. For example, if there were 7 observed deaths in a subgroup of men with an expected figure of 2.3, entering the Pearson and Hartley table for this mean figure would show that the cumulative probability of observing 7 or more deaths was 0.009 36. (Note: this may be obtained directly for some values of E by inspection of table 7, or by summing the individual values of table 39, which provides a finer gradation of values of E.) It must be remembered that the p-value is obtained from a one-tailed test, quantifying the probability of obtaining the observed or a more extreme value. The confidence limits are obtained in the way set out above, as this method is valid for expected values of any size.

10.5.3 Internal analyses in prospective studies

A very different approach is to use some form of internal analysis instead of calculating the expected mortality from national data. Oldham and Rossiter (1965) used a discriminant function to give a linear combination of eighteen measurements made on a sample of men; their results facilitated interpretation of the data, and did not appear to be very dependent on the distributional assumptions that were involved. A discussion with a number of statisticians on the appropriate analysis of occupational cohort studies (Liddell, 1975) distinguished: (1) *a posteriori* analyses (relating effects to causal variates) in order to determine the best hypothesis, with probability statements adjusting for simultaneous inference; (2) *a priori* analyses (relating hypothesised causes to subsequent effects) to obtain mortality rates for defined subcohorts; (3) summarised data in life-table form comparing subcohorts. This approach was used in a major study of asbestos miners in Canada reported by Liddell and colleagues (1977); they suggested that the conventional analysis was useful to place the cohort mortality-rates in the appropriate demographic context. The regression analyses, which were more complex to perform, provided absolute risks when the complete data set was used. Further analyses by the same method (McDonald *et al.*, 1980) suggested that the *a posteriori* analyses had the advantages that interaction between several variables could be examined and it avoided the requirement for external rates. Darby and Reissland (1981) developed a test for trend which examined the distribution of observed and expected deaths in exposure categories across age–calendar-period–time-since-first-employment subgroups. The expected values were calculated assuming a no-dose effect. They had to exclude subgroups where there were no deaths or where all the person-years in any given category was the only entry. The authors also carried out a conventional analysis using national rates and obtained comparable results from both approaches.

Alderson *et al.* (1981) were asked to see if control of the environmental exposure had reduced the risk of lung cancer in workers in the bi-chromate industry. However, because of the nature of the data available, those who had worked before the plant had been modified had in general a longer duration of work, and had been followed to older ages. There was thus confounding between duration of exposure, length of follow up, and whether or not the individual had worked before the plant modification. In order to disentangle these confounding factors a multiple-regression analysis was carried out using death from lung cancer as the dependent variate. Table 10.8 shows the main results for this analysis; duration of work and duration of follow up were associated with appreciable variation in risk of lung cancer, though an independent contribution did come from calendar period of employment (i.e. distinguishing the influence of modification). This internal multivariate analysis thus confirmed the suggestion that the plant modification had had an effect on risk of lung cancer, though it also indicated that duration of employment and duration of follow up were more important factors in determining risk of lung cancer.

Table 10.8 Results of multivariate analysis, showing the independent contributions of various factors to risk of lung cancer in chromate workers

Factor	Category	Contribution to risk of lung cancer*
duration of employment (years)	< 9	− 59
	10 −	+ 2
	20 +	+ 164
duration of follow-up (years)	< 9	+ 118
	10 −	+ 56
	20 +	− 88
period of employment	pre-change	+ 73
	pre/post-change	+ 50
	post-change	− 112
factory	Bolton	− 96
	Eaglescliffe	− 33
	Rutherglen	+ 62

Source: Alderson *et al.* (1981)

*The scores may be compared to indicate the relative contribution to the risk of cancer; they approximately indicate the percentage variation from average risk of lung cancer for all men in the study.

References

Recommended reading

McDonald, J. C. (1981). *Recent Advances in Occupational Health*. Churchill Livingstone, Edinburgh

Other references

Alderson, M. R. (1972). *Br. J. ind. Med.*, **29**, 245–54

Alderson, M. R. (1979). In *Perspectives and Progress in Occupational Health* (W. Gardner, ed.) Wright, Bristol, pp. 151–86

Alderson, M. R. (1980). *J. Epidem. Comm. Hlth*, **34**, 182–5

Alderson, M. (1981). In Banbury Report 9: *Quantification of Occupational Cancer.* Cold Spring Harbour Laboratory, New York, pp. 590–610

Alderson, M. R. (1983). *Job Titles as Surrogates for Exposure.* In press

Alderson, M. R., Rattan, N. S., and Bidstrup, L. (1981). *Br. J. ind. Med.*, **38**, 117–24

Axelsson, G., and Rylander, R. (1982). *Int. J. Epidem.*, **11**, 250–6

Bailar, J. C., and Ederer, F. (1964). *Biometrics*, **20**, 639–43

Baxter, R. A., and Henshaw, J. L. (1982). *Ann. occup. Hyg.*, **25**, 95–100

Blot, W. J., Brinton, L. A., Fraumeni, J. F., and Stone, B. J. (1977). *Science*, **198**, 51–3

Boyd, J. T., Boll, R., Faulds, J. S., and Leiper, J. (1970). *Br. J. ind. Med.*, **27**, 97–106

Case, R. A. M., and Lea, A. J. (1955). *Br. J. prev. soc. Med.*, **9**, 62–72

Cook, R. R. (1979). *J. occ. Med.*, **21**, 784

Cook, R. R. (1980). *J. occ. Med.*, **22**, 369–70

Council of European Communities (1979). *Official Journal*, **22**, C 89/6–9

Darby, S. C., and Reissland, J. A. (1981). *J. R. statist. Soc. A*, **144**, 298–331

Dean, G., MacLennan, R., McLoughlin, H., and Shelley, E. (1979). *Br. J. Cancer*, **40**, 581–9

Elwood, P. C., McAulay, I. R., and Elwood, J. H. (1982). *Lancet*, **1**, 1112–4

Enterline, P. E. (1975). *J. occ. Med.*, **17**, 127–8

Enterline, P. E. (1976). *J. occ. Med.*, **18**, 150–6

Epidemiological Project Study Group (1979). *Report on the Collection and Handling of Occupational Information.* Medical Division, Shell International, The Hague

Evans, H. J., Buckton, K. E., Hamilton, G. E., and Carothers, A. (1979). *Nature*, **277**, 531–4

Faculty of Occupational Medicine (1982). *Guidance on Ethics for Occupational Physicians.* Royal College of Physicians, London

Fox, A. J., and Collier, P. F. (1976). *Br. J. prev. soc. Med.*, **30**, 225–30

Fox, A. J., and Goldblatt, P. O. (1982). *Longitudinal Study: Socio-demographic Mortality Differentials.* H.M.S.O., London

Gaffey, W. R. (1975). *J. occ. Med.*, **17**, 128

Gilbert, E. S. (1982). *Am. J. Epidem.*, **116**, 177–88

Goldsmith, J. R. (1975). *J. occ. Med.*, **17**, 126–7

Harnes, J. R. (1980). *J. occ. Med.*, **22**, 364–9

Hemminki, K., Miemi, M.–L., Saloniemi, I., Vainis, H., and Hemmincki, E. (1980). *Int. J. Epidem.*, **9**, 149–53

Hoar, S. K., Morrison, A. L., Cole, P., and Silverman, D. T. (1980). *J. occ. Med.*, **22**, 722–6

Liddell, F. D. K. (1960). *Br. J. ind. Med.*, **17**, 228–33

Liddell, F. D. K. (1975). *Arch. envir. Hlth*, **30**, 266–7

Liddell, F. D. K., McDonald, J. C., and Thomas, D. C. (1977). *J. R. statist. Soc. A* **140**, 469–91

McDonald, J. C., Liddell, F. D. K., Gibbs, G. W., Eyssen, G. E., and McDonald, A. D. (1980). *Br. J. Ind. Med.*, **37**, 11–24

McMichael, A. J. (1976). *J. occ. Med.*, **18**, 165–8

McMichael, A. J., Haynes, S. G., and Tyroler, H. A. (1975). *J. occ. Med.*, **17**, 128–31

Medical Research Council (1973). *Br. med. J.*, **1**, 213–6
Mancuso, T. F., Ciocco, A., and El Attar, A. A. (1968). *J. occ. Med.*, **10**, 213–32
Marsh, G. M., and Enterline, P. E. (1979). *J. occ. Med.*, **21**, 665–70
Newhouse, M. L., and Thompson, H. (1965). *Br. J. ind. Med.*, **22**, 261–6
Office of Population Censuses and Surveys. (1973). *Cohort Studies: New Developments*. H.M.S.O., London
Ogle, W. (1885). *Supplement to the 45th Annual Report of the Registrar General*. H.M.S.O., London
Oldham, P. D., and Rossiter, C. E. (1965). *Br. J. ind. Med.*, **22**, 92–100
Ott, M. G., Holder, B. B., and Langer, R. R. (1976). *J. occ. Med.*, **18**, 171–7
Paddle, G. M. (1981). In Banbury Report 9: *Quantification of Occupational Cancer*. Cold Spring Harbour Laboratory, New York, pp. 177–86
Pearson, E. S., and Hartley, H. O. (1970). *Biometrica Tables for Statisticians*. 3rd edn., Vol. I, Cambridge University Press, Cambridge
Redmond, C. K., and Breslin, P. P. (1975). *J. occ. Med.*, **17**, 313–7
Registrar General (1855). *14th Annual Report of the Registrar General of Births, Deaths, and Marriages in England*. H.M.S.O., London
Registrar General (1971). *Registrar General's Decennial Supplement England and Wales, 1961. Occupational Mortality*. H.M.S.O., London
Registrar General (1978). *Registrar General's Decennial Supplement England and Wales, 1971. Occupational Mortality*. H.M.S.O., London
Rushton, L. (1982). *Lancet*, **1**, 1421
Rushton, L., and Alderson, M. R. (1981a). *Br. J. ind. Med.*, **38**, 225–34
Rushton, L., and Alderson, M. R. (1981b). *Br. J. Cancer*, **43**, 77–84
Rushton, L., and Alderson, M. R. (1982a). *An Epidemiological Survey of Oil Distribution Centres in Great Britain*. Institute of Petroleum, London
Rushton, L., and Alderson, M. R. (1982b). *An Epidemiological Survey of Maintenance Workers in London Transport Executive Bus Garages and Chiswick Works*. Institute of Petroleum, London
Sartor, F. A. (1982). *Am. J. Epidem.*, **115**, 144–5
Seltzer, C. C., and Jablon, S. (1974). *Am. J. Epidem.*, **100**, 367–72
Siemiatycki, J., Day, N. E., Fabry, J., and Cooper, J. A. (1981). *J. Natn. Cancer Inst.*, **66**, 217–25
Smith, A. H., Waxweiler, R. J., and Tyroler, H. A. (1980). *Am. J. Epidem.*, **112**, 787–97
Tough, I. M., and Court Brown, W. M. (1965). *Lancet*, **1**, 684
Tough, I. M., Smith, P. G., Court Brown, W. M., and Harnden, D. G. (1970). *Europ. J. Cancer*, **6**, 49–55
Vianna, J. N., and Polan, A. (1979). *Lancet*, **1**, 1394–5
Vinni, K., and Hakama, M. (1980). *Br. J. ind. Med.*, **37**, 180–4
Wegman, D. H., Peters, J. M., Boundy, M. G., and Smith, T. J. (1982). *Br. J. ind. Med.*, **39**, 233–8
Williams, R. R., Stegens, N. L., and Goldsmith, J. R. (1977). *J. natn. Cancer Inst.*, **59**, 1147–85
World Health Organisation (1974). *Report EHE/75.1*. W.H.O., Geneva.

11 Study Design and Inference

This chapter provides a few examples of the difficulty in identifying unexpected environmental hazards. This leads into a general discussion on study design. The points indicated in earlier chapters are reinforced by emphasising the issues that need to be borne in mind when planning an aetiological study. This cannot be translated immediately into a blueprint that will automatically provide all answers when considering a fresh study, but it is intended that sufficient guidance is given to cover the main dilemmas that arise when a new study is being considered. It is not quite so easy to compress the design of a study on a medical-care issue into a simple scheme, such as that advocated for aetiological studies. This is because of the very diverse nature of the issues that may be studied and the much wider range of disciplines and techniques that are relevant to such work. However, some points are provided that are appropriate to this field of work.

The chapter then turns to the issue of analysis and formulation of inferences. The statistical aspects are only briefly indicated (but further reading is specified), while some aspects of logic are set out that assist with interpretation of epidemiological data.

11.1 Monitoring for Untoward and Adverse Effects

In July 1972 the French Ministry of Health was informed that there had been an outbreak affecting children in various parts of France, who had a severe form of nappy rash, low-grade fever, and various neurological manifestations. The first such illness had occurred in the third week of March; all the children involved were aged three months to three years. They suffered from an erythematous rash in the nappy area with red, oedematous ulcerative skin lesions, moderate fever (occasionally exceeding 39 °C), irritability and vomiting; this was followed by drowsiness, alternating with excessive hypertonicity and startle responses. In the severe cases, convulsions developed, followed by weakness and lethargy. A quarter of the children went into coma, and one-fifth died.

The cases had occurred in four areas of France; there were 204 children involved, 16 of whom relapsed, while 4 had 3 episodes of attacks. Initial investigation of the children with this 'encephalopathy of unknown origin' failed to detect the cause. Many of the affected children developed symptoms in April, though other cases continued until August; some of the severely affected children were transferred to hospitals in Paris with special facilities, but the realisation that there was a new neurological condition was gradual. Attempts to isolate infectious agents from cerebrospinal fluids, blood, stool, pharynx and urine were unsuccessful, despite use of a wide variety of methods.

Epidemiological study in July revealed that the children had virtually no

314

contact with each other, despite the clustering of the syndrome in four parts of France; extensive interview with the parents revealed that most had used the same baby powder. Toxicological investigation of factory and store samples revealed no abnormal constituents; however, in August analysis of samples taken from the house of an affected child revealed 6.3 per cent of hexachlorophene. Detailed inquiry indicated that the majority of the affected children had been using the contaminated powder. The factory practice recovered spilt talc from the factory floor for reuse; it was supposed that this had resulted in the accidental contamination of the baby talc with hexachlorophene, which was used for other preparations made in the same factory. (This abstract is based on the paper by Martin-Bouyer *et al.*, 1982.)

There are some general points that stem from the consideration of the above example; how many of the diseases caused by accidental contamination will result in unusual symptoms, which help to alert the treating physicians? The distribution of the agent to several parts of the country and the limited number of children involved probably delayed recognition of the fact that this was a new and unexplained syndrome; presumably the reports of the severe nappy-rash helped the epidemiologists to identify that all had used the same baby powder (if the symptoms had been restricted to the nervous system this might not have been so easy an investigation).

11.1.1 Other sources of untoward effects

There are other examples where fresh hazards have unexpectedly occurred. For example, since May 1981 doctors in several parts of Spain have witnessed the evolution of an obscure disease; initially people of all ages and both sexes were affected, though there was a predominance of women. There was initial fever, headache, cough, dyspnoea, exanthems, pruritus, and myalgia; less frequent was nausea, vomiting, abdominal pain, clouding of consciousness, purpura, hepatomegaly, jaundice or pancreatitis. Later intense muscular pain, numbness of extremities and oedema developed. After three to four months scleroderma-like and other skin lesions developed, with severe muscular weakness and atrophy (these affected women rather than men). The epidemic particularly affected residents of working-class suburbs of Madrid.

Six weeks after the initial epidemic a link to adulterated cooking oil was established (denatured rerefined rapeseed oil was involved). Hormonal influences may have affected the sex ratio; there is also a clear genetic factor, with high frequency of particular H.L.A. haplotypes. The toxic agent has not yet been determined (Toxic Epidemic Syndrome Study Group, 1982).

Another topic area has involved attempts to identify adverse drug-reactions. Bulpitt (1977) has described the various ways of detecting such reactions, i.e.: clinical observations; collation of mortality trends with drug-usage data; long-term clinical trials; voluntary register of adverse drug-effects; routine collation of drug-prescription information with diagnoses for named individuals; detailed investigation of subjects after exposure to particular treatments. Since this article appeared, another approach to the topic has been the questioning of G.P.s about events occurring to certain patients known to have been given certain drugs (Inman, 1981). Bulpitt (1977) also indicated that the frequency of the adverse effect will affect the appropriate method for hazard detection; he distinguished between effects that occur more often than once in 300 treatments, from once in 300 to once in 3000 treatments, and less frequently than once in 3000 treatments (where a treatment is defined as either a short-term course, or therapy continued for a year in long-term medication). He reviewed the adverse effects that have been discovered in the past, and indicated the lead that provided evidence for there being a particular problem in each case.

The above examples indicate some of the problems involved in identifying untoward and unexpected effects of various chemical agents; it must be remembered that physical and biological agents can also provide threats to the health of mankind. The above examples relate to hazards from household articles, drugs and food; other sources may be changes in behaviour (e.g. the occurrence of Kaposi's sarcoma in homosexuals), alteration of the environment (e.g. is reduction of the ozone layer liable to increase the risk of skin cancer in the coming decade?), or introduction of new processes in industry (e.g. what impact has the growth of organic chemical production had upon risk of cancer in the workforce?). Alongside these 'problems' must be set the range of approaches used to monitor untoward effects (the chapters on mortality and morbidity statistics deal with some aspects of this, especially subsections 2.2.3, 2.2.4, 3.1.3 and 3.1.4). The ways of searching for adverse drug-reactions has been briefly introduced above, while chapter 10 has dealt with occupational hazards.

11.2 Study Design: General Principles

The challenge to any research worker is the generation of fresh 'ideas'; it is usually an issue of application of standard technique when planning a study to test out these ideas. From the point of epidemiology, the main issue is to suggest and investigate aetiological hypotheses. This is then followed by delineation of group or individual risk factors, the specification of the single (or multiple) agent, quantification of dose–response relationships, and then appropriate 'health-care' activity for primary or secondary prevention. As has already been discussed (see subsection 8.1.6), whenever any medical-care innovation is introduced, this should be followed by planned evaluation. The other two areas of work discussed in this book are (1) trials of intervention—of various aspects, ranging from prevention to therapy to medical care—and (2) medical-care studies. As a generalisation, the design of intervention trials and medical-care studies are conceptually simpler than the preliminary steps required in any aetiological study: the former study starts from a concrete issue (will the new drug have a different cure-rate, will a coronary care unit reduce case fatality?), while the aetiological studies start from a position of ignorance (what is the cause of schizophrenia, or what is the new cause of the changing incidence of malignant melanoma?).

This point is brought out not to denigrate the role of individuals involved in target-orientated studies, but to stress the difficulty of generating 'bright ideas' and to acknowledge that formal training and textbooks are not the source of, or guarantee of, generation of bright ideas. Obviously, application of intellect or innovative ideas can contribute to all forms of study (suggesting what might be studied, noting hitherto unrecognised applications for study, pursuading people to collaborate, ensuring valid data collection, using an ideal form of data analysis, and forming the correct interpretation of the data). Whatever the class of study, it is essential to bear in mind always that conceptualisation of the problem and the issues involved is the first and most important step.

Chapters 2–10 of this book cover a range of epidemiological and associated statistical techniques; how does one decide which is the most appropriate way to study any particular topic? In order to assist with consideration of this, figure 11.1 presents, in a highly schematic fashion, a pathway that may be followed in epidemiological studies. It must be emphasised that this is available to assist in considering the type of study that might be relevant, rather than as a blueprint that must be followed without deviation.

The study that seems most desirable scientifically may not be ideal for any particular issue; as indicated in the figure, previous knowledge must be considered. A research worker not previously involved with the field may be asked to carry out a study from stage 1 (i.e. an initial inquiry on a new topic), to work at stage 7 (intervention, when the knowledge exists upon which this may be planned). However, the type of study design and the detail of its development will also depend upon:

(1) The opportunities available for the study (agreement of collaborators and access to subjects, or retrievable data)
(2) The facilities available for the study (expertise for planning, trained supervision, field workers and interviewers, statistical staff, data processors and the resources they need, skills in interpretation)
(3) The time by which an answer is required
(4) The enquirer's assessment of the importance of the topic
(5) The research worker's impression of the degree of validity required in the results.

The framework in figure 11.1 is obviously not so clearly related to design of medical-care studies. The chapter dealing with this issue has emphasised that the epidemiological approach is only one discipline relevant to the exploration of these topics (others involved are the application of operational research, mathematical modelling, the social sciences, etc.). However, some of the work will involve either conventional epidemiological techniques, or modification of these techniques. Again, the figure 11.1 may help in considering the most suitable form of study. Bailey (1981) discussed a unified approach to the design of experiments, stressing the need for consideration of four aspects (a model, randomisation, combinatorial design, and analysis), rather than one in isolation to the others. The points of

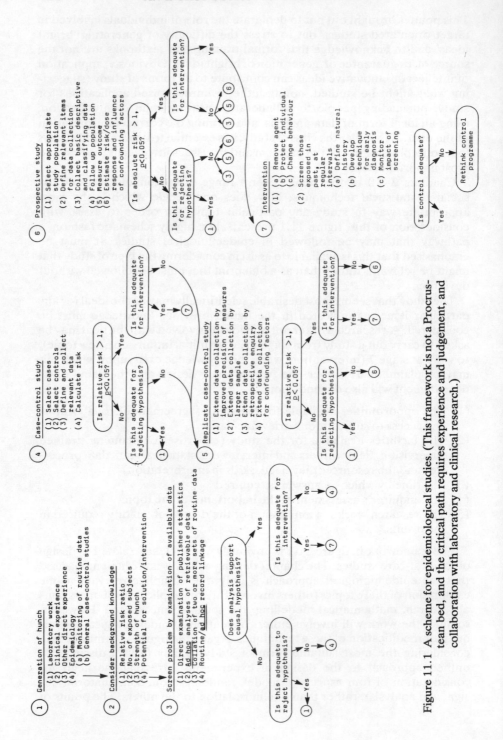

Figure 11.1 A scheme for epidemiological studies. (This framework is not a Procrustean bed, and the critical path requires experience and judgement, and collaboration with laboratory and clinical research.)

detail that he brought out were not clearly relevant to the general range of epidemiological work.

Several times reference has been made to the desirability of consulting statisticians. In the more global context of planning studies this needs to be generalised to consult someone with relevant experience, before an ill-founded study is launched. Where a grant has to be obtained there are two phases at which opinions may be sought, (1) in preparing the application and (2) during peer review. A greater risk of faults in study design being overlooked occurs when an individual identifies a topic requiring explora-tion and then plans, executes and analyses the study himself. It is well worth considering discussion of the project at least with colleagues, prior to initiating such work; this can often result in beneficial modification of the study. This suggestion is relevant both the inexperienced and the experi-enced worker; it is always easy to miss or ignore the faults in one's own study design, when readily finding the faults made by others—hence the value of peer review of any work.

Discussing medical science, Dollery (1978) drew attention to the pace of change of medical knowledge—with dramatic alteration in diagnostic methods and therapeutic procedures between 1938 and 1978, some occur-ring within a decade. He provided five examples of advances in therapeutics or clinical procedures (treatment for gout, peptic ulcer and hypertension, adjustment of fluid balance, and giving oxygen by mask). These examples indicated the interdependence of different branches of science; also, the initial work was not obviously relevant to health care of man; the examples did not indicate that targetted research was feasible in developing new lines of care. Dollery then acknowledged that targetted research to evaluate effectiveness, safety, or costs of treatment is perfectly feasible—but does not often get done.

Many authors have commented on the general aspects of study design, with particular reference to epidemiological studies (see recommended reading at the end of this chapter). However, as an alternative to consulting textbooks, scientific articles may be read to see how comparable problems were tackled in the past. This is especially useful if a report on a comparable issue can be found that has a full discussion on the reason for the selected design and a critical comment about the suitability of other designs. To reinforce the point that one particular study design may not be the sole way to tackle a particular problem, it is of interest to note the range of studies carried out by Poskanzer and his colleagues (1980) when investigating multiple sclerosis. They looked at mortality statistics in Shetland and Orkney over a hundred-year period, and the incidence and prevalence for more recent years. The influence of demographic change, migration, and case ascertainment was examined. A clinical study (including aspects of progression of the condition) was required, to see if the disease was comparable to that occurring in different parts of the world. Case–control studies were mounted to check on (1) the history of lifetime events, (2) histocompatibility differences, (3) variation in viral antibody titres, (4) the interrelationship of histocompatibility and viral titres. A sociological study on migration was also carried out.

11.3 Inference

It is a rather abrupt step from consideration of study design to the stage of interpretation or inference. The reason for the jump is that chapters 2–10 have dealt with the intervening aspects of study method, up to the stage of limited consideration of basic statistical techniques. Inference involves three interlocking aspects; (1) application of appropriate statistical technique, (2) logical appraisal of the results of this analysis, and (3) judgement. This section endeavours to provide guidance on the first two of the three aspects; it was felt that a textbook was not the place to expand on the application of judgement, but the emphasis should be upon the steps of probing and marshalling the facts and subjective impressions stemming from a specific study.

11.3.1 Statistical techniques

The limited statistical sections in each of the chapters 2–10 provide a foundation upon which statistical analysis of epidemiological data can be based; such analyses then lead on to discussion of the results and inferences. There are a number of special techniques that may be reconsidered, e.g.: multivariate analyses of routine data, the quantification of risk in case–control studies (with the production of appropriate confidence limits), and the distinction between relative and attributable risk (such as can be most readily performed in prospective studies).

One example of disagreement involves consideration of the environmental factors associated (causally) with variation in ischaemic heart disease mortality (water hardness, water calcium, other climatic and socioeconomic factors). Leger and Sweetnam (1979) suggested a particular technique to facilitate judgement (use of standardised regression coefficients in a regression equation based on logic transformation of death-rates).

Dales and Ury (1978) point out that when considering the possibility that a covariable may confound the study results (e.g. smoking, in a study of alcohol intake and bladder cancer), it is inappropriate to test the case–control difference in smoking. It does not matter whether or not these smoking differences could have occurred by chance: the important issue is whether they could account for the alcohol-related findings.

Walker (1981) presented a technique for the analysis of interaction between two causes of a disease; this was based upon the additivity of attributable risk. It was argued that this was the appropriate approach when moving towards decisions about either personal risk or public-health intervention. An example was given of the risk of oral cancer in those who drink and smoke, indicating that the best approach was to reduce smoking in drinkers.

Goldsmith (1977) suggested that 'path analysis', by examining interrelationships between various factors following a conventional multivariate analysis, could facilitate the distinction between causal and noncausal relationships.

11.3.2 Multiple comparisons

Both the analysis of drug-monitoring data (Shapiro and Slone, 1979) and material on the association of H.L.A.-typing results and liability to a particular disease (Emery, 1976) share a statistical aspect with some aetiological studies. When many items have been recorded about individuals in an aetiological study, there is a tendency to continue cross-tabulating, analysing, and testing the results until an answer is obtained that is 'statistically significant'. The same process may occur when carrying out a correlation or other analysis of complex sets of material from collation studies (see subsection 2.4.2). The difficulty is that the results from conventional statistical testing do not immediately convert to p-values where multiple comparisons have been performed.

The conventional tests of significance were designed for application in the very different hypothesis-testing situation (sometimes referred to as *a priori* examination of data). It is usually argued that if 20 tests of significance are performed, one of them is expected to be significant at the $p = 0.05$ level purely by chance. Various approaches have been devised for adjusting the initial p-value, to take account of the number of comparisons made. One approach is by using the Bonferoni inequality:

$$\hat{p} = p \times \frac{1}{n}$$

where $p =$ original p-value and $n =$ number of comparisons made.

However, the desirability of such a method is not unanimously accepted; Cole (1979) and Miettinen (1979) both felt that the results obtained by the initial calculations of p-values were independent of the number of comparisons made. This was in contrast to Shapiro and Slone (1979), who stressed that the system for generating the hypotheses and the number of comparisons made should be clearly described in any publication. Jones and Rushton (1982) discussed the 'partial solution' to this problem and concluded that greater emphasis should be placed upon estimation methods, with less reliance on significance testing. There are a number of statistical manoeuvres that have been suggested for alleviating the problem of multiple comparisons and the above paper may be consulted for further details.

11.3.3 Derivation of inferences

In order to interpret any piece of work, the following are required: the aim of the study; relevant prior scientific literature; study design; estimated power of study; source of subjects; response rate; errors and biases in the data; potential limitations from confounding; results including significance and confidence limits; relationship of results to the literature.

It has been pointed out that epidemiological studies can be descriptive or hypothesis testing or experimental (that is, with intervention). It is particularly the hypothesis-testing situation that causes the greatest problems in the derivation of inference.

In the nineteenth century, Claude Bernard (see Ryle, 1948) suggested that a physician was a person who reasoned experimentally even though he undertook no experiments. Such a person observed a disease in different circumstances, reasoned about the influence of these circumstances and deduced the consequences that were controlled by other observations. A number of authors have more recently supported this argument (Yule, 1924; Topley, 1940; Hill, 1953; Dudley, 1970). The opposite point of view was put by Platt (1952), who observed that the major advances in knowledge are the fruits of careful experiments planned in advance to test specific hypotheses. He also stated that data recorded, other than as part of a specific research project, would be of little value. Acheson (1967) suggested that these two extreme propositions are equally absurd.

How does one progress from a position of ignorance, through a hunch to a tentative, but testable, hypothesis that can be explored by preliminary and detailed studies? The most difficult stage in this recursive cycle of investigation is the identification of hunches that warrant further study. The question is, can the examination of routine data facilitate the identification of such hunches? Published work describing advances in knowledge often fail to reveal the source of the basic hunch.

Hogben (1940) stressed that the Hindus and Arabs had needed a means of reckoning in their commercial undertakings and this practical application was a stimulus to the development of arithmetic (which was of more value to them than the 'armchair' theories of the Greek mathematicians). Sherrington (1922) quoted Pasteur, who said that 'to have the fruits there must have been cultivation of the tree' and then qualified this by pointing out that there is merit in appreciating the possibilities of earlier work, but this is only a preliminary to the main achievement. Spence (1953) suggested that the recognition of a new phenomenon only takes shape in the mind endowed with imagination and insight, but he also stressed the need for skill in collecting and systematically treating the knowledge.

Medawar (1969) discussed two conceptions of science. Firstly, truth takes shape in the mind of the observer and it is his imaginative grasp of what may be true that provides the incentive to finding out. Secondly, truth resides in nature and is to be got at only through the application of scientific method. He pointed out that these two opinions contradicted each other, but that anyone who has actually done, or reflected on, scientific research knows that there is a great deal of truth in both of them. Popper (1972) discussed the 'bucket theory' which suggests that before we know anything about the world, we must first have sense experiences (that is accumulated observations). The 'bucket theory' further proposes that the examination of these observations will lead to hypotheses. Popper disputed this and said that the correct approach was the 'searchlight theory'. According to this, only by the formation of scientific hypotheses is it possible to identify what kind of observations ought to be made. These observations then play an extremely important role in testing the hypothesis. One of Popper's main arguments was that a topic becomes a science when its hypotheses can be tested. Jacobsen (1976) has suggested that Popper's denigration of the place of inductive methods is harmful to epidemiology. Jacobsen argues that there is widespread confusion between deductive and inductive logic and this creates difficulty in the understanding of the role of statistical inference in epidemiology. Himsworth (1970) emphasised that, in general, one only registers the experience that one expects and if one's attention is circumscribed by a mistaken idea, there is a tendency to remain unreceptive to the significance of events outside these views.

August (1976) has described how Mill's canons were based upon Herschel, and advanced as 'four methods of experimental inquiry'; though usually referred to as 'four', there was a fifth: that of 'the joint method of agreement and difference' which is usually ignored. Susser (1973) set out certain strategies for the derivation of inferences, based on Mill's canons:

The method of difference

This is the mounting of a classic experiment, such as has been discussed in chapter 7.

The method of agreement

This second approach is such that considerable support for a particular hypothesis is obtained from multiple studies carried out in different countries, by different groups of research workers, using different methods and yet all approaches show the same general relationship.

The method of concomitant variation

This method takes into account the association between the aetiological factor and the disease in a number of situations in which the intensity of the aetiological factor varies. For example, smoking has varied over a period of time, between the sexes and in different countries. In all these situations its variation has been paralleled by mortality due to lung cancer.

The method of residues

Having removed variation due to all known causes in an experimental situation, one is often left with a residue of incidence or prevalence of disease due to other causes. (Thus by studying nonsmokers, and so excluding the effect of smoking, it is possible to examine more precisely the influence of environmental pollution and its impact on the prevalence of respiratory disease.)

Hill (1965) discussed the distinction between association and causation when examining the relation between environment and disease. He indicated nine different aspects that should be considered. These were: the strength of the relationship; the consistency (has the finding repeatedly been observed by different persons, in different places, circumstances and times?); specificity (is the association limited to particular sites or types of disease?); temporality (is the particular change in the environment followed by the disease?); biological gradient (i.e. dose−response); plausibility (though it was emphasised that what is biologically plausible depends on the knowledge of the day); coherence (the causal interpretation should not seriously conflict with the generally known fact of the natural history and biology of the disease); experiment (does change in exposure result in change in risk of the disease?); and analogy (are there other comparable examples of a cause-and-effect relationship?). Having considered these aspects, Hill then emphasised that no formal tests of significance can answer the question. Such tests could and should remind one of the effects that the play of chance creates and they will instruct one in the likely magnitude of those effects. However, beyond that they contribute nothing to the 'proof' of the hypothesis.

This topic has also been discussed by Wynder (1966), Yerushalmy (1966), Burkitt (1971) and Lilienfeld (1976). The formalisation of decisions through analysis of (1) prior knowledge and (2) value judgements has been discussed briefly by the Lancet (1982) and more extensively by Wulff (1976).

Occasionally, the focus of interest will be on negative associations that are causal. For example, there is hard evidence of the protective effect of fluoride on dental caries, the suggestion that those having higher intake of vitamin A are at reduced risk of certain cancers, and the unexplained lower risk of Parkinson's disease in smokers. The obverse of identifying causality is the issue of demonstrating that a suggested hazard does not exist. Strict scientific method indicates that it is impossible to prove that a relationship does not exist—studies only demonstrate that they have not found any indication of an actual (or statistically significant) effect, the philosophy being that the next study may generate findings that, for the first time, there is a positive (causal) relationship that is unlikely to have occurred by chance. Much as consistency in different positive studies is thought to add considerably to the weight of evidence, so will repetition of 'negative' findings indicate that no hazard has been inadvertently missed because of some local or chance factor. This is particularly so when different workers have used a variety of methods in several countries.

There is a statistical aspect to the issue of negative findings. It is possible to calculate the smallest actual hazard that any given study is likely to have missed; this depends partly upon the frequency of events occurring in the general population, the increment in deaths possibly caused by the hazard, the size of the population studied and the period over which the deaths are studied.

Earlier chapters have discussed the calculation of attributable risk (see subsections 5.5.5 and 6.5.1). This is really only appropriate after the conclusion has been reached that there is a causal relationship between the agent and the disease. However, consideration of relative risk is only one of the important elements in excluding a confounding effect (where the main agent–disease association is very strong, it is unlikely that this is due to confounding with another agent associated very strongly both with the factor of interest and the disease). Consideration of the attributable risk can then lead on to a social evaluation of the problem and an appropriate programme of prevention (see Arrow, 1976; Kates, 1978).

References

Recommended reading

Fisher, Sir R. (1966). *The Design of Experiments.* 8th edn, Oliver and Boyd, Edinburgh

Other references

Acheson, E. D. (1967). *Medical Record Linkage,* Oxford University Press, London
Arrow, K. J. (1976). *Social Choice and Individual Values.* Yale University Press, New Haven
August, E. (1976). *John Stuart Mill.* Vision, London
Bailey, R. A. (1981). *J. R. statist. Soc. A*, **144**, 214–23
Bulpitt, C. J. (1977). *Br. J. Hosp. Med.*, **1977**, Oct., 329–34
Burkitt, D. P. (1971). *J. Natn. Cancer Inst.*, **47**, 913–9
Cole, P. (1979). *J. chron. Dis.*, **32**, 111
Dales, L. G., and Ury, H. K. (1978). *Int. J. Epidem.*, **7**, 373–5
Dollery, C. (1978). *The End of an Age of Optimism.* Nuffield Provincial Hospitals Trust, London
Dudley, H. A. S. (1970). *Lancet*, **2**, 1352–4
Emery, A. E. H. (1976). *Methodology in Medical Genetics: An Introduction to Statistical Methods.* Churchill, Edinburgh
Goldsmith, J. R. (1977). *Int. J. Epidem.*, **6**, 391–400
Hill, A. B. (1953). *New Engl. J. Med.*, **248**, 955–1001
Hill, A. B. (1965). *Proc. R. Soc. Med.*, **54**, 295–300
Himsworth, H. (1970). *The Development and Reorganisation of Scientific Knowledge.* Heinemann, London
Hogben, L. (1940). *Mathematics for the Million.* Allen and Unwin, London
Inman, W. H. W. (1981). *Br. med. J.*, **282**, 1216–7
Jacobsen, M. (1976). *Int. J. Epidem.*, **5**, 9–11
Jones, D. R., and Rushton, L. (1982). *Int. J. Epidem.*, **11**, 276–82
Kates, R. W. (1978). *Risk Assessment of Environment Hazard.* Wiley, New York
Lancet (1982). *Lancet*, **2**, 911–2
Leger, A. S. St., and Sweetnam, P. M. (1979). *Int. J. Epidem.*, **8**, 73–7
Lilienfeld, A. M. (1976). *Foundations of Epidemiology.* Oxford University Press, New York
Martin-Bouyer, G., Lebretin, R., Toga, M., Stolley, P. D., and Lockhart, J. (1982). *Lancet*, **1**, 91–5
Medawar, P. B. (1969). *The Art of the Soluble.* Penguin, Harmondsworth
Miettinen, O. (1979). *J. chron. Dis.*, **32**, 111
Platt, R. (1952). *Lancet*, **2**, 977–80
Popper, K. (1972). *Objective Knowledge—an Evolutionary Approach.* Oxford University Press, London
Poskanzer, D. C., Prenney, L. B. Sheridan, J. L., and Kondy, J. Y. (1980). *J. Epidem. Comm. Hlth*, **34**, 229–39
Ryle, J. A. (1948). *Changing Disciplines: Lectures on the History, Methods, and Motives of Social Pathology.* Oxford University Press, London
Shapiro, S., and Slone, D. (1979). *J. chron. Dis.*, **32**, 105–7
Sherrington, J. (1922). *Brit. Med. J.*, **2**, 1139–40

Spence, J. (1953). *Lancet,* **2,** 629–32
Susser, M. (1973). *Causal Thinking in the Health Sciences—Concept and Strategies of Epidemiology.* Oxford University Press, London
Topley, W. W. C. (1940). *Authority, Observation, and Experiment in Medicine.* Cambridge University Press, London
Toxic Epidemic Syndrome Study Group (1982). *Lancet,* **2,** 697–702
Walker, A. M. (1981). *Int. J. epidem* **10,** 81–5
Wulff, H. R. (1976). *Rational Diagnosis and Treatment.* Blackwell, Oxford
Wynder, E. L. (1966). In *Controversy in Internal Medicine* (F. J. Ingelfinger, A. S. Relman and M. A. Finland, eds.) Saunders, Philadelphia, pp. 649–58
Yerushalmy, J. (1966). In *Controversy in Internal Medicine* (F. J. Ingelfinger, A. S. Relman and M. A. Finland, eds.), Saunders, Philadelphia, pp. 659–68
Yule, G. (1924). *Report of the Industrial Health Research Board No. 28.* H.M.S.O., London

Definitions

There has been a recent advance in this field, with the preparation of *A Dictionary of Epidemiology* (J. M. Last, ed.), Oxford University Press, London. This provides, often followed by brief comment and discussion, for about 1500 of the terms used in epidemiology—bearing in mind the overlap with related disciplines such as genetics and statistics. There may be variation in the definitions used by different workers: it is obviously desirable, for the sake of ease of communication, that use should be avoided of one term where another is that more generally applied by the epidemiological community.

The following definitions cover a range of specific terms that have been used throughout the text. These represent the key expressions used in epidemiology; their use has been indicated in the text, but it has been thought advisable to collect the formal definitions into this list. This is not to indicate that such definitions should be learnt by rote, but to provide a precise expression of the meaning of each of these terms for reference purposes.

Concepts Involved in Epidemiological Studies

Descriptive study   Such studies delineate (1) the distribution of disease in a population and the factors associated with presence or absence of disease in individuals, (2) the natural history of a particular disease, (3) the distribution of health care resources and (4) the met demand of the health care system (the 'workload').

Hypothesis testing study   Investigates an hypothesis stemming from judicious interpretation of descriptive studies, or from direct clinical observation or work in laboratories. Such a study is planned to collect data relevant to testing the hypothesis.

Intervention study   A planned study, with appropriate control, which alters the exposure to aetiological factors (or introduces some form of prevention) and quantifies the influence of this change.

Method study   A study with the specific aim of developing new data-collection methods or analytical techniques.

Methods of Epidemiological Studies

Cross-sectional study   A study in which data are collected at one point in time from respondents by questioning, examination or investigation. The results may be used for descriptive purposes, or some limited forms of hypothesis testing.

Case–control study   An hypothesis-testing study in which data are

327

collected from (1) patients with the disease being explored and (2) an appropriate sample of control subject (who may be matched for sex, age or other attributes).

Retrospective study   An hypothesis-testing study that collects information about past events by direct enquiry from respondents. This, and other data, are then usually related to the distribution of disease in the respondents.

Prospective study   Investigation and categorisation of a sample of individuals, who are then followed over a period to detect the subsequent incidence of disease among them. The analysis predominantly examines the relationships between variation of the initial measured variates and incidence of disease.

Cohort study   Investigation of a group of individuals, who share some common characteristic (year of birth, place of residence, place of work), and follow up of these individuals over a period of time.

Rates

Reproduction

Birth-rate   The number of live births in a geographical area during a time period divided by the estimated population of the area. It is usually expressed per 1000 persons per year.

Fertility-rate   The number of live births in a geographical area during a time period, divided by the female population of child-bearing ages (usually 15–44 years) in that area. It is usually expressed per 1000 women per year.

Distribution of disease

Incidence rate   The number of patients developing a particular condition in a geographical area during a time period, divided by the estimated avarage population at risk. It is usually expressed per 1000 persons per year.

Prevalence   The number of persons with a particular condition (or abnormality) present at a point in time, divided by the estimated population at risk. It is usually expressed per 1000. This is technically a point prevalence rate; an extension of this is a period prevalence rate, which is the number of persons with a particular condition identified over a stated period of time, divided by the estimated average population at risk. It is usually expressed per 1000 per unit of time.

Sickness in the community

Inception rate—spells   The number of spells of sickness that start during a defined period divided by the average number of persons exposed to risk during that period.

Average duration per spell The total of the entire durations of all spells of sickness ending during a defined period divided by the number of spells ending during that period.

Hospital discharge rate The number of discharges from hospital during a time period, divided by the estimated mid-year population for the hospital's catchment area. It is usually expressed per 1000 persons per year. The denominator for a discharge rate can be the beds rather than the population, to give an indication of the use of beds, where the rate becomes the number of discharges per bed per year. The rate can be specific, for example the number of discharges of children under 15 per 1000 children in the catchment area per year.

Mortality

Crude mortality-rate The total number of deaths in a geographical area during a time period, divided by the estimated population of the area. It is usually expressed per 1000 persons per year.

Age- (and sex-) specific mortality-rate The number of deaths for a given age (and sex) subgroup of the population during a time period divided by the estimated population for the same age (and sex) subgroup. It is usually expressed per 1000 men (or women) of the specific group per year.

Standardised Mortality Ratio (S.M.R.) The number of deaths, either total or cause-specific, in a given population, expressed as a percentage of the deaths that would have been expected if the age- and sex-specific rates in a 'standard' population had applied. An S.M.R. can be calculated for persons working in a particular occupation, those living in a particular locality, or for other defined subgroups of a population.

Stillbirth-rate The number of stillbirths divided by the number of live and stillbirths in the same time period. It is usually expressed per 1000 total births per year.

Perinatal mortality-rate The number of stillbirths plus deaths in the first week of life in a geographical area during a time period, divided by the total number of live plus stillbirths. It is usually expressed per 1000 total births per year.

Neonatal mortality-rate The number of deaths in the first 28 days of life in a geographical area during a time period, divided by the number of live births. It is usually expressed per 1000 live births per year.

Post-neonatal mortality-rate The number of deaths between the 29th day and the end of the first year of life in a geographical area during a time period, divided by the number of live births in the same time period. It is usually expressed per 1000 live births per year.

Infant mortality-rate Number of deaths under the age of 1 year occurring in a geographical area during a time period, divided by the number of live births in the same time period. It is usually expressed per 1000 live births per year.

Cause-specific mortality-rate The number of deaths from a specific cause divided by the estimated mid-year population at risk, expressed per 1000 per year.

Case fatality-rate   The number of patients dying from a specific condition, divided by the number developing the condition; it is usually expressed per 1000 affected persons. For hospital inpatients this statistic may be the rate of patients dying prior to discharge from hospital.

Road accident rate   The number of injured persons in a geographical area during a time period, divided by the estimated population at risk, expressed per 1000 persons per unit of time. This accident-rate may be based on the number of fatally injured, the number of seriously injured, or the total number of fatally plus seriously injured persons. The accident rate may be calculated as an age- and sex-specific rate; instead of using estimated population at risk, the denominator may be the number of vehicles registered, or the number of vehicle miles travelled.

Need and Demand

The following five categories of need and demand are interrelated and there is overlap between one category and another. These items are not subdivisions of a continuum and there is no necessity for a patient to pass through one stage before attaining a subsequent one.

Health need—unperceived   A condition that is unrecognised by an individual or his family, but is potentially discoverable by a practitioner on careful investigation of the total physical, mental and emotional wellbeing of the individual, using standard techniques and accepted criteria. Such a condition may warrant intervention (when it is thought that prevention, management, or specific therapy will be of benefit), but will also include those diseases for which currently available forms of intervention are of little benefit to the patient.

Health need—perceived   A health-care need is perceived when the individual or his family identify an 'abnormality', which they acknowledge is usually brought to the attention of the medical profession. Subsequently, they may (1) take no action whatsoever to seek medical care, (2) make use of one of the informal agencies including self-medication, or (3) contact one of the conventional branches of the health service. Not all perceived need will be accepted by the medical profession as being correctly identified; in certain circumstances this may be labelled as over-demand or neurosis.

Demand—stifled   Perceived health need that is not translated into overt demand due to 'bottlenecks' in the provision of facilities.

Demand—unmet   Requests for health care that have not been fulfilled at a point in time. These are most easily identified as waiting lists and other forms of queues for care. However, they will also include events where the patient's expectations have not be fulfilled.

Demand—met   A health need, however identified, that has been handled by one of the branches of the health service.

Index

331